Those Who Touch

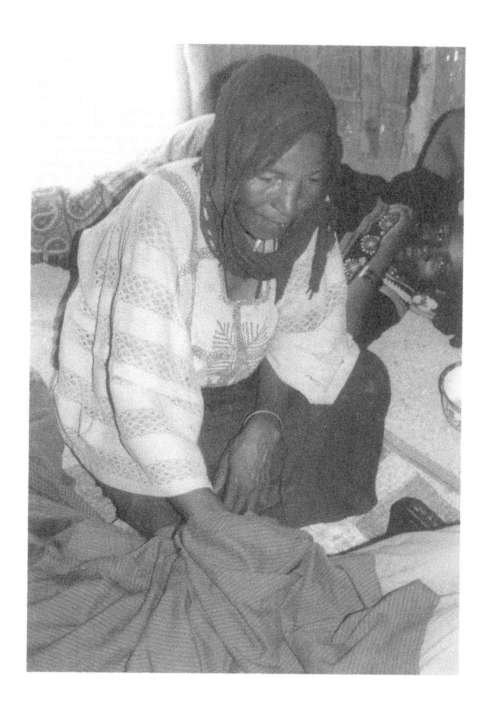

Those Who Touch

Tuareg Medicine Women in Anthropological Perspective

Susan J. Rasmussen

NORTHERN

ILLINOIS

UNIVERSITY

PRESS

DeKalb

Library of Congress Cataloging-in-Publication Data

Rasmussen, Susan J., 1949–

  Those who touch : Tuareg medicine women in

anthropological perspective / Susan J. Rasmussen.

     p.   cm.

Includes bibliographical references and index.

ISBN-13: 978-0-87580-610-5 (pbk. : alk. paper)

ISBN-10: 0-87580-610-4 (pbk. : alk. paper)

1. Women, Tuareg—Medicine. 2. Women, Tuareg—Ethnobotany.

3. Women, Tuareg—Rites and ceremonies.

4. Muslim women—Niger. 5. Women shamans—Niger.

6. Women healers—Niger. 7. Herbs—Therapeutic use—Niger. 8.

Traditional medicine—Niger. I. Title.

DT547.45.T83R384 2006

615'.321'08993306626—dc22

2005020691

Contents

Preface   vii
Acknowledgments   xi

Deconstructing and Recasting Female Healing: Preliminary Remarks   3

PART ONE

Departures—Herbal Medicine and Local and Authoritative Systems of Thought   11

  1. The Vexing Problem of Difference and Classifications in
     Anthropology and the Local Ethnographic Setting   15

  2. Herbalism, Medicine, and Curing—Medicine Women's Concepts of
     Wellness, Illness, and Healing   30

PART TWO

Touch and Word—Learning and Transmitting Medicine   53

  3. Touch, Body, and Senses   57

  4. Word and Deed—Oral Traditions and the Mythico-History of
     Herbal Medicine   80

  5. Medicine Women, Gender, and Physical and Social Reproduction
     over the Life Course   96

  6. Natural Imagery (Arboreal Tropes) in Herbalism—Plant Uses in
     Nature and Culture   117

PART THREE

Medicine Women and Wider Systems of Power   133

  7. Medicine Women, Sacred Places, and *Al Baraka* Ritual Benediction   135

  8. Medicine Women and Islam—Relations with Marabouts   148

  9. Medicine Women and Other "Shamans"—Herbalism, the Spirits of
     the Wild, Divination, and Power   166

  10. Changes in the Wind—Medicine Women's Relations with
      Established Biomedicine   179

Conclusions—Herbal Healing, Modes of Thought, and Gender   193

Notes   197
Works Cited   203
Index   213

Preface

"My mother died after I had learned everything, it was time. If your parents authorize you, you can do it (healing) anytime. The ones who do this best here, however, are the old women of the Bagzan (Massif), which is the origin of our medicine. According to our knowledge, they do medicine. It is the *al baraka* (blessing, benediction) of the mountains that contains all sorts of medicinal trees."
—Herbal medicine woman, Aïr Mountains, northern Niger

When I questioned Lala, the most senior herbal medicine woman on Mount Bagzan, about how Tuareg herbal medicine began, she explained: "Inheritance of herbal healing from (our ancestress) Tagurmat is like a secret. The medicine of *tinesmegelen* ("medicine women", sing. *tanesmegel,* from *amagal,* or medicine) is like 'living milk herds,' (*akh huderan*): it is transmitted to, belongs to, and is practiced and managed by women, like property."[1] Lala, like many medicine women, learned her profession from her mother, apprenticing while she was young, but waited until her mother's death before practicing full-time herself. Another elderly herbalist, Ana, put it this way: "Only women know trees. My medicine is inherited from the mother of my mother."

This book examines predominantly female herbalism in seminomadic, Muslim Tuareg communities of Niger and Mali, most extensively practiced in the countryside by specialists widely called *tinesmegelen*. The book is not, however, an ethnobotanical or bio-cultural study. Rather, it addresses healing-related issues in the anthropology of religion and modes of thought in relation to gendered practice. Medicine women come from diverse backgrounds, though many are of noble origins in their traditionally socially stratified system. These specialists work with leaves, barks, and roots from trees that are believed to contain spirits with matrilineal ancestral significance. However, their practices include diverse healing techniques that transcend herbalism. Many local residents emphasize that knowing trees is a necessary but insufficient criterion for practicing this profession—medicine women must receive their medicinal knowledge from founding culture heroines and must obtain authorization to practice from older relatives. Thus the pharmacological aspects of their work are not the central focus here. Rather, the emphasis is upon what herbalism and medicine women have to contribute to wider cultural studies of African and other, indeed all human philosophies—including those conventionally considered part of Euro-American biomedicine—as "cultural inquiry" (Karp and Masolo 2000).

Herbal medicine women inform cultural anthropological issues of representing "other" imaginative worlds and creativity. These creative worlds do not occur in a void but are animated by the contexts of practice. "Healer" is a somewhat inclusive and elusive term in anthropology. In currently fashionable studies of plural medical systems, it is often used as a gloss to refer to many roles—midwives, shamans/mediums, and herbalists. This book ponders the broader theoretical significance of a local healing specialism for the anthropology of religion, medical anthropology, gender, and African modes of thought. Yet the analysis here is also grounded in an ethnographic context that offers intriguing insights, but also perplexing contradictions, concerning the interplay of researchers? and local residents' logical categories and classifications of health and illness. More broadly, this book asks: what is herbalism in the local cultural viewpoint, who are these herbalists, and how do these healers "speak" more generally to the magic, religion, and science conundrum in anthropology? In this respect, the present book differs from some previous studies of Tuareg healing that emphasized local veterinary science, plant and animal lexicons, illness taxonomies, spirit possession, and sociopolitical practices surrounding medical pluralism (Bernus 1969; Hawad 1979; Fiore and Wallet Faqqi 1993; Nicolaisen and Nicolaisen 1997; Noel in Claudot-Hawad 2002; Rasmussen 1995, 2001a).

Herbal medicine women diagnose by touch, treat predominantly stomach ailments with tree barks and leaves, set bones, and sometimes practice psychosocial marital counseling. A few conduct complex mediumistic divination as well. Most of their patients are women and children, although men, also, see them. Herbal medicine women must be mothers, yet preferably of older, post-childbearing status. Among some Tuareg groups, for example, clans in the Kel Ewey confederation in the Aïr Mountains of Niger, medicine women trace the origins of herbalism matrilineally to a pair of female twin daughters of their founding ancestress, named Tagurmat. In their accounts of this mythico-history, these healers related how these twins emerged from their mother's stomach after she was killed by her jealous husband. The twins began curing because of their inheritance from Tagurmat of natural substances used in healing (namely, wood), as well as knowledge. This origin of female healing—in alleged violence in the remote past—appears paradoxical in a community where rape and wife-beating are now rare, and it led me to delve more deeply into these herbalists' art and science.

How did life-saving and medicine originate in murder and death? Curiously, in a society where many women generally hold high prestige and there is relatively free social interaction between the sexes, the origins of female-centered healing are in a man's physical violence toward a woman. On first scrutiny, this mythico-history (the central motif of stories related to me by many other medicine women) appears as a variant or even inversion of the now-classic "myth of matriarchy" in anthropology, of alleged past female dominance suppressed or overthrown, now critiqued yet still intriguing (Bamberger in Rosaldo and Lamphere 1974; Lepowsky in Goodenough and Sanday 1995). In the Tuareg case, there are suggestions that more is at play than literal or organic healing with plants, though plants, in particular trees believed empowered with spirits, are also significant. Most important are gendered mythico-historical groundings of herbalism and, as Davis-Floyd and Sargent (1997) have termed it, "authoritative knowledge."

The present book examines how healing knowledge is conceived of and conveyed in herbal healing ideology and practice in an effort to yield critical insights into gender, authoritative knowledge, culture as praxis, and what anthropologists have generally conceptualized as "biomedicine," and "medico-ritual" or "magico-ritual" healing systems. In keeping with medicine women's and their patients' own emphases in local exegesis, I contemplate, through these specialists' voices and actions, the interface between religion and medicine.

The Tuareg case, while not necessarily representative of universal bedrock truths, hopefully builds on efforts to disrupt some anthropological generalizations. I argue that medicine women, in their historically commemorative and socially mediating roles, are mnemonic and mediating figures, who bridge modes of thought that are often represented in anthropology as separate and discrete (Malinowski 1948; Tambiah 1990). While modern anthropologists have for some years correctly argued for equally logical systems of thought (Evans-Pritchard 1950; Horton 1967, 1993), many theorists nonetheless have attempted to "fit" other imaginative worlds into clear-cut categories according to a priori Western logical classifications—for example, "science," "nature," and "culture," and "organic" vs. "nonorganic" illness. It is not my intent here to "beat the dead horse" of structuralist binary oppositions, already justifiably critiqued in anthropology, gender studies, and African studies (MacCormack and Strathern 1980; Mudimbe 1988, 1991; Karp and Masolo 2000). Nonetheless, I firmly believe that there is a need to further deconstruct and recast some of these categories which, while no longer considered hierarchical, ranked oppositions or dualities, still tend to be represented according to our own classifications. This trend—of thinking in terms of ranked, dual oppositions—is also characteristic of some studies of Tuareg healing. Previous brief references to Tuareg medicine women in the literature tend to classify organic illnesses requiring plants from nature as the sole domain of medicine women and their treatments. In a useful but very brief pamphlet on Malian Tuareg illness concepts (Fiore and Wallet Faqqi 1993), the authors distinguish two illness domains—organic and nonorganic. One—that of herbal medicine women—is, they argue, "close to nature and feminine, and the other close to culture and masculine. . . ." One is based on "a view of illness as an imbalance between two opposed principles of hot and cold, the other, on a view of illness as invasion into the natural order by a superhuman or unnatural being or sign" (Fiore and Wallet Faqqi 1993:54). One treatment needs knowledge of herbs and medical skills from plants, the other of incorporeal beings (spirits), writing, and sacred (Qur'anic and other Arabic) texts.

In the present book, medicine women's voices and patients' cases, including my own experiences of their treatments, reveal finer distinctions, and suggest an intertwining of these different strands of knowledge (of the stomach, the head, and multisensorial healing) within the same domain of herbal medicine. Upon closer scrutiny, over my approximately twenty years of cultural anthropological field research in Tamajaq-speaking communities of northern Niger and more recently, Mali, on healing systems, ritual, gender, and the life course, I found medicine women's theories and practices to be far more complex and nuanced than the few references to them in the literature imply. My findings suggest that medicine women, their knowledge, and their practice cannot be compartmentalized according to any neat version of "body/mind" dualism or rigidly opposed to Islamic scholars' more "mental" (and by implication, "scientific") work with nonorganic illnesses; these divisions impose too rigid an opposition. The present book explores overlaps and contextual variations on these principles in herbal medicine women's theorizing and practicing of wellness, illness, and healing, and shows how medicine women also deconstruct additional binaries and reifications.

Some other anthropological studies of healing in different societies, while insightful and valuable, nonetheless also tend to establish rigid dualities or polar oppositions between authoritative knowledge systems, albeit of a different order. In a provocative study of plural healing systems in southern Africa (Green 1999), Green constructively warns against ranking Western biomedical and other healing systems. This author chides many anthropological studies for giving the latter inferior status merely because these studies distinguish other systems, such as those in Africa, from Euro-American established biomedical systems. Clearly, this can be an unintended consequence of such thinking (Horton 1967, 1982, 1993; Tambiah 1990). In my view, however, there is an alternative to these opposed and circular debates. Difference, whether within or between cultural systems, need not imply mutual exclusiveness or a hierarchy of categories. What, then, is the nature of difference? Some differences between systems, both within and between societies, may be complementary; indeed, this is the way many peoples view distinctions within their societies, whether social statuses, gender constructs, or modes of thought.

In wider anthropological efforts to avoid "exoticism" (Said 1978; Mudimbe 1988, 1991), with which I am in sympathy, there arise additional problems. I do not believe so-called culturalist explanations inevitably result in ranking and hierarchy; for that matter, more global emphases do not always avoid these consequences, either. Cultural distinctiveness may constitute a rich source of human imagination and creativity. As many anthropologists recognize, furthermore, even within one healing specialty there are fine nuances of knowledge, including contradictions, rather than a unitary or monolithic system of thought.

Fundamental to any comparative study of modes of thought and healing systems, therefore, is the recognition that all systems are characterized by an internal range of thought. Tuareg medicine women's healing art and science cannot be reduced to solely naturalistic or organic illness treatment, although of course they do unquestionably diagnose and treat illnesses of some sort—I first ask, what is the nature of these illnesses, medicine women's treatment of them, and wellness, in their own viewpoint and practice? In the chapters that follow, I show how the boundaries between "organic" and "nonorganic," and "natural" and "cultural," and "body" and "mind" are very fluid and porous. While this is not uniquely a Tuareg cultural characteristic—indeed, not news in anthropology—its connection to local elaborations of logical categories of thought and gendered practice need to be further explored, and they are teased out here, hopefully contributing to perspectives on female healing specialties and medico-ritual processes. Nor can medicine women's practices be reduced solely to "supernatural" or "superhuman" medico-ritual powers or even "personalistic" theories of illness. The present book does not argue for one or another overarching gloss or category. Rather, it analyzes cultural elaborations of these processes by focusing upon the multiple levels of significance to herbal medicine women's healing. Medicine women in their ideology and practice suggest more constructive directions in which to take some heretofore circular arguments in anthropology and African studies concerning gender, healing, and comparative modes of thought.

Acknowledgments

As always, I am overwhelmed with gratitude when I recall the kind assistance of all friends, consultants, colleagues, and other persons—both at home and abroad and over the long term—who have made this work possible. Many local residents of northern Niger and Mali offered me generous hospitality and contributed in many ways to my studies of Tuareg healing systems over the years. For reasons of confidentiality and safety, I choose here not to specify the real names of specific persons in the smaller rural sites of my research because of the precarious peace that currently prevails in Tamajaq-speaking communities of these countries—as of this writing, still fragile and uncertain despite efforts on all sides following the peace accords between Tuareg separatist rebels and central governments.

First, I extend my deepest gratitude to several of my field host families—who became my friends as well as assistants—blurring the boundaries between "objective" and "subjective" understandings, during my numerous and lengthy residences in the rural Air Mountains region around Agadez, and Agadez itself. Over the years since I first met them, the predicament of many persons in that region, sadly, has been one of "reversal of fortune"—in a series of droughts, the 1990–1996 rebellion, and political, social and economic turmoil—both recent and longstanding. I admire them for "enjoying the moment" in life, never remaining angry for long, and wasting nothing. Most recently, I am also indebted to others who hosted me during my first visit to the Adagh-n-Ifoghas Mountain town of Kidal and a rural community in its vicinity. The latter groups had recently returned to their homes following refugee flight, and only slowly were regaining their property and health and overcoming their fear following the political violence in that region during the 1990s. As a stranger and new guest in Mali, I appreciate their warm reception, generosity, and trust. I am also grateful to several persons who patiently instructed me in the Air and Ifoghas dialects of Tamajaq.

Additional persons who have facilitated my studies, and/or contributed to them in countless other ways, include family and friends at home, and in Africa, the directors of the IRSH research center in Niamey, Niger and the CNRST research center in Bamako; the director of the IRSH branch library in Agadez; the director of the library at Radio Kidal; and other supportive staffs. Over the long term, other scholars have also inspired me to explore anthropology of religion, symbolism, gender, healing systems, the life course, ethnographic analysis issues, and African and Tuareg ethnography. They include Johannes Fabian, Roy Wagner, Robert Levine, Ivan Karp, Paul Stoller, Dominique Casajus, Helene Claudot-Hawad, Alitinine Ag Arias, Mohammed Ag Erless, Alhassane Ag Solimane, and others. In support for my field research projects, I am grateful to Fulbright Hays, the Social Science Research Council, Wenner Gren, and the National Geographic Society. I am also grateful for the constructive suggestions of readers of this book in its manuscript form—Edith Turner,

Barbara Tedlock, and my editor at Northern Illinois University Press, Melody Herr.

Finally, I have always been inspired by, not solely exotic stories of "far-off" lands, but also familiar stories told by my own relatives. Some tellers are now, regrettably, gone. Tuareg medicine women remind one of the need to listen to those still alive, before they pass on, leaving their stories unfinished and questions unanswered.

Those Who Touch

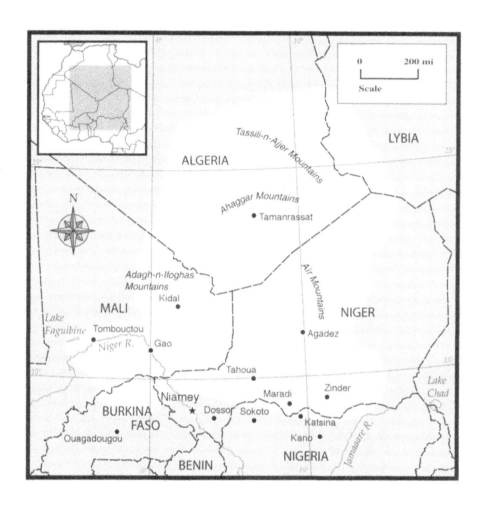

Deconstructing and Recasting Female Healing

Preliminary Remarks

Many scholars (McClain 1989; Sargent and Brettell 1996; Winkelman 1992, 2000, 2001) have argued that midwifery, shamanism, herbalism, and other medical occupations permit women to achieve status or prestige outside their domestic lives. In many of these studies, healing is interpreted as serving women's economic or political self-interest or as an avenue for women to participate in central cultural institutions of significance to both sexes (McClain 1989:1–2) otherwise denied them. In other studies, healing is seen to embody cultural images of femaleness as nurturing, or as mediating between realms of existence, for example, nature and culture, the living and the ancestors, purity and pollution (McClain 1989:2). Among Tuareg, while some women belong to maraboutique (Islamic scholar) clans and actively participate in Islamic rituals and pilgrimages, particularly upon aging (Rasmussen 1997), nonetheless women tend not to specialize professionally as much as men in Islamic scholarship, in contrast to some neighboring Hausa peoples (Hutson 1997). While some previous data (Nicolaisen 1961; Bernus 1969; Fiore and Wallet Faqqi 1993; Rasmussen 1992, 1995, 2001a; Noel in Claudot-Hawad 2002) give the impression that Tuareg Islamic scholars (called *ineslemen* or marabouts) tend to specialize in treatments focusing upon the head, and that herbal medicine women tend to focus most centrally upon the stomach, a closer scrutiny, undertaken in this book, suggests that this binary opposition should not be taken too literally or opposed too diametrically.[1]

I first heard about female herbal healers early in my field research in Tamajaq-speaking communities in northern Niger. Many described *tinesmegelen* as "women sorcerers, like Hausa *bokaye*" (*bokaye,* sing. *boka,* is the term among the neighboring Hausa for a healer who does non-Qur'anic healing, usually with perfumes, plants, and herbs, and sometimes includes mediumship) (Schmoll in Comaroff 1993; Rasmussen 1994, 2001a). Healers and patients stated proudly, "there are 99 *ilaten* herbal remedies on Mt. Bagzan in the Aïr region, which *tinesmegelen* mix and combine in various recipes for different illnesses. They know all the medicinal trees and plants on Mt. Bagzan." *Ilaten* denotes medicinal plants and also, nowadays, often is used colloquially to refer to vitamins. I became intrigued when other residents added, cryptically, "Nonetheless, medicine women do not heal just because there are many trees on Mt. Bagzan; rather, it is their inheritance."

Most Tamajaq speakers still live in rural communities, in the mountains and plains of the Sahara Desert and in the Sahel savanna areas along its fringe. These are regions that, while never isolated, are often of exceedingly difficult geographic access. In some regions, there are no roads but only clusters of tightly packed volcanic rocks, occasionally cross-cut by rough paths, where only donkeys and camels can pass. In others, trucks slowly ply steep, rocky, unpaved roads, winding upwards, over a "lunar" landscape. Except in the mountain massifs (Aïr in Niger, Ahaggar in Algeria, and Adragh n

Ifoghas in Mali), which offer somewhat milder conditions with their seasonal bursts of bright red flowers, valued herbs for healing, and grasses for pasture, the climate is among the harshest in the world. There is a very short and unpredictable rainy season, with occasional severe flooding (July–August). More usual are recurrent droughts and temperature extremes: up to 130 degrees F. in the hot season (April–July), and down to freezing (32 degrees F.) at night during the cold season (December–March), when there are also high winds, sometimes reaching 80 miles an hour, and sandstorms. In the northern regions, oases gardens require daily irrigation. There are, however, rewards for those who live and travel there: vistas of astonishing if austere beauty and unexpected moments of respite from discomfort. From the distance, I shall always yearn for the "orange sherbet" sunsets, the vast sky, its blanket of brilliant stars, and cool evening breezes.

I remember how, early in my research, upon my first arrival at sunset in a small seminomadic community, I was warmly welcomed, fed, and generously given a small conical grass building (called a *tettrem* in that region) where I could sleep until the hot season, when we all slept either in cooler nomadic tents or outside in the open. Even in that intricately constructed, strong shelter, however, I slept fitfully, awakened by the high winds, and I was obliged to chase after the door, which had become detached and buffeted about like a feather. I also remember the howls of jackals in the nearby rocks, and barking dogs, which ran in packs through the village after sundown.

These physical hazards, while undoubtedly more intimidating to me as an outsider, nonetheless can endanger anyone. Suffering cannot be prevented, but it can be relieved. Empathy and comfort are important cultural values. Although there is some regional variation in degree of specialization and emphasis upon inheritance, in many Tuareg groups, medicine women (*tinesmegelen* in the Niger Aïr dialect of Tamajaq and *tinesefren* in the Malian dialect) are respected and renowned for their integration of technical skills and religious devotion, particularly in rural areas. Even in towns, a few women still practice. Central to their practice is touch: many medicine women often diagnose and heal by touching the stomach after touching the earth, in their consultations with patients. Most medicine women treat with a combination of plants: women healers mix their own recipes and pass them down in their family or nomadic camp. The extent to which their learning and "certification" are formalized varies somewhat, but in general, most medicine women acquire their skills by lengthy apprenticeship with an older relative.

Although their close relationship to nature cannot be ignored, there are hints here of more complex and specialized practices, of healing illnesses that straddle organic and nonorganic categories as well as "natural," "personalistic," and "cultural" domains. Around Mount Bagzan, an Aïr massif where herbalism enjoys great esteem and herbalists are very numerous in certain descent groups, residents asserted, "*tinesmegelen* know all about women's pregnancy, childbirth, and health." In this book, I show how extravisual, textual and non-textual, and psychosocial medico-ritual knowledge are as crucial to their curing as medicinal trees. Also important is their medico-ritual healing paraphernalia: central to this is the medicine pot, called *ten* (or *tin*), ideally made of clay (not steel or iron). Many of their concepts of wellness and illness are difficult to translate exactly into Euro-American allopathic medical and English language terms. In fact, I argue, translation can only be approximate; indeed, seeking an exact equivalence only leads to "translation as treason." *Okuf*, for example, the local name for an illness of the upper respiratory tract that is difficult to translate exactly, illustrates in a preliminary way the complexity of these cultural elaborations. In the local viewpoint, this condition has very physical manifestations but is not caused merely by germs: for *okuf* also occurs "when one lacks something," the latter a more general condition designated by another term, *anoughou*. The remedy for *okuf* is a medicine that is inhaled, but its diagnosis often involves ritual divination to determine its possible range of causes. Therefore, while herbal medicine women, it is true, do often work with what Euro-American systems would classify as "natural (botanical/pharmaceutical) remedies," nonetheless, their work encompasses much more than this, and it more broadly inverts and reinvents natural and cultural categories and relationships. The present book explores these elaborations on universal themes of nature and culture in healing and religion from medicine women's viewpoint.

Many French-speaking Tuareg describe *tinesmegelen* as also being "like magicians." A medicine woman who has special mediumistic powers is called *tamanai* or *tamaswad*. Herbal medicine women who have acquired this additional divination skill are somewhat rare, and they must receive this from tutelary spirits in a calling, after an illness. Other medicine women specialize in bone-setting skills; they are called *tamadas* (pl. *timadasen*). Yet many herbal medicine women combine, to one degree or another, all these skills. Their occupation is learned, but is also usually inherited in clans. Many medicine women in the Aïr region northeast of Agadez, for example, originally come from a specific region: the area of Ajirou, near a dried riverbed (*oeud*) east of an old oasis and caravanning village that is also a holy center. At this site is sacred, consecrated, or "enchanted" land (*al hima*), surrounding a shrine of its past founder, a marabout from the East.

It is therefore difficult to generalize about medicine women and their healing in terms of biomedical, anthropological, or Western philosophical and ethnoscientific categories; for these are experienced in different ways by different healers, and many cure nonorganic disorders as well. Medicine women are fascinating because they do not fit neatly into any preestablished cultural or linguistic category in religion, healing, science, or "magic"—according to either occidental or local classifications. Thus the present study hopes to contribute to wider anthropological efforts to deconstruct and recast logical systems of thought (Crick 1976; Parkin 1990; Gottlieb 1992).

Medicine women also remind anthropologists of the need for caution against sweeping generalizations concerning mediumistic diviners and "shamans." In the standard anthropological definition, mediums are "shamanistic" healers found primarily in agricultural societies with political integration beyond the level of the small local community (Winkelman 1999, 2000). Although mediums engage in deliberate induction of ASC (altered states of consciousness) during training, they differ from the ASC of shamans. Mediums are selected through spirit possession and the spontaneous onset of afflictions. Mediums' initial ASC episodes leading to training are thought to occur spontaneously and outside their personal control. They involve possession experiences, episodes in which the personality of the individual is believed to be replaced by a spirit entity (Winkelman 1999:171). Although the initial ASC episodes of a mediums are spontaneous and out of control, they then engage in deliberate ASC induction procedures (for example, chanting and/or fasting), though they still have a possessing spirit.

In many though not all cultures, mediums are predominantly women and/or other persons who are generally assumed to be of " low social and economic status" (Winkelman 1999:171), or at least ambiguous, disputed status (Kendall in McClain 1989). The Tuareg case adds an interesting nuance to this. Despite social upheavals and property loss affecting both men and women from drought, nation-state law, and war (Claudot-Hawad 1993, 1996, 2002; Oxby 1990; Rasmussen 2001b; Keenan 2003), most Tuareg women still enjoy relatively high social prestige, and are now, through regional programs of cultural revitalization, peace, reconciliation, and repatriation of Tamajaq speakers, attempting to resuscitate their traditionally full socioeconomic independence (Murphy 1964, 1967; Worley 1991; Nicolaisen and Nicolaisen 1997; Rasmussen 2003).[2] Thus Tuareg medicine women refute many ethnographic and theoretical generalizations about gender and healing, and they open up new perspectives in the anthropology of religion. Medical anthropology, the anthropology of religion, and the anthropology of gender offer theories and concepts that illuminate herbal medical ideology and practice, but local specialists who do not conform completely to previous paradigms in these fields of study also have much to say to anthropology.

Through the years, I learned much from medicine women, and I am still listening. My strategy here is to convey their perspectives by opening many chapters with their own words (of course, these do not necessarily represent all medicine women; rather, I explore what can be learned from these women), and in narratives from interviews (structured and unstructured), guided conversations, and life histories. I intersperse these narratives with illustrative case studies and participant-observation because I believe in the value of contextual analysis of social practice (Ortner 1996; Ahearn 1998), as well as discourse. Following medicine women's voices, therefore, are others' voices as well (for example, patients' and marabouts'), interwoven into subsequent passages where these are relevant to a given context or illuminate more general principles of health, illness, and healing. Throughout, these discussions are interwoven with broader contextualization and analysis. I attempt to make sense of approximately twenty medicine women's perspectives as local theorists by situating them in wider socioeconomic, cultural, and healing processes, with some juxtaposition against my own experiences and categories during my field research in Tamajaq-speaking communities between approximately 1982 and 2002, predominantly in Niger and more briefly in Mali.[3]

My relationships with each medicine woman varied in depth and duration: I have been friends with some for over twenty years, with others, for less time, and I met a few recently, through local friends and field assistants. Hence the variation in depth and intimacy of data for each. Several central "core" figures offer rich insights in longitudinal histories and cases. Others appear more peripherally, yet still offer valuable insights. My goal is similar to that of some other researchers who attempt, in so far as possible, to present local healers' voices (Olkes and Stoller 1987; Perrone, Stockel, and Krueger 1989; E. Turner 1996; Stoller 1997, 2004; Trudelle-Schwartz 2003), albeit with awareness that some voices circulate more than others and a given selected voice does not imply perfect typicality or generalization (Crapanzano 1980). I hope to examine healing and ceremonial specialists in their full range of varying degrees of informal and professional dimensions. Many medicine women regard themselves as ordinary women who are unofficially recognized as proficient; indeed, in some regions, such as northern Mali, I found that many married women with children have some degree of medicinal knowledge, passed informally down from their mothers, particularly in more nomadic communities. These latter medicine women, however, tend to treat primarily a small circle of kinspersons or members of their immediate camp or village. By contrast, other medicine women, in particular those around Mt. Bagzan in Aïr in northern Niger, are more specialized: these latter undergo extensive formal apprenticeships, receive authorization from mentors to practice, and become widely renowned over great distances, called upon to treat non-kin as well as kin.

Methods

My methods included guided conversations, participant-observation, and unstructured and structured interviews. Additional commentaries appear interspersed throughout the chapters. Commentaries and narratives are followed by social contextualization with life histories, case studies, and ethnographic data interwoven with data from my own participant-observation—although I did not choose to practice herbal medicine myself, for reasons having to do with medicine women's required older and maternal status and my status as a younger and childless woman.

I analyze tropes, the metaphorical and metonymical significance of "natural" and "social/cultural" elements—indeed these cannot be separated—and relate them to patient's conditions, albeit with medicine women's commentaries and practices hopefully "tempering" my own analysis. I analyze how symbolism, ritual, and social practice persist and change according to different curing contexts. I combine some life history approaches with other anthropological techniques for the analysis of healing and ceremonial specialists (Perrone, Stockel, and Krueger 1989; McCarthy-Brown 1991; Trudelle-Schwartz 2003). Like Edith Turner (1996:xxvi), I attempt to usually allow the medicine women with their commentaries to "lead me," rather than to force their commentaries into a rigid index of categories, although of course it would be impossible to avoid completely my own culturally and academically grounded overarching concepts. The important point here is to illustrate how these latter are contingent, and never completely congruent with those of Tuareg medicine women.

The goal in the present account is to draw attention to how healers construct their experiences into both personally and culturally acceptable pathways in their roles as, in effect, artists, scientists, and mothers at once. This involves the acceptance of medicine women's accounts of their origin ("etiological myth" variants—the Tagurmat "motif") as, not just "folktales," but as a kind of mythico-history, in which the boundaries between myth and history are porous. Indeed, to medicine women, these "myths" are history: medicine women take them very seriously as truth. Yet there is the problem here that not all local residents take them equally seriously, and also, forgetting is equally important. Thus I find it also necessary to integrate these more subjective experiences and perspectives with wider events and situations that constrain and influence herbal healers' lives and professions, primarily in the latter portions of this book. I analyze these disagreements, however, more in terms of how medicine women view them: as not so much competition or rivalry or oppression, but as complementary. I attempt to show how this integrative process occurs in Tuareg herbalists' lives.

I do not claim that each medicine woman represents all such healers; nor indeed do these medicine women collectively represent all of them. I do not attempt to establish sweeping generalities or the representativeness of all these ritual practitioners. While medicine women do not work in a vacuum, my primary focus here is not medical pluralism among the Tuareg—such a study, emphasizing semiotic and sociopolitical processes surrounding medicine and diverse healers in wider infrastructures, has already been written (Rasmussen 2001a). No single work, of course, represents the "final word" on any topic. What is important is that a given healer's story be told in a form meaningful to the healer herself (McClain 1989:136). I would add here, however, that this narrative, at least in part, needs to be given expression in a way that reaches the reading audience, as well. All personal names are pseudonyms, in order to protect the anonymity, privacy, and safety of subjects. Place-names of regions, already-famous places, and large villages and towns are actual names; those of very small camps are fictionalized, modified, or omitted.

In early sections of this book, I analyze the relationship between herbal medicine, ritual, and other processes in medicine women's healing in order to critically deconstruct the concept of "medico-ritual" and related categories used to designate others' modes of thought and healing practices. Subsequent sections discuss interactions between medicine women and several other authorities and knowledge systems: their intense relations with local marabouts and, since the peace accords and repatriation programs following the armed rebellion, their more distant, yet looming relations with state and NGO-sponsored Western biomedical clinic staffs. The conclusions sum up and reassess classifications of herbalist and medico-ritual practitioners in logical modes of thought (art, science, religion) in terms of current concerns about anthropological constructs or glosses. Finer nuances are revealed in medicine women's specialty.

Organization of this Book

There are three major parts to this book. Part I consists of Chapters 1 and 2, in which I engage theoretical and ethnographic issues relevant to medicine women's work. Chapter 2 explores herbal medicine women's concepts of wellness, illness, and healing; there are narratives, vignettes, and a case study, with a focus upon the counteractive humoral "hot/cold" medical system many medicine women emphasize as well as its relation to other illnesses and treatments.

This material leads into the theme of Part II, learning and passing on the profession and wider cultural memory/knowledge systems, in particular, the senses, beginning with Chapter 3, in which the focus is upon touch and the body; in Chapter 4, emphasis is placed upon aural traditions, listening and sound, leading into herbal medicine women's mythico-history and position vis-à-vis cultural memory. Following this, in Chapter 5, I develop these ideas as they impinge upon the connections between herbal medicine, gender, and age and medicine women's mediating roles in wider processes of physical and social reproduction. In Chapter 6, I explore the metaphorical significance of arboreal imagery against the backdrop of herbalism and revisit the "natural" in relation to the "cultural."

Part III, on Power, consists of Chapters 7 through the Conclusions. These chapters emphasize the relationships between herbal medicine women and official authorities: specifically, in Chapter 7, there is an exploration of the practices of herbal medicine women in sacred spaces and their deployment of a power commonly more associated with "official" leaders: *al baraka* ritual protection. This material leads into Chapter 8, which examines medicine women's relationships with Islam and marabouts; Chapter 9 examines medicine women's mediumistic powers and divination practices within the framework of issues in "shamanism"; Chapter 10 briefly examines their relationships with state and NGO–sponsored clinic personnel and programs influenced by Western established biomedicine or allopathic medicine, and ways in which they cope with these forces. Finally, there are Conclusions regarding the wider significance of herbal medicine women's healing ideology and practice for modes of thought, gender, and healing in the anthropology of religion, medical anthropology, gender studies, and African studies.

Although I do not seek to force my data in this book into any previous theoretical paradigm, I acknowledge my debt to pioneering and current contributions in three major areas of inquiry: 1) modes of thought, particularly African systems of thought (so-called "magic, science, and religion" and philosophy debates); 2) gender and healing, specifically female practitioners; and 3) feminist critiques of science or "authoritative knowledge" (gender and science issues). I now situate my own work in these efforts.

Part One / Departures

Herbal Medicine and Local and
Authoritative Systems of Thought

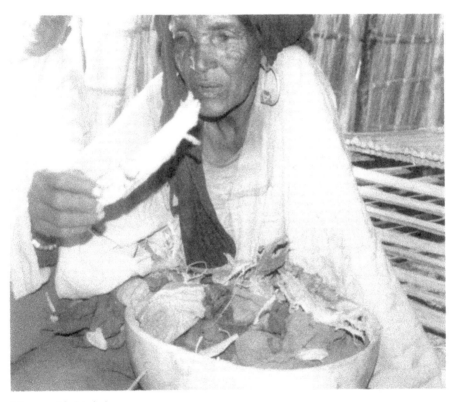

Woman with dried plants

12

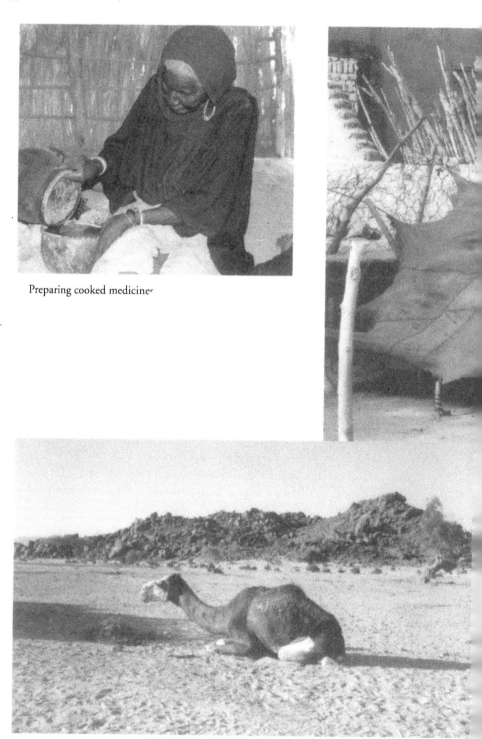

Preparing cooked medicine

Rural Saharan regions

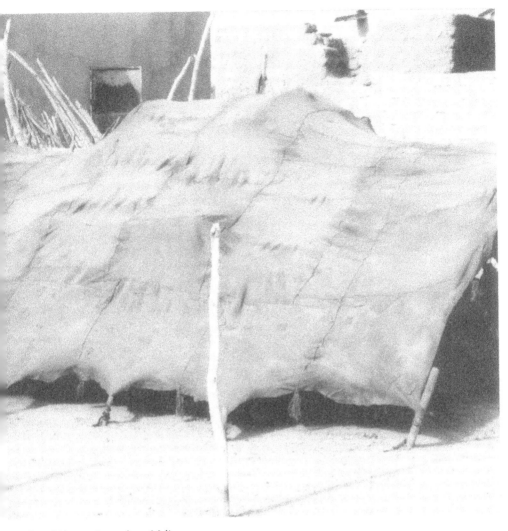

Goat-hide tent in northern Mali

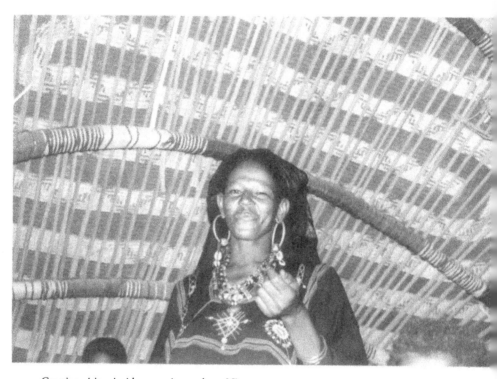

Greeting visitor inside a tent in northern Niger

1–The Vexing Problem of Difference and Classifications in Anthropology and the Local Ethnographic Setting

Local Modes of Thought–"Ours" and "Theirs"

In my view, Tuareg medicine women's work alerts one to the problem of two extremes of error in anthropology: on the one hand, exoticizing "others'" modes of thought and medico-ritual practices, a practice now justifiably critiqued by a number of scholars (Horton 1967, 1982; Hollis and Lukes 1982; Douglas 1966, 1975, 1996; Tambiah 1990; Herzfeld 2001)—and on the other, an equally problematic strategy intended as a corrective to this: assuming that others' beliefs and practices must be exactly like ours in order to be "logical" or "rational" (Malinowski 1948; Green 1999). The latter position assumes that equal must mean equivalence, or that two systems must function exactly alike, or else they are implicitly ranked. Unfortunately, the latter position has resulted, however inadvertently, in condescending attempts to remake others in our own image. Here, I follow Levi-Strauss somewhat, in arguing for understanding modes of thought in their own terms, as all coexisting and representing a universal human mental logic, although with distinctive permutations (Levi-Strauss 1962), although I do not endorse this theorist's abstract structuralist method or binary oppositions, or his insistence upon clear-cut distinctions between "our science" vs. "bricolage."

While I eschew the more insidious and sinister connotations of rigid classification orders, I nonetheless believe that, in order for meaning to be salient, an entity or action must in fact be in some way distinctive. As Parkin (1991) points out, for example, for a region to be designated as "sacred," it must be somehow distinct from other regions, and these latter must also be distinctive from the former, in somehow being different from "sacred." Following Lyotard's concern with *la différence,* Joan Scott (1994) has noted that equality need not imply sameness or identicalness. Local modes of thought are distinctive and interesting in and of themselves, as elaborations on universal themes, and need not be a taboo or polluted zone in anthropology today, as some theories of globalization tend to imply. While this book does not call for a return to older models of exoticism, Orientalism, or for that matter, its evil twin, Occidentalism (Carrier 1992), it seeks some alternative to the other extreme: of taking others' modes of thought too literally, for example, as being exactly like Western biomedical germ and contagion theories. Indeed, these latter are not even characteristic of all "Western" modes of thought (Martin 1994; Douglas 1966, 1996; Herzfeld 2001).

Currently, the challenge for anthropology, as I see it, is to avoid an overly globalizing, tyrannical modernistic bias, which can be just as oppressive and ethnocentric as older evolutionary paradigms. The goal of this book is not to show how "scientific" Tuareg herbal healing is in an outsider's viewpoint, or simplistically that "women, too, do their own science." Nor is my goal to force an African variant into models neatly based on our philosophy or biomedicine. In the relationship between the "West and the Rest," "Others" do more than simply "chime in" after Us; there is more to their modes of thought than merely an echo of our own. The present book analyzes Tuareg herbal medicine in its own right, as a local elaboration on universal human themes.

Indigenous healers provide at least 80 percent of medical services used worldwide (Green 1999:7). As Green correctly warns, by ignoring or dismissing indigenous and personal medical theories, health policy makers miss potentially key insights into improved characterizations of illness and rule out the possibility of understanding them and their continuing importance to many local residents. More problematic is the unintended consequence of these arguments: to force these indigenous medical theories into our own categories of thought, as for example, an "indigenous contagion theory" or "ICT" (Green 1999:7). There are useful questions raised here concerning assumptions about "our own" theories and categories. Are these latter, in fact, so "logical" that to exonerate ourselves from exoticism, we must show "others' categories" are just like ours? Local medical theories and practices do address critical global health promotion/disease prevention issues. Similarly, anthropological theories themselves contain local ethnographic data (Davis 1983; Martin 1994; Herzfeld 2001).[1] It is true that different languages may call the same thing by different names. Although ICTs often frame issues in terms alien to biomedical health providers (for example, as "pollution"), some specific ICTs have approximate biomedical equivalents as different sets of knowledge that address the same health promotion/disease prevention issues (Green 1999).

Notwithstanding the value of these insights, in my view they do not solve problems of translation, context, or even power. Rather than being obsolete in globalization, these problems have, if anything, become more acute. Some idioms (Crick 1976; Crapanzano and Garrison 1977; Parkin 1991), furthermore, resist exact translation. There is indeed the need to open effective lines of communication and coordination between biomedically trained people who direct global health promotion/disease prevention efforts, local healers, and client populations. Yet in this rush to find exact parallels and equivalences, there are also dangers of creating composite meanings and dismissing additional nuances important in local residents' own viewpoints. No biomedical or medico-ritual system is monolithic or a tabula rasa; all contain some elements that do not fit neatly into any category in any classification system. I do not believe the logic of a given system of thought need be validated by finding ways in which it mimics that of the researcher's or dominant system of authoritative knowledge.

Additional valuable studies (Arens and Karp 1989; Mudimbe 1991; Karp and Masolo 2000), alternatively, recognize that just because there are extra-biomedical, extra-human, or "supernatural" powers of creativity at work in a given medical or philosophical system, even under a rubric of "medico-ritual," it is not in any sense less logical than our own, though neither is it exactly like our own. Power, for example, may be conceptualized and may operate entirely differently from in our prevalent Weberian understandings of it. Also, cultural interpretations need not neglect analysis of power relations. The present book draws out the implications of these observations, as a reminder that equivalent status does not necessarily confer equality, and equality does not necessarily require sameness, or imply no difference. As Joan Scott (1994) observes, identicalness or sameness can in fact be used to oppress.

Recent scholarship has critically deconstructed and recast "magic," "religion," and "science" as themselves culture-bound distinctions and Euro-American classifications, and it has questioned efforts to make any system conform neatly to one or another of these categories (Jackson 1989; Tambiah 1990). Inspired in some cases by the works of Carlos Castaneda emphasizing the "separate reality" known to Yaqui Native Americans of the Mexican highlands, they have considered "magical" phenomena as objectively real, whether or not they are explicable in terms of Western scientific knowledge (Jackson 1989; Olkes and Stoller 1987; Stoller 1989, 2004).

I agree that calling apparently "magical" powers "rational" only by reference to the outside researcher's cultural formulation is just as problematic as calling them "irrational." Yet the outside researcher's formulation is difficult to dismiss from consciousness. This poses complex epistemological problems that affect the understanding of Tuareg medicine women's powers. Medicine women's treatments represent local theorizing, power, and elaborations on the general human theme of creativity, imagination, and problem-solving, thereby offering alternatives to all extremes (and circular arguments) of anthropological theorizing on modes of thought. Hopefully, this book about medicine women offers alternatives to, and constructive critical refinements of, some old tenacious categories that tend, despite their reworking, to persist and affect—indeed, infect and afflict!—medical anthropology. Medicine women remind us of the universal cultural penchant for classifying but also alert us to its limitations and dangers (Malkki 1995).

Hence the challenge of exploring the interface between religion and medicine. According to Green, "pollution" is most salient in its literal, empirically grounded sense; in contrast to theorists such as Douglas (1966, 1996) and Gottlieb (1992), he does not emphasize its symbolic aspect, for example, as "matter out of place." However, in my view, this is an artificial distinction. For this latter aspect may be just as instrumental, meaningful, logical, and powerful—for example, in a state regime of classification (Malkki 1995)—or as one aspect of a more general belief, practice, or policy of fertility and lineage perpetuation (Gottlieb 1992). One must therefore beware of overly literalist readings of modes of thought, including our own, the latter analyzed by Sontag (1978, 1989), Martin (1994), Tambiah (1990), and Douglas (1996). It is true that environmental theories are sometimes based on the belief that elements in the physical environment can cause or spread illness, for example, the idea that contagious illness can be carried in the air or wind. For example, many Bemba of Zambia believe that tuberculosis is an illness in the air, spread by inhalation of unclean dust carried by the wind. The Bambara of Mali classify smallpox, measles, and other contagious illness as wind illness because only the wind has sufficiently widespread contact with the body to cause outbreaks (Imperato 1977:15). The Hausa, likewise, classify certain spirits, the *iskoki,* as of the wind (Nicolas 1975); however, not all spirits are of the wind, not all spirits of the wind cause illness, and not only some spirits of the wind cause illness, but other spirits do, as well (Masquelier in Comaroff 1993; Schmoll in Comaroff 1993). According to Green, the *tifo temoya* illness in the air is a general Swazi term denoting "illnesses that are contracted through inhalation" (Green 1999:14). Sound preventative practices are indisputably found in these theories.

Yet these and other illness-related categories should not be given an exclusively literal interpretation, or used to make these beliefs exactly coincide with our own. Instructive here is a widespread Tuareg belief reiterated by many medicine women: the belief that women who have recently given birth are particularly vulnerable to *ado*, a disease of the wind and its associated spirits (Rasmussen 1997). But other persons—namely, men—are not so vulnerable to this, and new fathers do not undergo women's forty-day protective medico-ritual seclusion for this reason. When Tuareg men do need protection, it is for other reasons, such as vulnerability to spirits when they first take up the men's face-veil/turban.[2] Moreover, many Tuareg also believe in additional malevolent forces, but these have specific referents that are not easily reduced to a general "hygienic" basis. Rather they have a social and/or spiritual basis: the belief, for example, in *tegare* (denoting approximately the "flying of the birds"), a malevolent force that flies through the air from the angry heart of a smith/artisan toward someone who has offended him or her by refusing the smith's request for compensation or presents.[3]

Clearly, components of contagion theory relate to perceived rules or laws, observed cause-and-effect relationships, the natural environment, and/or the involvement of material things. But so-called Western theories of contagion, conversely, also include mystical elements, such as pollution beliefs and social and moral concerns, for example in folk theories of tuberculosis, cancer, leprosy, and AIDS transmission (Sontag 1978, 1989; Douglas 1996) and in notions of disease resistance (Davis 1983; Martin 1994). Green argues that many African theories are "naturalistic," agreeing with Murdock (1980) here, but disagrees with Murdock's classification of contagion or pollution theories as "mystical" and suggests that pollution beliefs, as well as those relating to environmental dangers, are "naturalistic" or "quasi-naturalistic" (Green 1999:14). They involve an impersonal process of illness through contact or exposure; polluted individuals are not singled out for illness or misfortune by a human or superhuman force; they typically become polluted from mere contact, from being in the wrong place at the wrong time. Yet this situating of humans in a given place is also culturally constructed; indeed, as shown in many studies of gender, nature, and culture (Ortner 1974, 1996; MacCormack and Strathern 1980), the category of "nature" is itself highly variable across cultures. As I show in forthcoming chapters, Tuareg medicine women's positionings in this scheme—in particular, their relationship to and actions in ritual spaces—are complex, variable, and contradictory.

Why invoke these classifications at all? Why force others' beliefs and practices into any of these categories? Herbal medicine women offer a precaution against anthropological tendencies to overgeneralize, overcompensate, or ignore evidence that at least some illness and treatment systems involve more complex, difficult-to-classify etiologies, diagnoses, and cures. In my view, the solution is to recognize that some etiologies in each local system include diverse types of explanation and modes of thought, including some from global encounters—and also possess their own, equally rational and effective bases of logic and power. The present book explores what these are and proceeds by exploring how these logical systems are elaborated and what their consequences are for local practitioners and for anthropology. This endeavor, in my view, seems to be the valid goal of anthropology and ethnography; to experience a way of life radically different from one's own but also characterized by some common themes in unexpected places.

Perhaps isolation, avoidance, or social marginalization of people in polluted states does serve to quarantine those who, in fact, could be a health threat to others because of their contagiousness. But there is the need to recognize a combination of logics here rather than sweepingly label or rigidly classify entire etiologies in "water-tight cabinets." To many Africans, health workers seem to supplant local explanations and theories with what sound to them like "scientific mumbo-jumbo" (Green 1999:15). The question raised here is an interesting one. How important is what we call a given system of disease etiology, even if we call it "indigenous contagion theory" rather than "pollution"? Just because a people do not have a term for something, that does not imply they lack a concept of it. On the other hand, because two concepts may be given an approximately similar translation, this does not imply their senses are identical.

In my view, the solution here is two-fold: to redirect analysis to this wider issue of local theories of causation, power, and logical interconnections; and to recognize the presence of the unknowable or a "separate reality," for example, pollution theories of illness, in all human modes of logic and power, not solely in healing and biomedicine, but also in anthropological theories of them and in everyday life (Jackson 1989; Martin 1994; Douglas 1996). These debates have reverberated throughout more specialized studies focusing on particular aspects of healing, for example, mediumistic shamanism. Winkelman (2002:1876) correctly observes that the nature of shamanism has been confusing because of a range of meanings and denotations associated with the concept of the "shaman." These stem from shamanism's origin outside of Western cultures and its similarity to worldwide practices involving the use of ASCs (Winkelman 1992, 1999, 2000, 2001). Although healing featuring spirit possession/mediumship/trance of specialists is found in many cultures, most anthropological studies of those healers glossed as "shamans" (a term deriving from Siberian languages) are based on data from Siberian, Arctic, Native American, and East Asian peoples. The meaning of shamanism as a total social phenomenon and as the point of articulation of the three levels—psychological, sociological and religious—of power, in which it is expressed, has been much studied by symbolic anthropology (Saladin d'Anglure 1994, 1996:507). The shaman appears, from this perspective, as a mediator who transcends these levels in a complex and dynamic fusion. Many Tuareg herbal medicine women, somewhat like shamans, are able to overcome contradictions between binary oppositions (man/woman, humans/animals, humans/spirits, living/dead) through playing with ambiguity, paradox and transgression, in order to manage crises, disorder, and change.

In fact, the exact nature of shamanism is in dispute, but the idea that shamanism is cross-cultural or universal was widely accepted before systematic empirical research established the commonalities. Yet much evidence from mediumistic healing is also nonempirical (Stoller 1989; Taussig 1987; E. Turner 1996). Thus the anthropological concept of "core shamanism" (Harner 1990; Winkelman and White 1987), while useful, still does not resolve the problem of nonempirical, subjective, and experiential data, problems of translation, and cross-cultural variations on this common theme. Despite different cultural backgrounds, however, Winkelman argues that shamans in hunter-gatherer societies have substantial characteristics in common and differ significantly from other types of "magico-religious" practitioners (Winkelman 1992). Cross-cultural research shows shamans are found among hunter-gatherers and slightly more complex societies with limited agriculture or pastoral subsistence patterns. These societies often lack political hierarchies and have leadership limited to the local community, where the shaman is a charismatic leader with informal political power (Winkelman 2002:1877).

The Tuareg case partly conforms to and partly contradicts these observations. The precolonial social order was stratified and hierarchical, but leadership was not strongly centralized and lacked absolute authority.[4] Whereas most Tuareg medicine women tend to conduct their healing in private, shamanic ritual was a most important group event, structuring relationships of individuals to the collectivity and cosmos (Winkelman 2002:1878). The present book will show these elements to be present in modified form in Tuareg medicine women's massage and diagnostic touch, cleansings and purgings, and plant medicines.

Rather than asking whether shamanism exists among the Tuareg, in some herbal medicine woman's more specialized skill in mediumistic divination and healing, I ask: what forms and meanings do "shaman"-like activities take among some, though not all, Tuareg herbalists? Some shamans' symbols are recognized and understood in "magical" or religious ritual, but others are arbitrary, carrying specific meanings assigned by the user and given by speech, nonverbal motions, or even just thoughts. For example, some other (non-herbalist) professional Tuareg *bokaye* diviners, predominantly men, often wear the color blue, associated with spirits, and red henna, associated with fertility and marriage, symbolizing their metaphorical marriage to spirits in their pact (Rasmussen 2001a, 2003). Symbols can be transformed from one ritual context to another. Objects used in rituals can be used in "magical" ways, their power intended to motivate the natural forces, or as a defense against malignant spirits or against forces directed at a person by the malign magic of another.

Tuareg medicine women, in particular those with mediumistic powers, appear to use "magical" principles, albeit similar to those of psychotherapists in processes of seeking hidden (occult) information about past, present, or future events, whether directly from spiritual beings who have information, or by tapping into the natural program in which traces of all events are permanently recorded. Both request and response are transmitted and interpreted symbolically, but among Tuareg medicine women, as I show, these techniques tend to be more enacted or embodied than verbalized or represented visually.

Many central nation-state regimes and missionaries have tried to restrict, if not abolish, shamanic and other mediumistic healers in this process, for example, in the former Soviet Union. These systems of authoritative knowledge and worldview relegated certain other kinds of orientations and activities—for example so-called pagan religions and their magical rites—to an inferior position, assumed to be superseded by others in evolutionary fashion. Yet multiple systems of thought can coexist in all times and places. Mudimbe (1988, 1991) has shown the coexistence of oral and written traditions in the same time and place; and Levi-Strauss (1962) has argued for the coexistence of the engineer and the *bricoleur*. The present book explores how herbal medicine women represent both at once, and suggest, in their own theorizings, another alternative that blurs all these contrasts, traversing different intellectual terrains. Here I share some scholars' position that African philosophy, and indeed any philosophy, is above all a cultural inquiry (Karp and Masolo 2000: Introduction).

Gender and Healing Specialisms

Anthropologists have over the past quarter century increasingly focused more criti-cally on the broader social and cultural implications of women's healing. Many are questioning previous essentializing tendencies toward portrayals of "universal woman" and advocating more nuanced and contextual gender-oriented perspectives (Di Leonardo 1990; Mikell 1997). The present book hopes to contribute to this growing concern. I ask how recent conceptual schemes in feminist anthropology concerning gender and science, and in the anthropology of religion concerning systems or thought (specifically, the magic-religion-science conundrum), inform Tuareg herbal healing, overwhelmingly practiced by women. I also ask, reciprocally, how Tuareg medicine women's healing either supports or refutes conceptual schemes in the anthropology of gender and anthropology of medico-religion. The life histories and case studies of medicine women and their patients I collected illustrate the ways in which women's healing articulates with particular features of gender relations, gender ideology, and practice in the social and cultural contexts of Tuareg communities.

Classifications assume more than they explain. Yet feminist constructs, for example public/domestic, continue to bear directly on many studies of gendered healing (Strathern 1981; Rosaldo and Lamphere 1974; Rosaldo 1980; MacCormack and Strathern 1980; Ortner 1974, 1996). Personal attributes may differ from gender con-trasts, however (Strathern 1981). The "public/domestic" has been shown to take on different meanings historically and across cultures (Brenner 1998). Valuable studies show that practitioners are often ordinary women whose obligations include the care of other household members, children in particular (Finerman in McClain 1989:24–42; Bledsoe 2002). Also, alternatively, some women who become ritual or other specialized practitioners of medicine, in this process are liberated from their domestic obligations, and infuse powerful female symbolism—including tropes of maternal nurturance—into their healing practice (Wedenoja in McClain 1989:76–98). A central focus in the present book is the gendered healing significance of these tropes, their use in social context, and their consequences. I argue that Tuareg medicine women's healing, while alluding to motherhood and nurturing roles, nonetheless constitutes more than an ex-tension of their domestic roles. I also argue that Tuareg medicine women's practices do not represent solely a "compensation for" or "liberation from" otherwise restricted gen-der constructs in their society.

Also of interest in this book are critical reformulations of "natural and cultural" tropes. While the old "nature/culture" argument is now recognized as much more com-plex than its classical formulation as a duality, and I do not "beat this dead horse," I do seek to explore local cultural elaborations of nature—for after all, medicine women do work with natural substances. Issues of nature/culture in anthropology (Levi-Strauss 1962; MacCormack and Strathern 1980; Ortner 1974, 1996), and female "pollution" (Douglas 1966; Goddale 1980), have received much attention. Recent work has shown that nature and culture contrasts differ from society to society, that different societies juxtapose gender symbols with those of nature and culture in distinct ways, and that Euro-American definitions of nature and culture may have little to do with contrasts that other cultures use to order the world. But I do not intend to set up a "straw man."

I am well aware that many works have shown cross-cultural contrasts and variations in nature/culture formulations, which often include neither such dichotomies nor gender-linked attributes, and have argued that these particular dualisms are therefore Western and modern. Nor do I intend to perpetuate a circular argument by debating the nature/nurture conundrum among the Tuareg. Rather, what interests me in this discourse, what I believe can be salvaged, are the natural and cultural substances and tropes in local epistemologies and practices of herbalist healing, and the local uses of gender symbolism to conceptualize and reconceptualize nature and its culturally extended meanings of reproduction and generation.

The idea that women are positioned not between culture and nature, but between different social worlds, persists in medical anthropological literature, for example, women's symbolic marginality is a central explanatory theme in female divination among the Zulu (Ngubane 1977). Among the Tuareg, neither most women nor most herbalists are exactly "marginal" or associated with pollution, although they do mediate different domains. Tuareg herbal medicine women must, in fact, be exemplary members of the social community. As we shall see, many are preoccupied with the need to expiate themselves from "sin" (abaket), and they observe certain ritual and social restrictions.

Hence the value of the Tuareg data for a critique of conventional categories and classifications in medical anthropology, feminist anthropology, and the anthropology of religion, gender, and science. The question is, exactly what forces shape women's dominant position among Tuareg herbalists? Somewhat like Zulu diviners (Ngubane (1977:88), many Tuareg medicine women in effect communicate with ancestors and thus are structurally similar to mothers and chief mourners (also women) at funerals. In both roles, women are marginal, in the sense of being positioned at a boundary between society and the world of ancestors. It is through birth in female bodies, and death through females symbolically, that people move between the two worlds (Ngubane 1977:88). The point here is that marginality can mean being positioned as bridges between different worlds, as culturally constructed in the local universe, rather than being outsiders.

I show how medicine women, ritual specialists who communicate with ancestral spirits on behalf of their living descendants, are marginal, albeit neither in the sense of nature/culture mediators of the old binary opposition, nor in the sense of compensating for "low status," pollution, or exclusion from "official" domains, as argued in some early functionalist explanations of female possession.[5] Where spirits with whom women healers communicate are socially important, for example in Haiti, women ritual specialists are also socially important (McCarthy-Brown 1991). Among the Tuareg, those spirits remain important, but are seldom explicitly referred to verbally, for several reasons. In some contexts, I show, they are threatened. In others, they are muted in name teknonymy from respect and reserve due to wider age and ancestral-related statuses. Herbal medicine women commemorate these statuses and guard the childbearing statuses of the next age cohort.

Important works have addressed the confluence of gender, aging, and healing in analyzing women's status in terms of the specific age at which recruitment to a female healing role occurs and reasons for this (McClain 1989). In some studies, it has been argued that menopause releases women from the symbolic associations, social obligations, and restrictions of fertile women, and that post-menopausal women enter the public domain, exercise authority, and acquire prestige in the same way men do (Brown and Kerns 1992). Here, the symbolic associations of "the domestic" become intertwined with other female symbols (McClain 1989). In the present book, I show how Tuareg medicine women act in some respects as exaggerated or hyperbolic grandmothers, rather than solely androgynously, or as men. All women, moreover, are associated with home, which is represented among Tuareg as the female-built and -owned tent, with which women are strongly identified in ritual, symbolic, economic, and kinship contexts. Yet their roles extend beyond this domestic space. Female healers therefore need not always acquire male attributes or "official" profiles in order to be powerful and/or prestigious in healing.

"Shamanic" Healing. Gender. and Power

Somewhat like the Serbian *bajalica* described by Halpern in McClain (1989) who cures fellow villagers with oral charms and conjurings, Tuareg post-menopausal women who predominate as herbalist/diviners, although past reproductive age themselves, are not opposed symbolically or in practice to mothering. Maternal and other feminine metaphors pervade their mythico-history and practice. Like Ngubane's (1977) Zulu diviners, Serbian *bajalica* (Kerewaky-Halpern in McClain 1989), and Korean *mansin* (Kendall in McClain 1989:139), Tuareg medicine women healers are closer to society's boundaries and thus are imbued with social powers that they embody and enact in healing rituals.

Some feminist anthropologists have noted that midwifery, curing, shamanism, spirit possession, mediumship and other medico-ritual activities can permit women to achieve status or prestige outside their usual social roles (Boddy 1987; Kendall 1989; Tsing 1993; Bledsoe 2002). Many of these scholars interpret healing as serving women's economic or political self-interest, or as an avenue for women to participate in central cultural institutions of significance to both sexes. In other works, healing is seen to embody cultural images of femaleness as nurturing or as mediating between realms of existence, the public and domestic (Rosaldo and Lamphere 1974; Chodorow 1974; Reiter 1975), and the pure and polluted (Fitz Poole 1981; Douglas 1966). Since these dualities are now critiqued by many anthropology of gender theorists as problematic and culturally constructed binaries (Buckley and Gottlieb 1988; Di Leonardo 1990; Rasmussen 1991; Brenner 1998; Wood 1999), the issue arises here of exactly what is mediated, how, and why, in herbal medicine healing. As mediators, Tuareg medicine women cross symbolic, social, and medical boundaries, particularly those separating the human world from that of spirits or ancestors, and intervene with the latter on behalf of their patients or clients. They also mediate wider forces that cause illness when the body experiences imbalance: namely, hot or cold, excess emotion like fright or anger, and harmful natural qualities like the wind.

Anthropologists are increasingly emphasizing the broader social and cultural implications of women's healing, for example, in agency, practice, discourse, and power. Many theorists are also questioning previous essentializing tendencies toward portrayals of "universal woman" and advocating more nuanced and contextual gender-oriented perspectives. Sargent in McClain (1989:204–18) describes how Bariba women's control over childbirth was usurped by the Benin government maternity services, a change that removed a traditional source of reward and achievement for mothers. Traditional midwifery is dying out in Benin towns, which thus removes one of the few avenues for social prestige open to women. In the latter portions of the present book, I explore the extent to which this is true among the Tuareg, by analyzing some medicine women's encounters with two more powerful official healing forces: namely, Islamic scholar/marabouts and biomedically trained clinic staffs in sedentarized and urban settings. In these contexts, the issue of authoritative knowledge is of central relevance.

Authoritative Knowledge Construction, Gender and Science, and Feminist Critiques of Science

Jordan (in Davis-Floyd and Sargent 1997:55–80) discusses the notion of authoritative knowledge, noting that, for any particular domain, several knowledge systems exist. Some of these, by consensus, come to carry more weight than others, either because they explain the state of the world better for the purposes at hand (efficacy), or because they are associated with a stronger power base (structural superiority), and usually both (Jordan 1993, in Davis-Floyd and Sargent 1997:56). For example, wise women in Anglo-Saxon medieval medicine were "shamanistic" in their regard for the unity and life of all things, and in their attempt to use the forces of nature for healing purposes. They knew herbal remedies and incantations. For example, they used belladonna like modern chloroform. They also relied on ritual therapy. These women healers, however, became restricted by the shifting paradigm of science: in the new worldview encompassing the scientific method, "all that appeared irrational and intuitive was subject to being purged in early modernism" (Achterberg 1985:69). Yet women's science and women's medicine were prime targets not solely of the developing Newtonian worldview and biomedicine but also of already established religion, namely the Church.

In other situations, however, equally legitimate, parallel knowledge systems exist, and people move easily between them, using them sequentially or simultaneously for different purposes. Yet frequently, one kind of knowledge gains ascendance and legitimacy. A consequence of legitimation of one kind of knowing as "authoritative" is the devaluation—often the dismissal—of all other kinds of knowing (Jordan 1993, in Davis-Floyd and Sargent 1997). Among Tuareg as elsewhere, the constitution of authoritative knowledge is an ongoing social process that both builds and reflects power relationships within a community of practice. Participants come to see the current order as a "natural" order.

Drawing in part on Davis-Floyd and Sargent and Jordan, I approach authoritative knowledge as an interactionally grounded notion. I discuss how participants in particular environments make visible to themselves and to each other what the grounds are for their proceedings. I show how, in some situations, some kinds of knowledge count and others don't, regardless of their relative "truth value." Jordan (in Davis-Floyd and Sargent 1997:59) describes how midwives, who in the environment of hospital-based training courses often appeared stupid, illiterate, and inarticulate, showed a completely different face when engaged in work in their own communities, where their skills were acknowledged and respected (Jordan 1997:60). In the latter portions of this book, I show how some Tuareg medicine women in more sedentarized and urban communities stand in effect between several worlds—where they encounter wider authorities of official Islam (marabouts), and nation-state and international NGO biomedically trained staffs—and I explore how medicine women manage these encounters, which present opportunities, but also dangers.

The Setting: Local and Wider Contexts of Tuareg Wellness, Illness, and Healing

I am convinced that it is impossible to convey the full complexity of human cultural experience in a few "introductory" pages of a single book. Thus I present much additional historical and ethnographic data in dispersed form where relevant to a given context, throughout the ensuing chapters and footnotes.

Before proceeding, I wish to clarify my stance concerning culture and ethnicity. While I admire recent efforts in anthropology to resist essentializing portrayals of "the Other," and I agree that one must be aware that cultural and ethnic categories have often been constructed in wider infrastructures asserting Euro-American authority (Said 1978; Carrier 1992; Urban 1998), I nonetheless believe that it is a mistake to completely abandon the concept of a certain unity in common themes of experience. Indeed, many local residents would be insulted by the opposite extreme, of denying them an identity. The challenge here is to avoid totalizing perspectives but still salvage useful elements in the culture concept that coincide with many (though not all) local viewpoints. Many contemporary European and American scholars emphasize the internal diversity of Tamajaq-speaking communities (Rasmussen 2001a; Bouman 2003), yet also their sharing of common themes. Many local Tamajaq-speaking scholars and ordinary local residents place great emphasis upon the salience of "Tuareg" as a cultural grouping (Dayak 1992), albeit one that is never static, isolated, or monolithic. Many insist upon the importance of temoust (denoting "identity," and sometimes, "culture"), based upon the Tamajaq language, and critique some older French uses of "l'ethnie," a term which they associate with folk notions of race. Therefore, although Tamajaq-speaking communities are characterized by considerable social and occupational diversity, as well as longstanding interaction through trading, migrations, and intermarriage, I emphasize in this section their shared commonality (though not uniformity!) for purposes of bounding my topic, clarifying my argument, and honoring local residents' and scholars' perspectives.

Most Tuareg (also sometimes known as Kel Tamajaq, after their language) today live in the northern regions of the nations of Mali, Niger, Burkina Faso, and in southern Algeria, and Libya, although many have migrated south, others have traveled across the Sahara on caravan trade, and a few, more widely on labor migration and other itinerant trading. They are believed to have originated in the central Saharan Fezzan region of Libya, although some groups trace their origins farther back to Yemen. Some Tamajaq speakers from Mali and Niger have fled from recent drought and war to refugee communities in Mauritania and Burkina Faso. In addition, many men travel extensively on the caravan trade of salt, dates, millet, and household supplies to Nigeria and as labor migrants to Nigeria and increasingly, now, to countries beyond Africa, where some sell artisan works and a few reside long-term, but tend to leave their wives at home (Rasmussen 2001b).

Tamajaq (alternative spelling: Tamacheq) is a language in the Berber group of the Afro-Asiatic language family. As elsewhere (Urban 1998), there is inconsistency of terminology, orthography, and insider-outsider labels, and much disagreement concerning names, labels, and orthography. Some political leaders, especially in Mali, prefer the name "Kel Tamajaq" ("People who speak Tamajaq"), underlining the centrality of language in cultural identity. Yet many others describe themselves as "Tuareg" in the presence of outsiders and do not consider the latter term pejorative, although it was imposed by outsiders.[6]

A number of sources—oral traditions recorded by Rodd (1926), Bernus (1981), and Nicolaisen (1997), Saharan rock art, and Arab chronicles—relate the early origins and migrations of various Tuareg confederations or "drum groups," the basic precolonial political unit. The Tuareg arrived from the North African Fezzan in the Saharan and Sahelian regions in successive waves between the eighth and fourteenth centuries.[7] By the fourteenth century, the Tuareg had become prominent as stock breeders and caravanners on trading routes that led to the salt, gold, ivory, and slave markets in North Africa, the Middle East, and Europe. Later, however, caravans declined when much trans-Saharan trade was diverted to the West African coast, and nineteenth-century European exploration and military expeditions in the Sahara and along the Niger River led to the incorporation of these regions into French West Africa and French West Sudan by the early twentieth century (Claudot-Hawad 1993; Decalo 1996; Rasmussen 2001a).

Before the advent of French colonialism in the early twentieth century, Tamajaq speakers were organized into hereditary, hierarchical, specialized occupational groups or social strata who were also, in principle, endogamous. Inherited social stratum affiliation once corresponded to occupation and prestige. Nomadic nobles (called *imajeghen*) controlled large livestock, managed the caravan trade, and protected and collected tribute from peoples of varying degrees of dependent status: tributary *(imghad)* and servile *(ighawalen* and *iklan)*, some of the latter on oases. Nobles practiced mutual client-patron rights and obligations with their attached smith/artisan *(inaden)* families.[8] There were, however, limits to nobles' powers, for example, subordinates enjoyed usufruct rights as fictive kin. In rural communities, elders and Islamic scholars adjudicate local-level disputes (Rasmussen 2004). Yet there has been considerable regional and class variation, and also flexible negotiation, in subsistence and stratification patterns.

The precolonial political structure included local drum chiefs who headed noble clans or lineages, who elected the sultan *(amenukal)* or their larger regional confederation. In many groups, the drum chief office was inherited through matrilineal descent, although personal qualities were also important. Under the domination first of the French colonial administration and later of nation-state governments, Tuareg political leaders experienced modifications in their powers.[9]

In the bilateral system of kinship, matrilineal ancestresses of the descent groups have been important in myth, rites of passage, and non-Qur'anic healing. Although there are regional and class differences in terms of their consequences for gender, it is generally agreed that most women enjoy high social prestige and considerable economic independence, and there is much free social interaction between the sexes.[10] Many Tuareg groups have been bilateral or bilineal since conversion to Islam between the eighth and eleventh centuries. Older matrilineal institutions have until recently served to legally protect women. In most groups, these institutions have become submerged within patrilineal institutions introduced by Arab-influenced Qur'anic law, as well as more recent colonial and postcolonial nation-state laws (Murphy 1964, 1967; Oxby 1990; Worley 1991; Claudot-Hawad 1993; Nicolaisen 1997; Bouman 2003; Keenan 2003). In some regions, such as southern Algeria, decline of the significance of the matriline is more marked, from influences of pan-Islamist reformist forces (Keenan 2003).

Nowadays many rural communities are becoming seminomadic. Many household compounds are enclosed by a tree-branch fence or adobe mud wall and contain adobe mud houses, usually owned by men, and the more traditional nomadic tent, owned by married women. Alternative forms of property transmission, in pre-inheritance gifts called "living milk" *(akh ihuderan),* in which some property (herds, date palms) is reserved for sisters, daughters, and nieces, are intended to compensate women for Qur'anic inheritance *(takachit),* in which sons receive twice the amount daughters receive. While living milk property once constituted women's primary source of economic independence, its future is now uncertain since the advent of nation-state laws and Qur'anic rulings, which tend to favor patrilineal inheritance, and also in the wake of recurring droughts, which have diminished many women's livestock herds, traditionally the primary source of their wealth (Keenan 2003; Oxby 1990; Worley 1991). These trends have produced some tensions between the sexes (Figueiredo 1996; Keenan 2003; Rasmussen 1995, 2000, 2003). There are cultural contradictions between rituals and symbols that continue to evoke matriliny, and legal and political processes that frustrate it.

Medicine women and their work emerge on one level, I argue, as a kind of mnemonic evoking the memory of these ancient matrilineal institutions. Many of their healing rituals, paraphernalia, and mythico-history clearly promote this cultural memory. Yet at the same time, my data suggest, the effectiveness of this mnemonic role socially and politically is uncertain and its future viability difficult to predict. More broadly, medicine women's roles confirm, following Connerton (1989), that how societies remember is indeed important, selective, and socially constructed. But I would add a caveat here: medicine women also warn that memories are not enough, and the effectiveness of these memories in practice is open to debate. On one level, then, this book explores the tensions between medicine women's work as mnemonic figures and social mediating figures, and competing claims to authority against these historic and contemporary backdrops of conflict.

There are also wider regional economic tensions. The French colonial administrators disrupted many local systems of adaptation and the natural ecological balance of the Sahara and Sahel.[11] Independent states inherited the effects of their uneven development of different regions, in particular their neglect of northern Niger and Mali. Some postcolonial governments also inherited the anti-nomadic bias of previous colonial administrations and tended to deploy "nomad" as a gloss for what were, in reality, multiple forms of subsistence practiced by diverse Tuareg groups (Bouman 2003). Colonial and postcolonial state governments placed restrictions on the trans-Saharan caravan trade and periodically sealed borders (Camel in Claudot-Hawad 2002; Keenan 2003).

In addition to droughts and unemployment, political tensions, such as a 1963 tax revolt in Kidal, Mali, have caused many Tuareg men to leave for Libya to find work, where some were also trained in military camps (Bourgeot 1990, 1994; Decalo 1996). Following the 1990 and 1991 massacres of Tuareg civilians at Tchin Tabaradan, Niger, and at Lere, Mali, parts of the northern regions of these countries were cut off economically during the Tuareg armed rebellion, until the 1995 and 1996 Peace Accords. Success has been variable and uneven; many say guardedly, "there is a fragile peace." There have been ongoing efforts to compensate many returning refugees for their losses.[12] Central governments have attempted to integrate more Tuareg into the national infrastructures (in ministries, militia, and education), but they are plagued by low budgets, crushing debt, and weak control over militia in peripheral zones.

Implications

These events raise interesting questions regarding gender that are relevant to the focus of this book. Herbal medicine women, as already noted, are overwhelmingly women, and treat predominantly (though not exclusively) women and children, and many trace their professional pedigree back matrilineally. Most Tuareg women retain high social prestige in ideology, although in social practice, men's attitudes in fact vary—for example, while male and female community leaders often point out with pride that "Tuareg respect women," some younger men have returned from exile with different ideas concerning gender and relations between the sexes. Many marabouts, oasis gardeners, and merchants practice polygyny, traditionally opposed by most women, and there is evidence of marriage of women at younger ages. Women, it is true, have played vital roles in much local cultural revitalization ideology—of both nationalist/separatist and current post-rebellion repatriation discourses. Both women and men sing songs exalting and critiquing members of the armed resistance, a traditional source of pride for men. It is uncertain exactly what role women will play in the future. They continue to control men's reputations in oral art (for example, in women's songs praising or critiquing current regional leaders). Yet bases of women's power in property and work appear to have suffered, since, as observed, they have lost many animals. On the other hand, many women have always participated, albeit indirectly, in men's itinerant trading and are now active in the burgeoning international NGO–sponsored cooperative projects (Rasmussen 2001b). Gender constructs and relations have therefore been affected by pressures to settle down in more sedentarized villages or towns and by lengthier than usual male exile.[13]

Many individuals still appeal to prestigious noble origins to justify certain conduct. Chiefly noble and maraboutique, particularly the special *icherifan,* clans who claim descent from the Prophet, still attempt to arrange endogamous, politically advantageous marriages between close cousins. But some other noble families are marrying off their daughters to non-nobles: Arab merchants and marabouts, and occasionally, prosperous ethnic outsiders and descendants of slaves, for purposes of economic security. Many husbands now pressure wives to bear more children to assist with gardening labor, and some women tend to resist husbands' polygyny less than they did in the past because of either parental pressure or their own need for economic support nowadays following droughts.

Since the mid-twentieth century, government and international NGO aid agencies have encouraged oasis gardening.[14] Land shortages, particularly in the Aïr region of northern Niger, compel many men to plant gardens farther and farther away from home, attenuating the usual initial uxorilocal postmarital residence custom and separating their wives from their own kin. Women must graze their dwindling herds farther and farther out to find good feed. In other regions, such as the Azawak middle regions of Mali and Niger, there has been greater resistance to oasis gardening because of the low water table and long-standing reliance on larger livestock herds.

These subsistence problems cause tensions between the sexes that are given gendered imagery: for example, some men blame women for allegedly "draining off" *al baraka* Islamic blessing/benediction from lands, gardens, and herds (Rasmussen 2004). In the more nomadic culture, women's reproductive biology was given imagery from herding: the womb was referred to sometimes as "the child's tent" and sometimes as a "leather sack"; and men were openly recognized to sometimes be at fault for a couple's childlessness (i.e., sterile). Most women in seminomadic rural communities bear approximately six to eight children. There are indications that with increased sedentarization, many families prefer more children to assist with oasis gardening. Precise statistics from large samples are not available, but many local residents indicate that "in the past, nomadic lifestyles discouraged having many children and there were efforts to space children." Nowadays, women fear that husbands may contract polygynous marriages if they are infertile. In more sedentarized contexts, there is increasing association of the womb with men's property interests, and wives are increasingly blamed for husbands' misfortunes, from poverty to childlessness: for example, if a normally industrious and prosperous man's livestock start to die off, sometimes his friends and relatives blame certain women and their families (matrilineally defined by emphasizing mothers, sisters, and daughters as passing on this tendency), who are alleged to "cause men to become poor" (Rasmussen 2001a, 2004). Land is becoming more important in communities that are becoming more sedentarized. However, rather than a bastion of security, land is as vulnerable to danger as livestock. While men inherit and own most gardens, women's reproductive powers, once associated with the tent and livestock herds, are increasingly linked to the fertility of humans and the blessing of land. Some dynamics of herbal medicine women's healing are directly related to these conflicts. Herbal medicine women will be shown to play important socially mediating roles in providing marital counseling in these conflicts between men and women. Nonetheless they do not view themselves as attempting to overturn the structure of gendered relationships in a Euro-American "feminist" sense.

Ideally, cultural values emphasize sharing and giving, obedience, modesty, respect, reserve, restraint in eating, verbal reticence, and caution in praise. There is a widespread belief in the need to constantly protect oneself from malevolent human social and superhuman forces; these fears are related to those values of modesty and reserve, expressed in two details of Tuareg dress: the men's face-veil and the women's head-covering (scarf).[15]

The Tuareg converted to Islam under the influence of Sufism Almoravid marabouts (Norris 1975, 1990). Many Arab explorers disapproved of what they perceived as Tuareg "laxness" in Islamic observances, in particular, for not secluding women. In many groups today, Islamic scholars are very respected and play important roles in ritual, healing, and politics (Nicolaisen 1991, 1997; Rasmussen 1995, 2004). Yet local cosmology and mythico-history antedating Islam, as well as many "popular Islamic" beliefs and practices, interweave with more "official" Islamic ones, both in the wider culture and in the specialized work of medicine women. This is shown in overlapping spirit pantheons in Islamic and local cosmologies: for example, Qur'anic spirits called *eljenan* or *djinn* and non-Qur'anic spirits called the People of Solitude or the Wild *(Kel Essuf)*. Persons may become possessed by these spirits, and they undergo special rituals to cure them.[16]

2—Herbalism, Medicine, and Curing
Medicine Women's Concepts of Wellness, Illness, and Healing

Medicine Women as Mediators, Facilitators, and Gatekeepers Who Challenge Both "Bricoleur" and Scientist/Biomedical Doctor Typifications in Anthropology

A *tanesmegel* is a curer who uses tree bark to cure, though she also obtains medicine from the market in Agadez. I have been a medicine woman all my life. I learned this from both my father, a marabout, and my mother, a medicine woman. The profession is inherited [in a *tawsit* or descent group]. I do not know my age. I am practicing curing because my relatives do it. I treat stomachaches and *tuksi* ("hot") illnesses; these cause sores on the stomach and swelling of the body. All types of people come to me. Women are more prone to catch the hot illnesses, however. Their causes include sweets and macaroni in the diet. The treatment is with special wood barks, cooked in water, and drunk in an infusion.

These comments are from Houna (pseudonym), a medicine woman who resides on Mount Bagzan in the Aïr region, during conversations I had with her on several occasions in a small caravanning village at the mountain's base. We usually sat outside on the embankment of a small dried riverbed or *oued* near the pastures where she was herding her goats. As we chatted, Houna coaxed her goats to browse for vegetation by calling *"Kru, kru, kru,"* to them as she nudged leaves off high tree branches with her long staff. At the beginning of my research, a small (preadolescent) schoolboy was also present, who assisted informally by translating some terminology. We often sat in the *oued* as we chatted. Houna was born on Mt. Bagzan. She was married; her husband traded on caravans to Kano and Bilma, and gardened as well. Houna had six children as of 1983; by 2002, she had several more children and most were adults (married and parents themselves).[1]

Houna and many other medicine women often expressed concern with food and eating patterns, particularly those of women. They attributed many illnesses to a lack of balance in the body from "eating bad things." Local diets vary according to degree of sedentarization and urbanization, and have changed over the past half century. In more nomadic camps, the principal foods consumed are millet and dates from caravan trading, a few vegetables from gathering, and, when rains and pasture are sufficient, dairy products such as milk and cheese from goats, sheep, and occasionally camels. Houna and many other herbal medicine women asserted that, "in the past, many plants gathered were eaten regularly as foods, but now these are only consumed as medicine (*amagal*, or *ilaten*, the latter denoting herbal remedies).[2] Meat tends to be eaten only at festivals, religious holidays, and rites of passage. But many women attempt to consume meat and milk more often if they have the means. Meat and milk are believed to make one fat, fertile, and attractive to husbands. Attitudes about millet are ambivalent. Although millet is important as a daily staple in parts of northern Niger, some more nomadic nobles, particularly those in northern Mali, associate it with former slaves and having "hard" flesh, and believe that milk, by contrast, makes the flesh soft and beautiful. On oases, additional foods consumed are maize, wheat, barley, potatoes, onions, tomatoes, and a few citrus fruits. Additional products obtained less regularly from trade and, more recently, food relief aid agencies and some small shops, include macaroni, manioc flour, rice, peanuts, and beans. Some foods have always been reserved as famine foods: the core of the doum palm and thorns of various species of trees, pounded and grilled. To assuage hunger pangs, many drink thick, strong sugary tea in shot glasses, though tea also is important in sociability.

Since the early 1990s, the traditional cereal staple, millet, usually obtained through caravan trade with neighboring peoples, has become increasingly expensive in many Tuareg communities because of droughts in regions where it is grown; thus an important cereal source of high protein has become more difficult to obtain. In some cases, this is now supplemented or replaced by store-bought manioc or refined flour. If this trend continues, it has ominous implications for local nutrition. Herbal medicine women lament this trend, recognizing that much processed food is less healthy. Medicine women are also aware that periodic droughts threaten many of their medicinal plants and trees, which traditionally constitute a rich local pharmacopoeia, particularly in more mountainous regions. Yet some medicine women nonetheless resent the intrusions and restrictions of some state and private NGO environmental policies.

Medicine women and other elderly persons are aware of the double-edged effects of these ecological and economic trends on health, though they also unconsciously express cultural values influencing ways of coping with them. Popular food tastes remain closely linked to social stratum and gender constructs. Medicine women are aware that the increasingly available, store-bought, processed and refined foods in boxes are avidly sought after by some people for purposes of status and for their convenience, but they are also less nutritious and more expensive. Many medicine women asserted to me that, "food was scarcer and less varied in the past, but healthier. It was necessary (then) to move about more often in order to find food (in nomadism and some hunting and gathering)." They indicated that, "although foods today are more abundant since one can find many sold in shops, such (boxes of processed) foods are not only less nutritious, but also require much money. In the past, the wild plants and grasses eaten by many people here were free, but also unpredictable and sometimes scarce."

Another medicine woman, whom I shall call Tana, from another small nomadic camp in the Aïr, stated,

> I am about 65 years old. My small clans are [the closely related] Kel Agatan and Kel Igurmadan. I was born in this camp/village (eghiwan). I am married. My husband is a caravanner. I have three living sons and three dead. One is about 31 years old, one is about 28 years old, and one approximately 25 years old. I do herbal medicine in order to cure people and earn money, also. I touch and I do medicines. I am not a diviner. I do what God taught me only: [with] medicines

from here and from the South [i.e., Hausaland]. I inherited this work from my parents, on the side of my mother. My father did cauterization *(tchiquat)*. I learned from my mother. I learned with God's help, and also I inherited that from my parents.

My "first *ten*" [referring to both the pot or calabash of medicines and metonymically, more generally, to treatment] was when I treated Hamid [a son], who was very young and my only son then. At that time, I worked also, I was young, I led goats and camels. I spent many years apprenticing [medicine]. When my mother was living, also, I did this, [but] we did it together. Many patients who see me are Kel Agatan. The origin *(arassal)* of all my medicine is from the Kel Agatan. One [We] can even identify a dying person. I diagnose the illness with the aid of my finger *(adade)*. I touch and sense something that is hard, especially around the bladder area.

One touches the stomach in order to be certain of [the patient's] health. It is the root. Also, the liver [sometimes] has illness [when it is pricked by something]. It is the stomach that protects all that the body contains. The liver possesses a medicine on the interior. I touch it, and I realign it when it is dislocated. There are also medicines for *tarzak* and for the liver. There is *tarzak* plain and simple (manifested in symptom of a back and shoulder problem, approximately between the trapezoids), *tchidguite* (a back illness that is more serious), *aghitiss (French translation, coupoure de sang*, or approximately in English, "cutting off of the blood"); its cause is a heavy burden. I also treat *tezoufnene* (difficult to translate exactly, but often described by assistants and French-speaking persons as a kind of indigestion; to medicine women, each color of vomit indicates a different illness type). . . . [In this], nausea is provoked by food and a lot of oil. There is vomit that is red, that which is yellow, and that which is green.

Often, the terms liver *(tessa)* and stomach *(tedis)* are used interchangeably in local descriptions of illnesses. In local cosmology, the liver and stomach are tropes for the matriline. In local anatomy concepts, these are classified as being all together in a sack. The stomach "is the person"—it is the point of attack of sorcery (antisocial thoughts, words, and actions) and also, along with the liver, attacked in certain phases of spirit possession (Rasmussen 1995). On the other hand, there is also the recognition that other stomach illnesses are caused by "bad" foods—impure foods, rich foods, and indigestion, and yet others are caused by smiths' alleged powers. *Tarzak* is usually a swelling of the back around the shoulder blades. In local cosmology, the back *(aghuru)* is a trope for authority, economic support, and the patriline.

One day while I visited Tana, she was treating a young woman from her camp and also her own small daughter. Her daughter had toted a full bucket of water to the well for her mother and hurt her right wrist *(amasur)*. Tana treated both patients over several days. The medicine woman touched the young girl's wrist and massaged it with a store-bought ointment. Her daughter, about four years old, also allegedly had a problem with her liver; Tana described it as "displaced" or "dislocated" from a fall. Tana rotated millet counterclockwise three times above the child, and touched her liver area. She then dangled the child upside-down. Tana also prepared internal medicines in advance in measures for sale for 100 CFA (approximately 20 US cents). She was very kind and soft-spoken but also sociable: she kept up a steady stream of pleasant conversation with patients during her treatments and invited me to visit her again.

These comments introduce some preliminary elements of medicine women's concepts of wellness, illness, and practice of healing. They are not necessarily representative of all these specialists, but neither are they completely idiosyncratic. Thus far, several key points emerge. First, as Tana points out, lengthy, careful apprenticeship with older relatives is important—usually, though not always, females and on the maternal side. Yet despite their specialized knowledge, these medicine women are modest and tend to minimize their own power, attributing much to God. They also continue other ordinary daily work—herding, upkeep of the tent, raising and educating their children. Their patients are often, though not exclusively, women and children. When they began healing, their early patients were close relatives. Their diagnostic procedures and treatments include both natural and ritual substances and actions; and the illnesses they treat straddle "naturalistic," "personalistic," and other domains. Religions— human and superhuman, the God of Islam, and non-Qur'anic spirits—are all significant in the afflictions and cures related here. The stomach, liver, back, and blood are important foci of these and many other herbal medicinal treatments. The women also appealed to multi-sensorial communication modalities in their examinations and remedies—not solely visual, but also tactile, gustatory, and aural.

Additional insights are offered by the another medicine woman, Tata. Her comments are followed by two brief vignettes, and then by a more in-depth and long-term case study.

Tata, very old and renowned, lives in a seminomadic oasis, herding, and caravanning village near Mt. Bagzan in Aïr. I have known Tata for approximately twenty-two years. We first met in 1983. Tata is now between seventy and eighty years old and has been healing for about twenty-five years. Although a herder, she lost many animals during droughts in 1984, 1990, and 2000. She is the older sister of the chief of a local descent group. She married at fourteen years old, but has been a widow for many years. Her late husband was a caravanner. Tata has six sons and four daughters, and she resides next door to her daughters, some cousins, and her younger brother, the chief. One son lives nearby; another resides in a village about five miles away.

Tata's relationship with her daughter-apprentice, Anta, and me revealed much concerning mother-daughter relationships in herbal medical practice. Although personable and kind, she was also reserved toward youths: for example, she took tea only with her age-mates. During our early conversations, interviews, and visits, perhaps because of my much younger age, Tata preferred to chat outside my tent and not approach too closely to where I sat. In the presence of youths, she held her head scarf up higher than usual for most Tuareg women, over her mouth.

By the 1990s Tata's daughter, Anta, was apprenticing from her mother, and, from respect, she refrained from practicing herbalism in a fully independent way. Until she grew older and/or received authorization from her mother to practice, she herded most of the time. About forty years old and divorced, Anta had one living child, and one was deceased. Yet despite Anta's status as an adult, married woman, and mother, she explained that she could not answer my questions regarding herbalists until she received permission from her mother. Tata responded to my questions for her daughter, rather than allowing Anta to respond directly herself. Tata allowed me to accompany her (but not Anta) on many healing consultations, and showed me her medicines, kept dry in a calabash, and an iron instrument used to cauterize. She purchased many medicines from women who gathered them and brought them down from the mountains.

Tata explained,

> A *tanesmegel* is a person who cares for [cures] people. I inherited this occupation from the mother of my father and from my father [i.e., in the matriline, though not entirely from women]. I learned the art [i.e., apprenticed] from my father's sister. The *tamadas* is a specialist within our *tinesmegelen* specialty. It is possible for anyone to be a *tanesmegel,* but they will do better if they have inherited this. I do not know how old I am. I practice curing because people like it. I was born near Agadez. My husband is now dead. He was not a curer. I treat illnesses such as *amerdio* (body bloating) and *tuksi* (a generic term for "hot" illnesses) with tree barks. Mostly women and children come to me. Illnesses that are typically caught by women include *anulem* (women's bloating). This is caused by eating too much sugar.
>
> To be in good health means to feel strength. Illness is something from God. It is caused by God. Women are weak. God causes this. Whether young or old, they are more often sick, [although this] varies according to individuals. Chance or luck is also necessary for attaining a happy life (*sa'a,* luck, from Hausa). There are certain places which are dangerous to the health, they are terrains called *tetekkes,* they cause illnesses. People must see a marabout before camping in them. The marabout dreams and divines. Misfortune also comes from God. Insane persons are those who are permanently ill.
>
> *Tuksi* ("hot illness") is that which provokes constipation. It enlarges the person, his/her anus opens. *Tessmut* ("cold" illness) is a sickness that prevents one from sitting still. Sometimes one urinates blood. It pricks the veins. Sometimes *tessmut* is hereditary; it can be inherited from the father or the mother. *Tazufnine* (indigestion) sometimes attacks the knees. There is also a sickness, *azera* (no precise translation available), a kind of indigestion or *tazufnine.* It is *azera* that can make one crazy, even marabouts cannot cure it.
>
> I inherited [*asstofara* or *gado,* the latter from Hausa, denoting "inheritance" and "bed"] my work from my father, but my father inherited his from his mother. Since I was small, I began my apprenticeship. I gathered medicines in the wild *(essuf).* My younger sister and my father both practiced medicine. When my father died, I continued to practice medicine. I was married, with five children. The Kel Agaten [from the mountain around Timia] and the Kel Bagzan [People of the Bagzan Massif], particularly the [Kel] Igurmadan, have many healing methods. Even our slaves practiced this. The related Kel Agaten, at first, they only touched. I also treat the respiratory illness *okuf.* Its medicine is a root of the *tachilchit* tree, and bark from the *aza* and, also, *amizou (Mitragyna inermes)* trees. In *okuf,* the nostrils close up. It is a type of hot illness or *tuksi.* Medicine for *okuf,* inhaled, causes sneezing. With the back and shoulder illness, *tarzak,* the body feels very heavy, as though from a burden. When you cut (with razor blade, in bloodletting), you pour out the blood, preferably around the middle of the month, for the following reason: two different bloods, one bad and the other good, are in the body. Each blood remains separate. The marabouts advised us about that. I touch the earth so I do not catch the illness

that I have touched in the patient. *Togerchet* (evil eye or mouth) is caused by a word and look, but this is less strong than *(ark) echaghel,* which is sorcery or poison. We herbalists obey the marabouts. Marabouts know medicines against *togerchet.* The moon causes another illness, *afa,* when its rays project on people. When a person is attacked by *afa,* he/she shivers.

Many herbalists and other women believe that sun's rays give a headache called *afa,* somewhat like heat stroke, but not exactly, because moonbeams and flashlight beams, also, can cause *afa.* Hence the difficulty of assigning too literal a thermal significance to this; it is not constructive to force these concepts into exact translation into English or biomedical (Western allopathic) labels.

Tata also introduced me to some ritual restrictions in medicine women's healing: "An unlucky day to travel is the last Wednesday of the month, since in the past the Kel Nad went to battle on that day and lost it, and never returned. [Kel Nad or People of Past or Before are believed, like Aligouran, the well-known Saharan culture hero, to have made the rock art in the Sahara.] The hour when the herbalist touches is important: the morning or the evening.

"For the child who drank milk of his small brother who has an illness called *laho* [a reference to the breaking of a postpartum sexual taboo by parents], that medicine consists of old droppings of cows from near the tombs of the [ancestral] Kel Nad [People of the Night or Past]. You have the child drink water with these medicines. You also dig a hole in the ground and place him/her inside it."

On one of her consultations, I saw Tata treat a child she diagnosed as afflicted with *laho,* although my research assistant believed that he suffered from tetanus *(tebes).* Tata returned once after initially treating him to see how he was. After three days, she removed the medicine (cow dung mixed with herbs) she had placed on his body.[3]

The important point here is that medicine women, in treating *laho* and many other illnesses, obliquely articulate and often treat the harm believed caused by violating sexual taboos: for example, birth defects and children's illnesses. In order to diagnose and treat these conditions, they create an atmosphere of intimacy during their consultations. Ideally, children should be spaced; it is considered shameful to bear a child before the older sibling is two years old. Thus recent pressures for more children to assist in gardens may well conflict with this tradition. Some couples' children's illnesses, such as *laho,* are attributed to the breaking of this taboo or to some other related ritual restriction. For example, conceiving a child before the end of the weeklong wedding celebration, when the couple is supposed to consummate the marriage, results in a child called *eljenagougou,* who may have birth defects such as slow learning or antisocial behavior. Or spirits may take a child away for additional reasons having to do with the actions of a parent. My field hostess, who was a trained first-aid worker, nonetheless believed the condition of a mentally deficient girl was caused by her mother having left her in a door frame as an infant: here, in this crossroads space of liminality, transition, and uncertainty, spirits were believed to have replaced the "real" (i.e., normal) child with the mentally deficient one. A child conceived under the moonlight, also, may suffer an illness of the spirits or perhaps die at birth. Ideally, conception is supposed to occur inside the married woman's nuptial tent, thereby encouraging ideal official marital endogamy and legitimate births.

In effect, therefore, medicine women remind patients of the importance of many taboos guarding maternal and matrilineal identity but also shield them from the shame of breaking them. This role was also apparent in another consultation, when Tata visited a man with a stomachache. Late one afternoon, placing a cauterizing iron in her medicine bag, she invited me to accompany her, explaining: "I prefer to avoid treating in the sun, for comfort's sake, although I cannot pass by some places too late, either, especially after sundown; for the tombs of prominent marabouts and ancestors along the route change into malevolent spirits under the moonlight. They may even cause the wind to shift and the sandstorms to cover up routes, disorienting unwary travelers."

So we set out around 5 p.m., as the burning heat waned but before the sun set, following the road linking two small seminomadic villages. I followed Tata as she walked swiftly past tombs of prominent marabouts en route. Tata's patient, a young man, seemed reluctant to discuss the suspected cause of his stomachache openly before young women such as myself, or even his female relatives. So I briefly withdrew. Later, Tata indicated that this man had a "hidden illness" for which the "stomachache" was a cover-term or euphemism *(tangalt)*, about which he felt shame *(takarakit);* thus the precise cause of his shame and his actual illness were not made explicit.

There are some illnesses that are specific to gender and sexuality in Tamajaq (Fiore and Wallet Faqqi 1993). Many of these illnesses involve some shameful actions or conditions. This may explain the reluctance of Tata's male patient to discuss his illness openly before young women. Tata spent the entire evening in this sick man's household, sleeping overnight in the compound in order to administer her medicines. This is one reason why many medicine women, to practice as full professionals and be sought out by diverse patients, should preferably be elderly and have had children. Male patients feel reserve toward younger women. Since I was of ambiguous status—married and of childbearing age, though childless—a few (though not all) patients, particularly young men, were not entirely at ease if I sat in on their consultations. Tata's frequent housecalls, during which she frequently ate and slept overnight with the family of the ill person, undoubtedly aided in diminishing the possible reserve sometimes felt by patients, in cases of "shameful" or "hidden" illnesses (i.e., of a sexual nature or involving antisocial actions or the violation of taboos). It is, in other words, "safer" to discuss these problems with the medicine woman more than with others. She thereby promotes hidden wishes, or alleviates psychosocial as well as physical pain—particularly in relations between the sexes, as shown in the next case, a more extended and longitudinal case study.

A Difficult Birth

In another consultation, along with several other elderly women, Tata was called to the home of a woman whom I shall call Fatima, who suffered from a difficult pregnancy and also experienced some stress in her marriage. Her household had experienced more general reversals. They had suffered many drought losses, and some men had been obliged to spend years away on travel that was more prolonged than usual (for example, not solely on the customary seasonal caravans to Nigeria, but also on longer-term labor migration to Libya and Algeria). Their mother had experienced a sharp decline in health. Many women in this family were active in the local spirit possession rituals as both singers and possessed persons.

During one rainy season, Fatima, the youngest of several sisters in this household whom I have known since the early 1980s, fell ill. She was in advanced pregnancy, but overdue. At one time, she reportedly had not urinated in three days. Her first resort was to try traditional herbal medicines, for she felt reluctant to travel to the nearest clinic, at that time located about twenty miles away in a large oasis. Thus older women in Fatima's family and also a few medicine women, including Tata, came to administer their medicines. Among them were herbal remedies, infusions she drank that the women in the household described to me as "mothers' medicines *(amagal n anna)*." These are predominantly red, and female relatives and medicine women often give them to new mothers, usually just following birth. However, in this case, they were given before birth, for strength. Medicine women referred to this treatment by a more technical term: they called it *tishi*. It includes leaves from many trees, including *bawre* (wild fig), *akakou, etafi, tuwila, anezum, arankat, afalo, tamat, teshghar, kuwurna, alanmawdragh, adaras, tedene,* and *audene.*[4] This infusion thus resembles female menstruation and fertility in its "key symbol" of the red color (Turner 1968). Situationally, this acted together with medico-ritual and more bodily focused healing practices to create a holistic healing force that infused the medicines' and the patient's identities. Some of Fatima's treatments appeared based on metaphor and metonym; others appeared counteractive. Metaphorical suggestion, or approximately what we might term "homeopathic medicine," pervades these key symbols, but group therapy also permeated Fatima's cure.

Yet even while treating women, the medicine women were obliged to observe some rules of reserve. For example, I noticed that inside Fatima's tent they wore their head scarves high over their nose and mouth (in the style similar to men's face-veiling in situations requiring much reserve or protection from contagion or pollution). Noel (in Claudot-Hawad 2002:155) reports that treatment for labor contractions consists of applying the palm of the hands to the kidney area and rubbing the woman from the feet to beneath the breasts with ashy fibers mixed with butter or commercial ointment. But even in this treatment, medicine women shun vaginal exams and the like, unless they are unavoidable in extreme cases requiring more invasive techniques. But these latter are usually a last resort locally and/or are left to Western biomedical gynecological and obstetric examinations in urban hospitals, to which many rural women are still reluctant to submit (Fiore and Wallet Faqqi 1993; Noel in Claudot-Hawad 2002; Rasmussen 1994, 2001a).

The herbal treatment of Fatima by Tata and other medicine women appeared to be effective in inducing labor; for shortly after these treatments, Fatima gave birth to a baby boy, who appeared healthy. Immediately afterward, women assisting the mother piled sand over the placenta and umbilical cord. Then the grandmother took the placenta and umbilical cord outside and buried them under three stones to the east of the compound. Female relatives, and in this case, which involved a difficult birth, herbal medicine women, then placed incense *(tafarchit)* in front of the new mother to protect her and her child from spirits. Fatima rested on the ground until evening, after an attached smith woman changed the bedding on her wood and mat bed. *Amzor,* the postpartum period of seclusion behind a windscreen following birth, began with its restrictions (practiced in some regions only until the name day on the eighth day, and in others, for the entire forty days): the new mother cannot go to the well, cannot visit, and cannot say bad words about anyone. If she breaks these rules, she will cease to have *al baraka* blessing.

However, this very protecting seclusion may itself transform into possession by spirits of the wild, in particular if the new mother is lonely and her husband is absent. Despite the successful birth of a healthy baby and the ensuing protective measures for mother and child, Fatima's illness, at first described by Tata the herbalist as "a fever" (tenede)—here both literally high body temperature and also a kind of local "hot" illness or tuksi—did not subside, and the young mother soon began also to suffer from something else. While on the surface her symptoms appeared to represent what Western biomedicine might term a "postpartum depression," there was need for caution here because in Tamajaq, there is only an approximate translation for this: tamazai, an "illness of the heart and soul." This may be, however, contracted outside childbirth, as well. In this local exegesis, the family and the medicine woman used this term to describe Fatima, who suffered from not only a fever or hot illness, but also tamazai. The latter is believed to sometimes lead to possession.

Fatima sat listlessly in her tent well beyond the initial forty-day seclusion required of mother and child to protect against jealous humans and spirits. She did not eat or sleep well, or bathe, even for the name day, when the new mother is supposed to bathe, have a smith wash and dress her hair in a new style, and dress in clean new clothing. When I enquired how she was feeling, Fatima only said sadly, "Essuf, essuf (the wild, the wild)!"

Eventually, Fatima went to the town of Agadez by agricultural cooperative truck, where she received six penicillin injections. Her fever appeared to be cured, and she rested for awhile there, staying at the home of a local smith attached to some noble families of her village. Soon, she returned to her rural village, but she remained depressed and did not emerge from her tent, not solely because of a mother's customary formal ritual seclusion but also because of her depression. Friends and neighbors worried that her head was now "in the wild or solitude (essuf)." In local possession etiology, there are numerous theories of this condition (see Rasmussen 1995). These include psychosocial and even plant-based theories of causation and cure; many Tuareg, for example, believe that ripening barley can make women fall ill with the Kel Essuf (People of Solitude) spirits.

Yet there are hints in this case of more sentimental considerations: barley becomes ripe and is consumed primarily during the cold dry season, precisely the season when many men are away on caravan trading or labor migration, before the hot and rainy seasons when relatives usually attempt to return home and assemble to renew kinship ties and hold weddings. Hence the significance—for Fatima's case, at least—of seasonal correspondence between this illness and psychosocial problems of loss, transition, and nostalgia—threats to the social person as well as the body—indeed, "nostalgia" is one meaning of essuf. Many Tuareg also blame love—in particular, unrequited love or love suppressed from being expressed (tarama) and shame (takarakit) for causing many psychological and physical problems. Boundaries between organic and inorganic illnesses are therefore hazy.

Fatima's relatives arranged a spirit possession exorcism ritual when her baby was about one month old. Her older sister explained Fatima's spirits as due to "inheritance (gado, from a Hausa term) from her mother." Her relatives, friends, and Tata the herbalist explained to me that the problem was that Fatima's husband was delayed on caravan trading expeditions to the South and had failed to return home in time for the child's name day. This is a vitally important rite of passage, in which the father and mother both play central roles in conferring names for the child and social personhood.

Many illnesses, notwithstanding their very real physical symptoms, are believed to strike at specific times in the life course and emanate from human and extrahuman agents. Upon transitions, jealous spirits and humans compete for and threaten the individual. This is why a new mother and her baby are sheltered and given special protective medicines by herbal medicine women and/or female relatives familiar with these recipes, as well as amulets made by marabouts and smiths.

Thus in many treatments, marabouts' amulets are necessary but insufficient; they must be supplemented by medicine women's preparations. In some cases of particularly difficult transitions such as Fatima's difficult pregnancy and childbirth, medicine women and marabouts refer patients to the spirit possession ritual practitioners: musicians who play percussion instruments and a chorus of young female singers who perform songs that "please" the spirits of solitude. Tata the medicine woman and others—primarily close friends and relatives of Fatima, as well as her father, a prominent marabout, recommended this treatment for her.

The important point here is that, although medicine women's baseline of treatment consists of touch and herbal tree medicines, they also collaborate and contribute to different phases of diagnoses, treatments, and referrals in cases transcending organic illness. Also, in many cases the boundaries between "organic" and "nonorganic," between illnesses of the stomach and the head, and between treatments of trees, treatments of Qur'anic writing, and musical ritual therapy are hazy. Many illnesses and treatments processually vacillate back and forth between these domains. For many, curing is a social process; social support goes along with more physiological treatment.

So following the administration of herbal medicines and injections at the Agadez Hospital, Fatima's friends and family arranged a *tende n goumaten* spirit possession ritual for her. This lasted from approximately midnight or 1 a.m. until 3 a.m. Soloists included her sisters, cousins, and supportive friends and neighbors. It was a small group, and the ritual space was a small stretch of land between Fatima's mother's home compound and her own home compound. [For the first few years of marriage, many couples reside uxorilocally, until bridewealth and groom-service obligations to the parents-in-law are completed.]. Around sundown, one of Fatima's sisters and a smith man assembled the *tende* drum, constructed from a mortar used daily to crush grain. During the ritual, they each played this instrument by turns; another (the oldest) sister played the *asakalabo* calabash. Fatima was led by close relatives from her tent into the ritual space before she entered a trance.

The songs were considered by local residents, who attend such rituals freely as the audience, to be very beautiful and well performed. Many of these songs referred metaphorically to tree branches swaying in the wind; indeed, this is the name of one of the drum patterns associated with possession (Rasmussen 1995). Fatima responded to the songs by rising from her initial prone position beneath a blanket and performing an elaborate head dance, called *asul*: this involves moving the head and shoulders, and sometimes the entire upper body from the waist, from side to side, more and more vigorously until there is collapse upon the ground. This latter motion is interpreted by local residents as becoming free of the afflicting spirits. There was much applause and encouragement from the audience, and men stood up and produced a distinctive sound in the throat, called *t-hum-a-hum*, believed to be the "sound of spirits." Fatima danced with abandon, twirling a sword borrowed from her father over her head and behind her shoulders. Yet she always remained seated, as is usual, and silent except for her hand gestures, which are used to indicate song preferences and drum patterns associated with particular spirits.

Fatima's mother fitted her with the white tassel over the veil; this is worn by women only during spirit possession, not every day, in contrast to the men's everyday veiling. Her mother gently rocked Fatima's baby in his cradle inside her tent while Fatima danced, almost in synchrony with her head-swaying back and forth. While mothers who sing in the chorus often bring babies to this ritual, the possessed, if a new mother, does not. The next morning, I asked Fatima if her neck hurt from dancing, and, to my astonishment, she said no. Although Fatima indicated that she felt better, her relatives, friends, and the healers stated, "She is not yet cured of her condition; her head remains in the wild."

Discussion

Clearly, Fatima experienced a concatenation and interpenetration of organic, nonorganic, and other conditions and cures that are difficult to translate or classify according to Western biomedical diagnostic systems. The physical, the social, and the psychological—not to mention the "medico-ritual" and various hints of pollution—all operated here in the different phases and treatments of her illness. Although I did not hear Tata or other healers mention any additional diagnostic categories in treating Fatima besides those mentioned above in her case study, in the Tamajaq language there do exist numerous terms for illnesses classified according to gender, age, and other factors. Hence the possibility of additional conditions and treatments that Fatima may have experienced, which local medicine women nonetheless did not pursue in Fatima's case. But their alternative treatments that I observed, combined with the hospital and ritual group therapy of the possession ritual, appeared effective, for ultimately Fatima was cured. As of 2002, when I most recently saw her, she was in excellent health. Her husband continued caravanning, but he returned frequently, and they had several more children.

The issue here is the local terms' translatability into English and other languages to adequately convey medicine women's and other local residents' concepts of wellness, illness, and healing. Another issue is the degree to which all herbal medicine women share specialized knowledge. Indeed, there may be regional and/or dialectal differences. In their brief pamphlet on Malian Tamajaq speakers' concepts of illness, Fiore and Wallet Faqqi (1993:47) list several illnesses specific to women and their treatments. These authors state that any woman with the knowledge can treat these illnesses informally, without official apprenticeship with an older healer or the latter's authorization to practice. Here I do not attempt to "match" or "fit" Fatima's and Tata's case study data simplistically into these categories, nor do I imply that these authors' findings are "inaccurate." Their work usefully lists selected illness and plant treatment taxonomies. But their taxonomies are detached from the dynamic contexts of use and transformations of meaning. While they are valuable as a source of Tamajaq "ethnoscience," there is still the need to proceed beyond these lexical terminologies and ethnomedical categories. Here I attempt to analyze the wider contexts, as well: more extended social processes and ontological bases of medicine women's healing.

In Fatima's case, there arise interesting questions concerning the specialization of medicine women's skills and their authoritative knowledge systems. My own data suggest that more serious illnesses, in particular, those that are associated with women and their more specialized and difficult treatments, require administration by not just any female relative, but a medicine woman with more specialized technical knowledge. I saw the medicine woman and other elderly female relatives administer several different herbal infusions to Fatima that she drank in a tea, and they also massaged her. Later, as noted, she underwent her possession ritual. Fatima received additional Western bio-medical/allopathic care—an examination and injections—while she was at the hospital. She indicated to me that she felt better but preferred the local herbal medicine and familial healing network, as she felt uncomfortable at the hospital.

Additional conditions may have also afflicted Fatima. *Tasemde ta n aressud* denotes approximately "the cold of pus," one local category of gynecological condition manifested by a flow of blood more often than in normal menstrual periods, followed by the flow of liquid and pus (Fiore and Wallet Faqqi 1993:47). One should bathe with a mixture of medicines from trees called *tebaremt* and *tajart*. The medicine woman then gives the patient a small amount of melted butter to drink after each bath. This first treatment lasts three consecutive days. Nine days afterward, one must redo the treatment. The patient must abstain from drinking a lot of water and must avoid chills. She must have her lower abdomen area and feet massaged often with melted butter. Her diet must be rich in boiled meat. In Fatima's case, the terms for this illness and its associated treatments were not explicitly mentioned; Tata and family members mentioned instead *tuksi* ("hot" illnesses), *tenede* (fever), and then *tamazai*, approximately a depression, and spirit possession. However, I noticed that gynecological treatments were also given. For example, Tata and other attending women massaged Fatima with oils, and at the name day celebration Fatima was given butter as well as liver and other parts of the meat from the slaughtered animal to consume for regaining strength. If families have the resources, new mothers are also given milk and goat cheese. Fatima was given a delicious and nutritious beverage called *eghajira* or *eghale*, popular around Mt. Bagzan: this consists of crushed millet, goat cheese, and dates mixed with water. Despite scarce pastures and livestock in recent years, Fatima's family was able also to sacrifice an animal for the name day, and its meat was given to her. But as noted, Fatima did not eat much of any of these dishes.

Another illness, *tasemde ta n amnennad n ehan*, "cold of the turning of the house" (*ehan*, uterus and tent), also merits consideration: this is characterized in the local viewpoint by a deformation or displacement of the uterus, caused by too early sexual relations. Its treatment requires a specialist (generally a man who has mastered the technique in veterinary science) examine the patient in order to discern the position of the uterus and proceed to manually put it back in place. Then one administers the same treatment as in the case of the preceding illness.

In fact, Fatima was married at a somewhat younger age than usual, about twelve years. Some noble families, impoverished from drought, are marrying off daughters at younger ages than in the past; this is corroborated by some other ethnographies (Keenan 2003). However, local residents told me that such early marriages do not usually include cohabitation; rather, the couple waits until after the woman is "more mature" (i.e., has regular menstrual periods) to consummate the marriage. Furthermore, at the weeklong wedding, except in cases of marriages between divorced, widowed, and/or elderly persons, a marriage should not be consummated until the eighth evening, until the couple "gets to know one another," although in many regions, there is very free courtship between the sexes (Murphy 1964, 1967; Nicolaisen 1997; Rasmussen 1997). Friends and assistants disapprovingly related to me a case concerning one man who was divorced by his new wife, very young, for trying to consummate their marriage too soon, and too roughly. Such conduct is condemned by both women and men. Marabouts ruled that the man was at fault, and he had to return the bridewealth.

Fatima did not have children until after she had been married for several years, and she appeared happy on most occasions when I saw her over many years of my research. Indeed, her unhappiness here derived from some combination of organic gynecological factors and her sadness of missing and loving her husband, rather than rejecting him. This suggests that she did not appear to have suffered from too early sexual relations.

Sum-Up and Wider Implications

It is not the goal here to exactly correlate the Tamajaq illness and treatment categories listed above—or for that matter, their English approximations in translation—with Fatima's illness and Tata's treatments. But I shall discuss some implications and more general themes emerging here. In sum, treatments included some, but not all, of the more specialized gynecological methods of treatment or modifications of them. As shown, Tata the medicine woman and other closely related older female relatives massaged Fatima's lower abdomen, administered to her the "mother's medicine," made sure she received nourishing foods such as butter and meat, and later, also arranged a possession exorcism for her. One should recall, furthermore, that Fatima visited the urban hospital once for shots.

Striking in these illness classifications and in the concepts and treatments in Fatima's and Tata's case are the presence of not solely organic but also nonorganic afflictions that sometimes coexist or "morph" into each other back and forth. Treatments, while initially emphasizing "natural" herbal and other substances, often also feature psychosocial support, such as not offending a person—in particular, a pregnant woman or new mother—or not denying them material, spiritual, or social resources and support. The full social network is activated, as well as nutritional and medicinal resources. Husbands, in particular, are pressured not to harm a wife physically or emotionally. The psychosocial dimension of Fatima's suffering emerged as central here, despite the very real physical pain and fever she also experienced. In particular, a husband's actions, if they cause distress to a pregnant woman (whose anger is given a special term: *tourgoum*), are believed to produce direct physical consequences—a difficult childbirth or even a miscarriage or birth defect. Medicine women articulate these problems in consultations and informal gossip, and as shown later, also nonverbally in many treatments.

Men of honor are in principle supposed to respect all women. Until recently, polygyny was rare, and in more nomadic settings women have tended to bear fewer children. While childbearing and motherhood are extremely important, so is fatherhood, and men, as well as women, may be blamed for a couple's childlessness (Rasmussen 1998a). In rural communities, wife-beating is still extremely rare. But women sometimes suffer other types of harm. There have been long-standing problems of loneliness, of separation from kinspersons and spouses, in caravanning, nomadism, and raiding, and more recently, in labor migration, war, and refugee flight. In more sedentarized communities, many prosperous male chiefs, marabouts, merchants, and gardeners are now contracting polygynous marriages if the first wife has not borne children, or if she is perceived as "becoming an old woman" (Rasmussen 1997, 2000).

Fatima's husband, as of this writing, had not contracted a polygynous marriage. His frequent and prolonged absences, however, undoubtedly placed a strain on Fatima, both psychologically and economically. Her own herds had been much reduced by droughts. She lived far from local wells, and her recently married brothers had moved their oasis garden, once a rich source of vegetables, to neighboring villages of their wives' kin, where most of the produce now went as contributions to their own affines' households.

The foregoing narratives, commentaries, vignettes, and longitudinal case study suggest important themes in medicine women's theories of wellness, illness, and healing. Organic or "natural" illness and treatments among Tuareg suggest several categories: organic or natural illnesses; seemingly "personalistic" illnesses due to malevolent actions or feelings or taboo-breaking by humans; and illnesses due to spirits. Yet the boundaries between them and their associated treatments are by no means clear-cut, and these conditions are not static but instead dynamic and transformative. Fiore and Walett Faqqi (1993:53) argue that women, and more rarely men, monopolize the domain of the organic or natural illnesses, whose exegesis emphasizes the rupture of internal equilibrium (contagion, bad diet, excess of hot *[tuksi]* or cold *[tessmut]*, etc.). Marabouts control treating illnesses due to spirits, whose exegesis emphasizes or focuses upon relations with the superhuman world (Fiore and Walett Faqqi 1993:53). These authors separate natural and spiritual illness treatments and specialists.

I found that classifications of some organic illnesses vary from one medicine woman to another. Other medicine women with whom I conferred, furthermore, gave somewhat different illness etiologies. Another medicine woman, Anta, for example, stated, "*Alafaze* is a condition caused when one falls or is stamped on by an animal or person. *Tuksi* (hot illnesses) are caused by food that contains much oil with tea, sugar, tomatoes, also. *Ezziz* is caused when you wash and you walk on hot earth, you burn, and you are attacked. *Tessmut* (cold illnesses) are caused by raw maize or corn. *Afa* can be caught in the moonlight or sunlight. *Anoughou,* another imbalance, is caused by a change in diet from food you are accustomed to, or if you change the time of eating. *Tezoufnine* (approximately indigestion or other stomach problems) is caused by foods that contain fat, especially cheese, oil, anything with fat or grease. Evil mouth or eye is caused if a person talks about you with the spoiled mouth (i.e., negative gossiping). An enemy does sorcery against you. A hospital can cure fever *(tenede)* that I cannot cure."

Other medicine women divided the major illnesses into several categories: hot, cold, allergy, wind, rupture of habit, and skin. Another category reported in the literature is *asikulu,* walking under the sun, which causes eye or urinary illnesses. Other classifications I collected emphasize additional causes: for example, *amaghres,* a rupture of the normal diet that differs from *anoughou* in provoking *amaghras* illnesses such as syphilis and eye illnesses. Thus *anoughou,* a category involving a related disruption of normal routine, seems less specific in its consequences; friends often diagnosed me with this when I appeared fatigued or mildly ill after travel. Other illnesses often mentioned are *tetawen,* attacking the eyes, among especially persons who nourish themselves only with milk or dairy products; and *ahus,* a poor diet that provokes stomachaches or coughs. Medicine women know the value of vitamins or nutrients, but they do much more than manage these "natural" or "organic" elements.

Many medicine women's comments and also some aspects of Fatima's illness and Tata's diagnosis and treatment allude to the classical "hot/cold" thermal/humoral imbalance, and the widespread counteractive medicine system; for example, the ambiguity in Tata's diagnosis of Fatima's fever *(tenede).* Certainly Fatima was literally physically "hot," with a possible postpartum fever. Yet more subtle conditions were also present. Related to this, as the medicine women described to me, is *afa.* This condition includes literal heatstroke from exposure to sun and even hot mats and also, as noted, extends into more metaphorical domains of exposure to moonbeams and even flashlight rays. Interestingly, many Tuareg asserted to me that "women can also get *afa* from men's flashlights during evening festivals. They should pretend to ignore them." Flashlights are often used by men flirtatiously at rural evening festivals (with no electricity); hence the hint here of some social control in this illness etiology, and the dilemma many Tuareg experience between free courtship between the sexes, on the one hand, and competing injunctions by Islamic scholars, on the other, to contain it.

Another ambiguous category is a condition from humidity and cool air, which causes *tilwayen* or bone pain, migraines, and *timazzujen,* or ear infections. Yet "heat" takes on multiple connotations. Of course, the presence of a fever postpartum has been frequently documented medically, as for example, what Europeans called "puerperal fever," which killed many women following childbirth in medieval Europe. In the Tuareg case, while Tata diagnosed Fatima as having a "fever" *(tenede),* it should be noted that such a diagnosis is given to describe, not solely a literal hot body temperature, but also by extension, a "hot" illness *(tuksi)* more generally. The thermal qualities of the hot/cold dichotomy have characteristics including, but not limited to, physical temperature, which I explore presently.

Here I do not seek to establish illness taxonomies, of greater and lesser inclusiveness in the older "ethnoscience" tradition in anthropology, or to translate exactly across languages and cultures. Rather, in my view, what is useful here is to try to refrain from literal translation yet still understand, to connect these concepts to context, as one does in the process of thinking in a different language rather than attempting to translate it in advance. Such an approach seems more productive for adequately understanding the Tuareg counteractive humoral medical system. Among ordinary illnesses, the basic categories of hot illnesses *(tuksi)* and cold illnesses *(tesmet)* were often mentioned to me by many herbal medicine women. In general, hot illnesses evolve quickly, and cold illnesses evolve so slowly that they are only perceptible at an advanced and dangerous stage. Cold medicines treat hot illnesses and vice versa; counteractive healing here operates similarly to the Moorish and Latin American systems. According to the mode of preparation or, more rarely, according to the dosage, the same product becomes a hot or cold medicine. One must also take into account the seasons in the diagnosis and treatment of illnesses: cold illnesses are more frequent during the cold season and hot illnesses during the hot season.

Much medical anthropological literature attempts to show a universal hot/cold classification system, translating these concepts into systems of digestive, neurological, and cardiovascular pathologies (Noel in Claudot-Hawad 2002). Some works establish distinctions regarding the causes of illness and classifying them into natural and supernatural (Lejean 1986). Others provide a historical overview of diverse interpretations since the colonial era (Hureiki 1999). One recent work lists taxonomies and lexicons of selected hot/cold illnesses, though without any context of use or discussion of meaning (Fiore and Wallet Faqqi 1993:54–55).

Medicine women with whom I conferred often emphasized classifications based upon these opposed principles, of *tuksi* ("hot") and *tessmut* ("cold") conditions, but also subsumed some other illnesses within each. These generic categories of heat and cold involve humoral balance and counteractive medicine, hot and cold in both literal thermal senses and metaphorical extensions beyond them. They are expressed in local conceptions of the universe. For example, villages are hot, dunes are cold, wheat and corn are hot, millet and *fonio* are cold. Despite some variation, in general, hot regions are rocky, mountainous regions, regions of riverbeds, zones of floods, urban centers, and forests. There are, of course, seasons that are hot, as is there a cold and dry season *(essemed* or *tajirist)* from December to February; the moderate season occurs from September through November *(harat)*. Night is hot. Hot foods are all foods eaten in their heated state, as well as certain foods unheated. Contact with hot soil, lack of water, not washing, overspiced and rich foods, all produce heat. Dunes, plateaus, and the countryside are cold places. Cold seasons are called (with slight variations by region and dialect) *hewelen,* from the first half of April to the last half of June, and they end when the Pleiades appear and the wind blows to the east; *akassa* (or in some dialects, *ejina)* is the rainy and hot season. Day is cold. Cold foods include rice, millet, cold milk diluted with water, curdled diluted milk, cow's butter, lamb or mutton, and gazelle meat. Too much contact with water, eating cold foods, and getting wet—all these states lead to the cold condition.

In Europe from the times of Hippocrates and Galen, this "hot/cold" classification scheme was also influential. In Aristotle's texts, for example, human beings were classified according to the two principles: women as hotter than men because of the formers' alleged abundance of blood, considered hot in their bodies. To the condition of heat were also associated certain emotions, for example, joy. While cold was connected to death and fear, heat was generally given a more positive connotation, and cold a negative one. From Greece, the classical theory was passed through Arabic doctors in Spain and then exported by Spanish conquistadors in the sixteenth century to America. This theory is also documented for West Africa, Australia, and New Guinea. However, the semantic domain of the two terms *hot* and *cold* changes according to the culture and within a culture, I would add, according to a specific context. Cooking, drying, preparation and transformation, and social processes as well modify the quality of things, so they become cold or hot. In a list given me by several herbal medicine women and other local residents, "cold" may include a urinary problem, which requires not bathing for one week and drinking warm water to reinforce plant medicines that the patient took beforehand. Some Tuareg explained, "*tuksi* is internal. Whereas *afa* and *ezziz* [the latter an illness from sitting on hot sand or on a warm mat] are external. But all three have to do with heat, and are 'hot' illnesses."

Cold foods include millet, rice, fonio, melted butter, water in which dates are boiled, fresh milk with water, lamb or mutton, rice, and all cereals that one pounds but does not cook. Hot foods include curdled milk, sugar, oil, milk without water, eggs, and tamarind. Moreover, all plants have two forms, heat and cold, which depend on the manner in which they are prepared. Additional hot foods include dates; all fruits of the desert; milk boiled with sugar; millet pounded to which one adds milk; the millet/cheese/date/water beverage *eghajira* or *eghale;* beef, goatmeat, chicken; and cooked butter; goat meat, cooked lamb or mutton; milk just milked; and some specified "a date without being steeped in water"; millet and rice with added spices; and fish. Hot colors include indigo and tinted (as opposed to white) percale. Cold places are streams, dunes, and uninhabited places. Hot places are hills, stones, streams with surrounding hills, and towns.

My assistants/consultants and friends used these categories not solely in diagnosis of organic or "natural" and nonorganic illnesses but also in describing personal character. A hot person, for example, refers to a person who gets angry and emotional easily. This designation of a "hot" character refers to someone who is easily excited. One young man in Agadez, Niger, for example, sensitive and a gifted poet, was considered by others to be very easily angered and upset, and he frequently fell into a depression. He was also a political activist, often harassed by the local police, and eventually went into exile abroad. While men are ideally supposed to be somewhat hot, many Tuareg believe that too extreme heat can be harmful for men. The Agadez man was not exactly shunned socially, nor was he reprimanded openly, but others somewhat apologetically referred to him as "not very calm." Cold types are nervous, pale, high-strung; hot types are smiling and agitated, and some are insomniacs. Fiore and Wallet Faqqi report that there also exist individuals who are two things at once: who have, for example, a hot stomach, whereas the rest of their body is cold (Fiore and Wallet Faqqi 1993:59). There are also divisions of the body in additional criteria, for example, into upper and hot (Ag Erless 1990), but one should not overgeneralize that all upper-body ailments or pains are always "hot" illnesses.

These beliefs in part explain the prominence of medicine women's diagnosis by focusing upon the stomach, the variety of distinct terms for vomit or "indigestion" (as *tizufnine* was variously translated to me), their complexity, and the prevalence of purging medicines I encountered in many medicine women's practice. Although many illnesses derive from imbalance between these forces of heat and cold, there are people who have *tuksi* in their blood, but it sometimes is not as an illness. In its own manner, this theory resembles our own biomedical idea of "carriers" or "asymptomatic" persons, or perhaps also our notions of recessive genes or heterozygous rather than homozygous traits. But many Tuareg state that such persons must be careful: "hot" persons must eat cold foods and not wash. A "hot" person does not like water, whereas a "cold" person washes and drinks a lot of water, eats very little, and enjoys fresh drinks and cool places; his/her digestive tract does not boil and the excrement is allegedly cold. Although medicine women examine that which comes from the body (blood, stools, urine, and in particular—as Houna, Tana, and Tata indicated—vomit), to know how to adjust their treatments, medicine women must also carefully discern, not solely one's literal thermal/temperature state but also a variety of additional factors having to do with personal psychosocial experience.

The basis of these thermal categories, therefore, is not solely literal but also symbolic, psychosocial, and interactional. Certain personal pathologies are believed to be caused by an excess of one or the other principle. Herbal medicine women treat these conditions with counteractive medicines. In many respects, therefore, well-being depends on equilibrium, which includes but also transcends literal humoral conditions. Many Tuareg do not like the food of the towns: the rural beverage taken by many caravanners and labor migrants on travel, *eghajira,* is balanced, cold and hot at once.

There are numerous debates concerning the wider significance of these classifications of hot/cold systems in diverse cultures (Randall 1993; Ag Hamady el Mehdi 1988). These debates reflect the problem of the so-called emic vs. etic perspective—many anthropologists now agree that this is a false distinction, however, and indeed, everything is "emic" because one cannot really see the etic; the hot/cold system illustrates these difficulties. Therapeutic techniques appear based on the dynamic of oppositions and equivalences organized around these principles of hot and cold, but as shown in Fatima's case, it is collective social experiences that determine the response to a problem. As Fatima's pregnancy and birth case revealed, a supportive community is mobilized. Here, participants encourage changes in conduct, and remedies are redefined and incorporated into collective knowledge. Thus local theories tend to become modified and diverge from rigid taxonomies, since they often expand these categories metaphorically into an individual's social relationships, thereby blurring organic and nonorganic illnesses.

Although hot/cold is known and utilized in popular knowledge, therefore, it is not the sole consideration, and it is difficult to establish a general rule, since healers do not share the same point of view on the classifications of hot and cold illnesses. In other words, there are divergences of knowledge on hot and cold. Tuareg classification into hot and cold illnesses and temperaments in traditional medicine is therefore used to interpret different situations, individual and collective. In counteractive medicine, when someone suffers from cold illness, one administers a hot remedy. This is not, however, an absolute rule, for in some cases, adding cold onto cold or hot onto hot can eradicate the illness (Figueiredo-Biton in Claudot-Hawad 2002:137). Thus a given remedy takes into account other parameters beyond the illness itself.

An attack of fever such as that of Fatima therefore represents an accumulation of overabundant heat, but an attack of spirits such as that also afflicting her, diagnosed, treated, and referred by Tata the medicine woman, and by the spirit exorcism ritual specialist, engenders a feeling of "cold" illness. As shown in the next chapter, gender typifications are relevant here, for women are ideally supposed to be somewhat "cold," though not too cold. Moreover, as observed by medicine women, this is an ambiguous classification here, and is difficult to treat with humoral medicine alone, for this attack is at once psychic and organic.

The point is that therapy for a given illness may take different forms. For a difficult pregnancy and birth, as Fatima experienced, sometimes a marabout intervenes, who interprets whether there are Kel Essuf present or an alternative cause. In Fatima's case, her father was a renowned marabout, widely sought after for Qur'anic divination and healing. But predominantly female herbal medicine women (relatives and nonrelatives) and possession exorcist specialists were ultimately called upon for her treatment, and later, also hospital and clinic staff. Thus Fatima's illness event set in motion different agents to intervene, though Tata's intervention cannot be isolated or oversimplified as only "natural" or "organic" in its focus. Knowing how to interpret the specific illness is the domain of specialists, but is also, to some extent, a socially shared knowledge, with a goal of reestablishing the general well-being of the person.

Hence the important role of medicine women in socializing or domesticating certain illnesses—as mothers socialize "difficult children", to bring the naturally "wild" or uncontrollable under human social control—but complexly, into a simultaneously natural physical and social cultural balance. Indeed, all illnesses everywhere have both natural (organic) and social, cultural, and spiritual elements. Ideals of conduct vividly show the central importance of this process: reserve; hiding one's wishes and weaknesses; and avoiding risk of social pollution or ostracism or ridicule.

Although some afflictions are believed to have more organic causes, etiology, and symptoms, which entail some physical isolation, for example, measles and tuberculosis, there are cures that call for varying proportions of ritual, herbal, and other medicinal treatments. While most medicine women and their patients recognize that some illnesses require pills (for example, antibiotics) and surgery, which local residents increasingly seek out at hospitals and clinics, nonetheless, other ailments are decidedly nonorganic, if not in symptomology, then in cause, and require ritual and social adjustments, either alone or in combination with biomedicines, to heal. These latter are exemplified by several beliefs and practices pertaining to personal well-being and social harmony— which are intimately connected, in the local view. For example, attitudes of coveting can be a cause of illnesses such as *togerchet,* caused by inconsiderate words, which are believed by medicine women and "lay" nonspecialist persons alike to make the victim more vulnerable to Kel Essuf actions. Medical knowledge interprets social relations to identify causes of dysfunction. For example, the art of speaking clearly plays a prominent role in the prevention of some illnesses. Words that leave the mouth have an effect upon one's bodily condition. Words can reach the soul of a person (can "drink the soul" of someone, equivalent to killing him or her), and even compliments can provoke ambiguous sentiments, jealousy, desire, and the risk of bringing evil eye or mouth *(tehot, teshot* or *togerchet),* and thereby creating disequilibrium (Casajus 1987, 2000; Noel in Claudot-Hawad 2002:147; Rasmussen 2001a).

Certain important cultural values in moral conduct, for example, *takarakit* or shame/reserve, and *imojagh* or dignity, are ideally supposed to impose limitations on conduct: too openly boasting, for example, invites coveting and jealousy. Many taboos, therefore, serve as "leveling mechanisms," limiting accumulation of wealth or power and moderating consumption by any single individual or social stratum. Ideally, they serve to restrain undisciplined or selfish conduct in an environment of scarcity that requires, ideally at least, balanced reciprocity, sharing of resources, and mutual aid. Their manifestations and consequences, whether in the form of organic or nonorganic afflictions, and regardless of whether they are defined in terms of human or superhuman causation, cannot be reduced to some "folk" version of biomedical contagion or "germ" models.

Thus concepts of health and the manner of maintaining it reveal the coexistence of different medical knowledge systems. Seeking cures takes an individual on the road between different models, each with a specific concept of condition of health and wellbeing. This was shown in the case of Tata's earlier male patient, whose affliction never came out into the open or received public ritual recognition or medico-ritual action. In concepts of health and well-being, local medical knowledge is constructed by collective experiences, but these are given individual subjective meanings with the collaboration of the medicine woman. Health is perceived as one aspect of the harmonious order between different worlds in balance: the visible world in part physical and in part social, and the invisible world of the other forces, the Kel Essuf, the spirits. These two worlds come together and form the social environment. The capacity for an individual's balancing these two worlds is one criterion of health. The act of healing is a movement toward reintegration of the individual toward his/her social environment. While I agree with some other researchers that there is generally a collective sharing of experiences that reinforces knowledge here (Noel in Claudot-Hawad 2002:147), I differ in that my evidence suggests that, in some contexts, certain knowledge (diagnosis, treatment) of illness is kept private, while in others, it is more collective; the outcome depends upon the context of medicine women's collaborative effort to define the illness.

In much of their logic of preventative actions, therefore, many medicine women refer, not solely to matters of diet and humoral balance, but also social/moral conduct Islamic and pre-Islamic (or popular Islamic), and additional cultural beliefs concerning gender: notions of pure and impure, hidden and open, precautions and their violation. Illness disrupts the envisioned ideal of balanced harmony between the visible and invisible world. The logic here is that since suffering *(tezzort)* is often hidden, it must be surmised according to the conduct of a person. Elsewhere (Rasmussen 1995), I have pointed out the significance of "hidden illnesses" among the Tuareg and the powerful influence of reserve and shame in healer/patient interaction. Observation is not focused solely on the body; the medicine woman also examines the speech of the ill person, what is said and not said, and his/her social rapport and integration into the group. She listens to the etiology of the illness, how he/she first noticed or perceived the illness. She observes the general appearance of a patient, especially the eyes, ears, mouth, and skin—its tone, texture, and temperature. Touch is done through the clothing, except on women patients' stomach.

Some illnesses medicine women diagnose and/or treat are caused by breaking social rules. These additional conditions that herbal medicine women treat defy neat classification into organic and nonorganic and have only approximate, rather than exact, translations into the English language or into Euro-American established biomedical paradigms, as shown next.

An Angry Person

One such illness, called *karambaza,* is a special stomach ailment believed transmitted by smith/artisans who are angry and resentful and activate (consciously or unconsciously) a malevolent force called *tezma* because nobles have not paid them for their work or because they covet a noble's property. In such cases, the smith's anger is said to fly from his heart to the victim. One basic divination ritual many medicine women use to diagnose *karambaza* is to rotate a pot over the fire, at the same time pronouncing the names of the foods or other items possibly craved by the smith in order to diagnose the cause; when the pot stops rotating, this indicates what angered the smith/artisan. Frequently there is tension between Tuareg smith/artisans and other Tuareg, in times of increasing social turmoil when smiths are acquiring new wealth from their work in the tourist trade and nobles, impoverished, are experiencing difficulty supporting them (Rasmussen 1998b). *Tezma* is believed to strike children and livestock in this way, in particular, precisely because they are so highly valued. *Karambaza,* which usually afflicts in the form of diarrhea, is believed to be caused by *tezma* powers, which are activated automatically. Its diagnosis and treatments include seeing an herbalist, gathering up the sand from the site of the smith/artisans' footprints, and throwing it into the fire, or alternatively, the suspected smith offender is required to jump over the afflicted three times. While a biomedical "reading" is possible here in certain respects, nonetheless local residents convey a more layered and nuanced interpretation of the problem, as the following case illustrates.

Once, during the cold, dry harmattan season, a wedding was held in one of the local chiefly and maraboutique families around Mt. Bagzan in northern Niger. My host family and I attended, and a woman brought back home some leftover meat from the feast. The child's mother had seen an herbal medicine woman recently for her own illness, a liver problem, and the medicine woman had stated that her liver was confronted with a sudden change (for example, not enough or too much food or food of a new type) and had been attacked, with the resultant condition called *anoughou.* The meat was distributed to members of the household, and adults and children all ate some of it. One child, a daughter approximately ten years old, developed stomach troubles from the meat. The girl's mother suspected a nearby smith woman of causing her daughter to fall ill. Normally, smith/artisans in the Bagzan region of Aïr perform wedding praise-songs for nobles, in particular at a couple's first wedding, and receive as part of their remuneration portions of the slaughtered animal's meat. However, at that particular wedding, the marriage of a divorced woman to a man who had also been previously married, fewer musical festivities were held, and smiths attached to that noble family therefore did not receive their usual compensation/gifts.

The mother took her daughter to an herbal medicine woman, who spun around a pot, calling out the names of the possible foods responsible for the girl's stomachache. It stopped at her mention of the wedding meat, thereby diagnosing the problem as *karambaza* caused by the *tezma* of a neighboring attached smith woman, who frequently stopped by their household bearing messages and dressing the women's hair. This smith was blamed verbally, though no physical retribution was taken against her. The mother gathered sand up from the place where the smith had left prints, and threw it into the fire. This ritual action and the disapproving gossip were followed, however, by another remedy: the mother also obtained some stomach medicine from a newly built local clinic. However, despite the added Western biomedical treatment, most family members continued to blame the smith as the primary cause of the child's illness, and as shown, additional "ritual" curative measures were also taken. Thus one must distinguish between local logical explanations of cause, effect, and treatment.

My first reaction—admittedly a culture-bound interpretation—was to attribute that child's illness solely to the leftover meat, which I suspected must have been tainted when the child ate it, after approximately forty-eight hours; or perhaps the child's immune system was weaker than others'.

Yet problems of spoilage and stomach illnesses are much rarer during the dry season than during the hot and rainy seasons, and, furthermore, it should be noted that we had all eaten this meat—including other, even younger children—and no one else, local adult, child, or this researcher, came down with the stomach illness. As also noted, a bio-medical stomach medicine was taken, and the pattern of blame and its prescribed rit-ual cure were also followed here, with social and cosmological bases remaining locally significant. Perhaps the mother did give her child pills, just in case these worked, though she never articulated the cause of the ailment in such biomedical terms. The point here is, regardless of the multiple remedies, causation (explanations of misfortune, af-fliction), the medicine woman's theories were taken very seriously. Also, while the body manifests symptoms whose origins may have been spoiled food, nonetheless, social rela-tions are also an important issue in discourse and social practice for many local residents. An approximately parallel example might be a case, in the United States, of a diagnosis of cancer, followed by a discussion among a family attempting to focus upon some possible causes—such as stress from recent disputes, marital disruption, etc.—since other relatives may not be struck down by it, regardless of genetic tendencies.

The important point is that, in disagreements, revisions, and contradictions of herbal medicine women's diagnoses and treatments, medicine women's treatment is not limited to the body, and their knowledge does not necessarily become muted or sup-pressed. Rather, their theories and practices become entangled with patients' more long-term problems and solutions to them. Many of these afflictions and cures, as shown, have only partially to do with actual biomedical "germ" theory and are not lim-ited to the body, or to "organic/naturalistic" illnesses or cures; yet at the same time, medicine women, like many healers, possess multiple theories of illness etiology and cures. In these processes, medicine women use multiple sense modalities in learning, practicing, and transmitting their healing forms. The next two chapters examine these sense modalities in relation to concepts of the body and person.

Part Two / Touch and Word

Learning and Transmitting Medicine

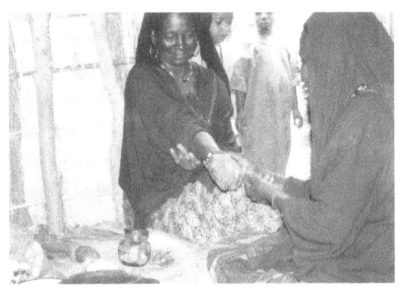

Touching to diagnose

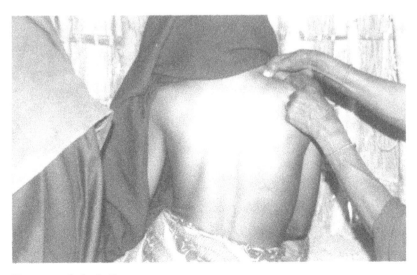

Treatment of a back ailment

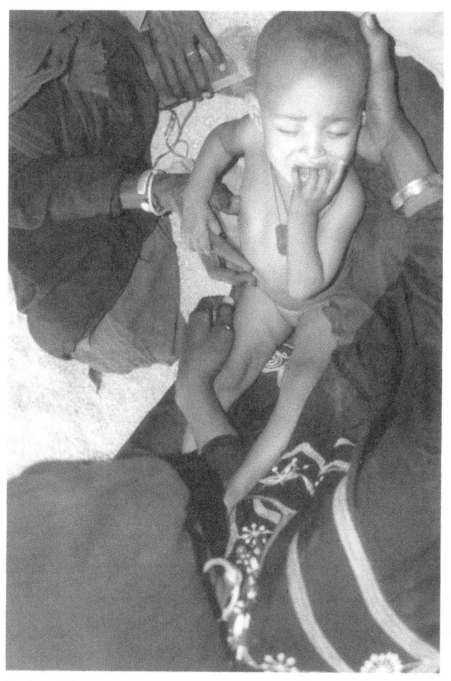

Treating a child

55

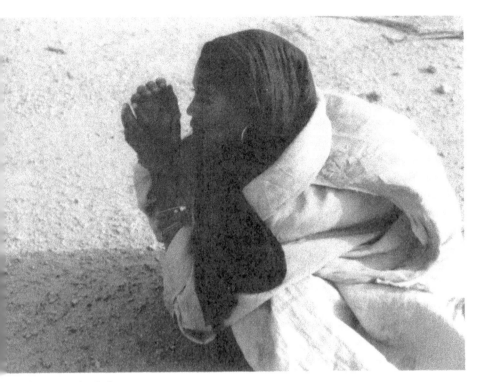

Woman praying before tree

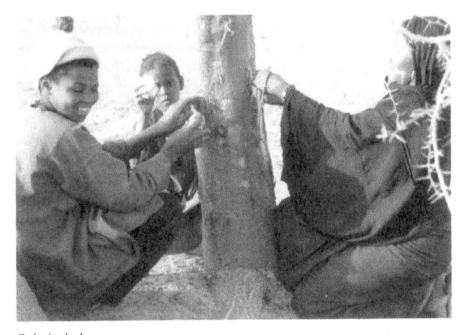

Gathering bark

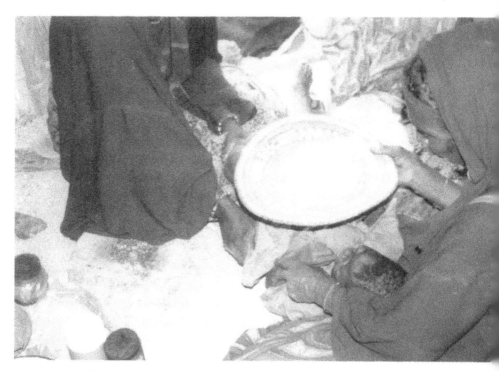

Passing millet over child

3 – Touch, Body, and Senses

My aim in touching the patient is to touch the illness in its place. I touch the ground because this is tradition, like a prayer. During a cure, I also pronounce certain words, such as *"Bismillah"* (Islamic blessing or benediction) and medicine names. I sometimes refer patients to the *tende n goumaten* possession ritual if they have spirits. My specialty's illnesses require touching by a medicine woman; those of the *tende n goumaten* possessing spirits require exorcising spirits, by drumming and singing, primarily. Marabouts treat very strong spirits who enter the mouth and make a person thin. To be in good health means to be nice and never to insult. God brings good or bad health. In my opinion, men are generally healthier [than women]; why? Because women eat bad things. People of all ages get sick equally often. [But] no one I have seen has a perfectly happy life.

These words are from Houna, a medicine woman we first met in Chapter 1. They introduce us to some basic principles of medicine women's profession: the central importance of touch and tactile-based knowledge and practice in medicine women's learning and teaching of their knowledge, their diagnosis/divination, and their treatment.

There are two major ways of preparing herbal treatments: by cooking them over the fire and by steeping them after they are dried, in water as a tea: the former is called *as-siwi*, the latter called *adir adir*. Cooking over the fire is the preferred technique for more serious illnesses. Some medicine women do only the steeping of teas. Some other medicine women do only the cooking of medicines; and others, such as Tata, do both. A few others, more renowned, know and practice all these methods, including divination by dreaming as well as the more usual rotating of a pot. Many herbal medicine women, like more specialized diviners, use combined touch and scent in divination/diagnosis, called *edes* or "touch" (Hawad 1979; Rasmussen 2001a).[1]

Other medicine women, in addition to practicing herbalism, set bones. Yet despite the special term *(tamadas)* for those in this sub-specialty, they, too, are classified more generally as a kind of *tanesmegel*. Tana, whom we met earlier (in Chapter 1), explained, "A bone-setter is a kind of herbalist, because she must know medicine first, in order to treat *(tigou amagal)*. It is as though the *tamadas* takes the temperature. There is a kind of touching *(arabaz)* that is accompanied by her own medicine: massage. The person learns massage. One does it to cure *tarzak* and *aghitiss*. The herbalist specialist is stronger because she knows all the trees, and in addition she knows *tarzak, coupure du sang*, illnesses."

In local classification, all these medicine women fall under the rubric of *tinesmegelen* (or *tinesefren* in the Malian dialect). Somewhat approximating the distinction in Western allopathic biomedicine between general practitioners (GPs) and specialists, medicine women vary in degree of specialization but share certain central skills, such as a basic knowledge of the body, touch, and medicinal trees and plants. What is important is expertise in these domains of knowledge and the ability to relieve suffering. One medicine woman, for example, was able to diagnose some eye problems, although she was without the electricity- or laser-based technical machines such as the light or laser beam or x-ray, and for these latter, she recognized the need to refer some cases to hospitals. Yet as noted earlier, translations here are only approximate. Medicine women also contrast to Western biomedically trained health personnel: the former place greater emphasis upon touch and sound than sight in their diagnosis and healing.

Amina, a medicine woman on top of Mount Bagzan, offered further perspectives on these processes; she said,

> If I receive a patient, I touch first to diagnose [know] the illness; if it is *tezouf-nine* (indigestion), for example. If it is *tessmut* ("cold" illness), the intestines are soft. But if I feel that which is hard, then, it is an illness caused by *tuksi*, "heat." The intestines swell when it is *tuksi*. I treat *tuksi*, indigestion, sprains, and illnesses from "cold" *tessmut*. I never dream to divine or diagnose. The *ten* (pot) of medicine recipes is composed of one hundred trees. One *atitaga teguiz* (mixes, stirs) in a pot made of red clay, you drink and chew that. Patients pay me *eguim* (denotes both 5000 CFA or US$10 and, more traditionally, seven forearms, a measurement) of cloth, or 2500 CFA (US$5). In the past, cloth measure was a currency; now, this measure has an equivalent in West African francs or CFA. But no one pays me with any object that is black because our relatives do not like that.

Amina's comments reveal that, although touch is an important technique, it is a preliminary step in medicine women's work, and the patient and herbal medicine women must collaborate in healing an illness; patients do not merely passively receive medicines, rather they must accompany the ingestion of medicines with additional ritual precautions and dietary restrictions. Medicine women also need to observe visual and tactile taboos, such as avoiding the color black and using only clay-based containers. She also indicated that some medicines are ingested, some inhaled, and others applied to the body in washing, though refraining from washing for a time is also sometimes required. There are also hints here that women's, men's, and children's medicines are distinct. Payment is flexible and variable.

Another medicine woman, Fana, provided more extensive insights into the interconnections between touch, the body, and herbal treatments:

> I do both touch and bark medicines. I inherited my work from both my mother and father. I learned from my mother, for about five years; I have been practicing now for about ten years. I began at the age of forty years old, after the death of my mother. My mother died after I had learned everything; it was the time. If your parents authorize you, you can do it anytime. The ones who do this best here, however, are the old women of the Bagzan, the place of origin of [our] medicine *(arasal n amagal)*. According to our knowledge, they do medicine. It is the *al baraka* of the mountain, Mt. Bagzan is blessed with trees that contain all sorts of medicines.
>
> In order to identify the illness, I touch. I treat by touch, also *adir-adir* (herbal teas steeped in water). I know all the medicinal trees, but I do not do all the

combinations (recipes) of the *ten* (the ensemble of all medicine recipes and a "pot"; thus metonymically, the medicine pot here stands for the herbal repertoire). . . . I do not cook medicines over the fire. Some illnesses attack the liver: a dislocated liver, for example, happens when there is much illness, and when one falls, also. The liver and the heart are the foundation of the person. The liver can suffer from *anoughou*, the sudden stress from disruption of the usual routine, or, when one falls, it dislocates. Everyone comes to me for treatment: women and men, everyone especially with liver problems.

Yesterday and the day before, I treated a woman and a child. Patients pay me what they can pay. I touch the earth because that is a benediction, as a goal or wish. I rotate medicines as an alms or offering. Sunday, Monday are good days for healing. The diviner divines by looking; the herbalist touches. All female healers touch the stomach. The stomach is the basis of many illnesses. Each place has its illnesses. The stomach is full of things. When I touch an illness, I feel a hard spot. Sometimes, if the healer touches someone, and the illness is serious, for example spirits, she refers the patient to marabouts. I touch in order to find these Kel Essuf spirits. When I feel them, they move in the stomach. I touched someone in whom I felt spirits, when he arrived he was crazy. I referred him to marabouts. He is now in good health.

Some liver illnesses are *tchidguit in tessa* (pricking of the liver) and *anoughou* (lacking something in a sudden change of routine). *Tegare n tessa* (literally, flying to the liver) is caused by evil eye or mouth *(togerchet)*, negative gossip, also. The liver is the person. When attacked by sorcery, the liver can be treated also by barks of some renowned herbal healers. They use barks against sorcery from the Bagzan; our most senior medicine woman, Lala, the head of herbalists on Mt. Bagzan, knows them, you must ask her.

Magical Hands: Learning and Transmitting Knowledge and Healing through Touch

More broadly, the foregoing comments of Houna, Amina, and Fana remind us that in therapeutic touch, the practitioner centers his/her own thought and is sensitive to receiving and sending nonverbal messages or energy through the hands (Kitzinger in Davis-Floyd and Sargent 1997:209–29). Within Euro-American cultures, great stress is usually placed upon the visual modality of the sensorium. With few exceptions (Douglas 1975; Olkes and Stoller 1987; Stoller 1989; Tyler 1987, unspoken elements in discourse tend to be trivialized or ignored (Kitzinger in Davis-Floyd 1997:209). Until recently, other modalities such as aural, olfactory, and bodily were neglected. Increasingly, works offer rich perspectives on these latter (E. Turner 1996; Classen 1997a; Rasmussen 1999:55–74, 2000; Stoller 1997).

Tuareg medicine women have long recognized that one important element in the interaction of human bodies is touch. Touch conveys messages, either conscious and purposeful or unconscious, with unintended but powerful consequences read differently by the receiver. Sometimes these messages contradict verbal communication (Kitzinger 1997:209). Sometimes they are mixed or confused.

Sometimes touch reinforces messages conveyed in the form of speech. It is not just a way of sending out arbitrary signals. Touch has its own—often intricate—language specific to a culture. In situations that are culturally significant, in particular transitions such as birth and death, touch given by those attending is often (considered to convey) authoritative (knowledge) (Kitzinger 1997:209).

Significantly, apart from healing, the contexts in which touch is important and deployed among the Tuareg are few, and touching in other social contexts is rather restrained. One reason for this is undoubtedly the great cultural emphasis, among persons of noble origin, in particular, upon dignity, restraint, reserve, and their feeling of some shame concerning bodily contact. Perhaps this is also related to the precolonial stratified system requiring formal conduct between certain persons. In the countryside, greetings tend to be highly formalized: there is a series of verbal inquiries with formulaic responses. Among marabouts, in particular, a stylized handshake consists of extending and withdrawing the fingertips of the right hand several times—the number of motions dependent upon such factors as the length of time the parties have been apart and their respective social statuses. Otherwise, bodily contact in greetings is fairly minimal, at least in public, between most persons. Hugs are rarely given in public, even between close friends and relatives. Instead, one's true sentiments—including affection—are usually veiled and expressed through indirect and subtle means. While verbal conversation is highly valued, nonetheless, in this domain, as well, noble cultural values emphasize allusion and metaphor.

Loud yelling, "vulgar" language, physical jostling, touching of garments and body, are disdained, associated with the conduct of smiths and former slaves—persons of ambiguous or lower social status—and avoided between those of noble background. Some physical mock wrestling *(tebillant)* occurs, but only between certain persons who practice joking relationships on specific occasions—for example, between nobles and smiths, and between women—almost always at rites of passage or during communal work projects such as tent-building and repair, in a humorously competitive spirit (Worley 1991; Nicolaisen 1997).

Gestures *(sikbar)* are used in much tale-telling performance, but again, these are surrounded by restrictions. For example, smiths and griots are expected to use them more effusively than others. Also, one must stop using gestures upon the approach of a parent or parent-in-law (Rasmussen 1995, 1997). Women, in particular, noble women are traditionally not supposed to make people laugh. Until recently, their physical movements were ideally supposed to be limited to some herding tasks, education of children, and playing musical instruments. Walking was supposed to be undertaken only for short distances, slowly, and with great dignity. Another purpose of this is to gain weight, toward the ideal of fatness, a sign of fertility, beauty, prosperity, and ability to have others do the hard physical labor—difficult for many to attain.

Hence the widespread importance of physical, kinesthetic, and verbal restraint and limitations upon touch among many, on most social occasions. Medicine women, I argue, counterbalance and provide relief from this cultural trend. In medicine women's healing, touch is one way of conveying knowledge and healing. There is in this context important physical contact, expressed not solely by stroking and holding but also by many types of named massages. Indeed, I argue, touch and dynamic manipulation of the body in Tuareg herbal healing counterbalances the absence of touch in many other domains. Medicine women in effect "cuddle," thereby compensating for this restriction and offering individuals comfort in a culture characterized by much public reserve, restraint, and distance between many persons, and also, many arduous tasks in a harsh physical environment, which stress the body and soul.

Powerful messages are communicated and received. In herbal medicine women's divination and treatment (especially those by the more specialized bone-setters), touch centers upon the stomach, liver, and sometimes, joints of the body such as the wrist. Joints of the body are by extension points of social articulation: joints in ritual are extended to represent kinship relationships. At memorial commemorative alms feasts, balls of *eghale* (made from crushed millet, goat cheese, and dates) are distributed as alms and in this context symbolize the kinship relations of the deceased (Rasmussen 1997). Perhaps also, the joints are significant in touch as a kind of human (manual) "polygraph" test, pulse-reading, "palm-reading," or psychoanalysis: I saw several instances of medicine women holding the wrist and making comments concerning the well-being and/or thoughts or problems of a patient.

This practice of touch is central and constitutes an alternative divination method. As a medicine woman I shall call Hadia explained, "Me, I [also] use barks. [But] the person who does not know touch does not know medicine. The person must know both trees and [how to] touch. I do not do dreaming divination (literally, "seeing," *asawad*). Those medicine women who do this have relations with spirits. I do not have relations with the spirits, I have relations only with my hand. I know each illness with it, because that is my work and it is my inheritance. I only look at God. Also, anyone whom I get along with, I treat; if not, I do not treat."

Touch has additional significance and uses. As in many societies, Tuareg medicine women's comforting body contact, skin stimulation, massage, and physical support are elements integral to the experience of birth. Through touch, for example, Tata in her treatment of Fatima acquired information about the position of the baby, the strength of the mother's contractions, and the progress of labor, and she was able to convey this tactile knowledge to others. Through touch, a medicine woman acquires information about the position and condition of the stomach and other bodily parts and afflictions, for example, of the bones, as well as psychosocial stress, and is also able to relax patients. Authoritative yet informal touch among medicine women thus constitutes a validated system of authoritative knowledge. Because touch consists of physical contact, it incorporates beliefs about the human body and about relationships between human beings and often, also—as we shall soon see clearly—social relations between humans, ancestors, and spirits. Comforting words of advice and concern occur at the same time as physical touching.

Another medicine woman named Zara, an elderly woman in the Kel Igurmadan descent group about seventy years old, and a member of a local chiefly and maraboutique family, elaborated on these points:

> A person touches the earth before touching the patient as a sort of ablution, for the sake of all the trees on the earth. [Zara demonstrated this, not solely verbally, but also physically by touching my assistant's hand.] Here is my hand [you see], you must touch in order to see what is wrong with the patient. That hand has a kind of pain [where] it is necessary to do cupping.

I have been curing for about thirty years, since around forty years of age. I did not do this before, because I did not have authorization. Also, a young girl is not given authorization, one does not allow her [to practice independently] because she is not yet complete. She might even use a medicine that is not correct [for the ailment]. . . . I began my apprenticeship when I had my first daughter, at about 25 years old.[2] One needs the authorization of all relatives. They do not authorize youths because they fear youths do not [fully] understand medicine [yet].

Zara considers herself to be both a *tanesmegel* (as noted, the generic term for medicine woman) and a *tamadas* specialist in massage. She once attended a training program for matrons in a large oasis about twenty miles from her village (around 1989), but she indicated that her own tactile-based techniques did not derive from that training program but from medicine women's own long-standing practice. She diagnosed primarily bone and joint problems, twisted or fractured bones *(amezeghi),* for example. She treated a sprained ankle with sheep fat and broken bones with rooster fat and massage. She demonstrated her techniques for me and my assistant by touching and massaging us. As she massaged, Zara touched the earth and murmured incantations in alternation. She indicated she also did cupping for twisted bones. She could not do this during a very cold season, however, because of her own increasing symptoms, her descriptions of which suggested arthritis.

Zara was married and widowed four times. Her four living children include one son who had a store in her small village and did business in Agadez. He was a polygynist: his first wife resided nearby, and a second wife resided in a neighboring village where the family's oasis garden was located. One of Zara's cousins was a former rebel fighter, who sometimes visited her, wearing his camouflage uniform with a green turban/face-veil. Before Zara gave birth to her daughter, she had lost a child who died very young. She named her next child Taklit, denoting "female slave," in order to detract the spirits from her and prevent them from taking this child away from her. Perhaps from gratitude to God for her daughter's survival to adulthood (though Zara did not state this motive so explicitly to me), she later arranged a marriage for this daughter to a prominent marabout, who already had an older first wife. Zara's daughter had been a renowned singer in her youth. Since her marriage, this daughter no longer sang in public because of her new social position as wife of the prominent marabout, in deference to some Islamic scholars' ambivalence toward non-liturgical music.[3]

Zara indicated some bilineality, and even more flexible ambilineality, in tracing her professional practice; she indicated she inherited this from her father, but she traced her recipes matrilineally, through women and the Kel Igurmadan (line). She explained, "The Igurmadan clan is more specialized in medicine. I learned to do medicine on top of Mount Bagzan with the late mother of the father of a cousin on my father's side. Among the Igurmadan women, raised by our relatives, as soon as she was born, our ancestral founder held a special box of medicines. Thus [medicine] is something innate, inherited. Our medicine is from Tagurmat, our ancestress. When Tagurmat was born, she began to make [herbal] medicines."

Most important in Zara's techniques, however, are touch and memory. "*Tinesmegelen* who are not bone-setters don't cut and don't touch the joints/bones. *Tinesmegelen* treat children. A *tanesmegel* who is also a *tamadas,* however, knows more: birth problems, for example—she can remedy a breech birth, better than just an herbal specialist. Yet since the *tamadas* uses fewer (tree) medicines than other more herbal-specialist *tinesmegelen,* they usually charge less money." Here Zara takes pride in her own specialty as prestigious and useful, despite its bringing less financial remuneration than selling herbal remedies.

According to Zara,

> It is with the aid of my fingers that I know the illness [while touching], even if it is in the stomach. Among the people of the Bagzan, there are others who, even if they merely touch you and you have confidence in them, that will cure you [without any other medicine]. This is called *tajiye n'assilimoumisse* (which denotes approximately "faith-healing," laying on of hands). For example, a man from Iferouan [to the north, near the Tamgak Mountains] had a snakebite, and an *echerif* from Mount Bagzan healed him in this manner. . . . I differ from other herbal healers in that I do razor cutting, I do bone-setting, everything. I touch children's stomachs. My hand can arrange the child [in the womb] from the exterior [can realign a child in breech birth]. But I have begun to become weak and old; I drank jackal's blood during the cold season to cure a cough, and I have problems with my eyes now. People come to me. They pay me anything, and choose their healer according to preference.

I visited Zara several times, both to observe consultations with her permission and to obtain treatment myself. I had known her for approximately twenty years. Zara held up her hand to me and explained, "My hand that you see, this touches the sick place. The head also calculates and gives the result. Hand and head communicate together. The *icherifan* treat only with words and hands, do not use herbal medicines. They are the descendants of the Prophet. Some herbalists and diviners can do this faith-healing, as well. The real [complete, greatly effective] treatment is like that.

"There exist rules and requirements for cures. For example, a woman who has her husband beside her, other herbalists do not treat her [i.e., when a woman has sexual relations with her husband, the medicine she has drunk does not work]. . . . Also, herbalists cannot treat women during the healers' menstrual periods." Notably, Zara mentions here that some conditions and medicines require that the patient actually refrain from touch: namely, female patients cannot have sexual relations with their husbands during treatment.

These ritual restrictions outside the immediate healing context, during the wider treatment, along with the centrality of touch by medicine women during immediate healing, suggest the need to protect the touch and medicines of herbal medicine women by keeping them separate from other contacts (in particular, sexuality and reproduction). In other words, the touch of medicine women must be kept separate from other types of touch. In this regard, these precautions recall some other efforts at ritual separation to ensure power, for example, the different fertility forces of humans and forest among the Beng (Gottlieb 1992). They also approximate the idea in Euro-American biomedicine that some antibiotics are mutually exclusive and "cancel out" each other if taken together.

The rule of touching is to touch the patient three times, in three visits, and three treatments, in for example, massage *(arabaz)*. Sometimes if you touch something, you must also touch the sand. But I refer women who have been torn by childbirth (in French, *les femmes fistues*) to the hospital. In my preparation of medicine, I cook the head of a sacrificed animal along with the medicines. When you serve medicine to a patient, you must take it off the fire, and when you give it, you increase the water in the pot, with the head of a ram or goat on the side. When the patient takes the medicine, they eat the head, also. If I treat a man, I slaughter a ram. If it is a woman, I slaughter a female goat. I do razor cuts on the fourteenth or fifteenth day of the month because there are two bloods, good and bad: the bad blood leaves on that day. I use herbs, cuts, touch, and massage.

Zara indicated that she cured less now, because she felt too old to travel far and gather plants; they are far away in the mountains, an uphill climb. So patients came to her. They paid her approximately 100 CFA (about 20 US cents), or a fee according to capacity, or gave her tea and sugar. Zara saw men, women, and children. Often, a patient stayed with her for three days; for many conditions are believed to require two follow-up treatments after the initial one, thereby bringing the total to three treatments, the same number of times the herbalist ritually touches the ground, murmurs "Bissmillallah," and circles alms over children.

I sought treatment for my own aches and pains, minor but ubiquitous in the exertions of travel and rural Saharan living. I was also prone to sinus and migraine headaches in the wind and sun. Zara touched the earth as she massaged my neck and shoulder area; when I inquired why, she explained, "the earth is significant because plants grow there. Also, our touching the earth conveys a blessing. Our rotating medicines indicates alms, an offering."

Zara diagnosed a bunion or hammertoe not as a genetic mutation, as in Western biomedical opinion, but as "an old fracture that did not heal properly." She also treated a "kink" in my neck and aches around my shoulder-blades, which I attributed to heavy lifting of water buckets, baggage, and equipment. In contrast to some other treatments, Zara did not suggest any additional underlying problems or causes of this particular affliction. She seemed concerned with more immediate tactile relaxation techniques rather than diagnosing long-term social processes that might have provoked this condition. She gave me a soothing massage *(arabaz)* on the upper back and neck, as I leaned forward in a seated position similar to the position Americans take in currently popular "chair massages." She lifted my blouse above my neck, never removing it entirely, and massaged—with long yet firm strokes (not "shiatsu-style")—my neck and shoulders with a salve from the Agadez market. I gave her 125 CFA and soap. I returned again the next morning and two more times, over several days. At each consultation, Zara massaged my back and neck and also applied the same salve from the Agadez market. She then murmured "Bissmillah," and touched the ground three times. Many residents explained that the herbalist touches the ground "in order to take the disease out of both patient and healer, and to throw away or take away disease; the ground absorbs the disease." Thus the spiritual and physical are treated as one, bringing in a compendium of skills.

Edez (touch) and the *ten* or medicine pot are central to herbal medicine women's medical knowledge and treatment. Yet not all those who touch and use massage know all, or the same number of tree medicines. Thus in local classifications, there are various degrees and finer knowledge specializations among different medicine women. The most renowned and respected medicine women know diverse treatments, however. Ideally, they know both massage and herbal tree medicines. Others tend toward one or the other; some know only touch or massage but have less knowledge of tree barks, leaves, and roots. The latter tend to learn more informally, and undergo less rigorous apprenticeships.

Tema, a woman in a seminomadic village of marabouts, gardeners, and caravanners where the chief of the Kel Igurmadan resided, exemplifies a medicine woman who was informally rather than formally trained. Her own career appears more similar to those of many other medicine women I met in northern Mali, who tended to view their profession in more informal terms and did not appeal to inheritance in clans as much as medicine women in northern Niger did. Upon asking if there is a medicine woman in a given vicinity, very often the question is phrased, "Is there someone who touches here?" Tema and her patients simply said, "I (she) touch(es)" to describe her profession.

Now in her mid-forties, Tema related to me how she had learned touch and massage, but not complex herbal remedy treatments, from her mother. She did not trace her practice formally to any founding culture heroine. Perhaps she did not mention Tagurmat because she was in a prominent local chiefly and maraboutique family; such families are very devout and tend to be more reticent concerning (though not intolerant of) myths about female founding ancestresses in general. Marabouts, of course, have a stake in preserving their own healing specialty, and, as shown later, herbalist/marabout relationships are the object of careful reflection among healers.

Tema married young in an arranged "family marriage" to a close cousin who caravanned. After about twenty years, he died, though after ten years of widowhood, Tema eventually remarried. When Tema gave birth, she was assisted by her mother, several cousins, and other female relatives. She had four living children, three daughters and one son. Two died, one son shortly following birth. I saw him upon a visit, and he had appeared of very low birth weight. Despite her respected status and prestigious social origins as a member of the chiefly and maraboutique families, Tema, like many other such persons, suffered from poverty: she had lost many herds and appeared somewhat malnourished.

Tema was somewhat unusual, though not unique, in that she inherited from her first husband an adobe mud house (usually built, inherited, and owned by men). Tema also retained her original female-owned nuptial tent. The land in her compound belonged to her and her children. She resided nextdoor to the local mosque, near a sheltering acacia tree in the center of the village, and also near the primary school *(École Nomade)* built in the late 1970s. A short distance away was a new clinic built around 2000 as part of promised policies to "develop" the northern regions, following peace accords between rebels and the government.

Around 1990, Tema became the second co-wife of the local primary school handyman, who come from Timia in 1981. While Tema was of noble social origins, her current husband came to her village initially as an escaped former slave. The school director at that time gave him shelter and offered him a job as handyman. Upon Tema's second marriage, she experienced some trauma and violence. Her husband's first wife became furious at his polygyny. She said little, but once, while the two women were out in pastures during transhumance, the first wife set fire to and burned down Tema's tent. A council of marabouts and elders ruled that the first wife had to repay Tema for the damage in money and mats. Though many local women opposed polygyny, they sympathized with Tema because they disapproved of the violent act of her co-wife. Most people favor "talking things over" before resorting to physical violence.

Despite jealousy over men's polygyny, furthermore, the major concern for Tema and many other women is with preserving their kin ties to female relatives and their economic independence. What really mattered to Tema was that, throughout both her marriages, she resided uxorilocally. Tema considered herself very fortunate to be able to remain next door to her mother and sisters, rather than moving away, as many women do nowadays as their husbands search for new lands to plant oasis gardens. Her current husband was unlikely to move back to his own region of origin because there, he was considered servile—if not officially, unofficially, in continuing low prestige and low-paid labor for his former owners.[4] He was also unlikely to travel on labor migration, since he had a salaried job at the primary school.

Tema's closeness to her mother and sisters undoubtedly facilitated learning herbal medicine, although unlike some other medicine women, she did not view her learning as a lengthy formal apprenticeship and did not receive formal authorization from a senior medicine women to practice. Her success resulted more from her social network: she was well liked and considered to be pious, kindly, and responsible. As of 2002, Tema had become the treasurer of a new women's agricultural cooperative in her village, though she continued to do some curing by touch and massage.

Tema was among the first local women to befriend me. She often offered to make up my face and assist me with proper dress for Muslim holy days and other festivals. She was outgoing, somewhat more accepting of me earlier in my research than many other local residents who, while never inhospitable or hostile, were initially shy, even fearful of an outsider. Tema's comments here reflect her experiences and concerns: she asserted, "a good life consists of obtaining clothing and food and having children. Children are useful because they help later when you are old. A first birth is a promotion for the mother (tinout). After (the woman's) periods cease, there is less strength and no need of men. As a woman becomes old, she becomes like a man because she is free, she can come up beside the mosque, but her husband sometimes looks for a new wife." In this statement, perhaps she was obliquely referring to the position of her co-wife, her husband's first wife, who was older.

Tema had participated in a first-aid training program in a nearby village and derived some knowledge from that. She stated, for example, that "a pregnant woman should avoid heavy work and sexual relations with her husband, or else there is illness. If women have a child each year, they lose blood, and also may get knee problems." Yet she also continued to believe in some long-standing Tuareg concepts of the body; she stated that, "if conception occurs at the first menses, a child can be (born) crazy because the mother's period has not yet come out of the body." In other words, as shown earlier, there are cultural measures to protect too-young girls from sexual exploitation. When Tema first had her period, she indicated, "I was afraid because that was something new." She then paraphrased, but translated into local cultural terms, some concepts she had learned in the training program: "During one's period, vessels attached to the back flow after filling with blood."

Negative Gossip

Thus in some respects, Tema mediated between local and biomedical concepts, though she did not render these concepts in "hybrid" form. For she also continued to emphasize many medicine women's integration of body/mind and organic/nonorganic illnesses and treatments. Tema's mediation between local and biomedical systems of knowledge and also between social factions in her community became evident to me as she gave me a diagnostic massage. One day, after a few minutes of massaging my back, suddenly she paused and stated that she had found a hard spot that "told" her something. She interpreted this as follows: "this means that someone is doing *togerchet* (evil mouth or eye; negative gossip) against you. You should protect yourself with marabouts' amulets." When I inquired how she identified this, she explained that her hand had weakened suddenly while touching that place on my back. To this advice, Tema also added that I needed to pay her, or she would catch my *togerchet*. She also advised me to protect myself by giving alms to a small child, preferably on a Friday (the Muslim prayer day), before obtaining amulets. As if to comfort me that I was not the only person suffering, or perhaps to warn me of possible complications if this condition went unremedied, Tema added to this news that the local chief's granddaughter had Kel Essuf spirits, and a marabout was treating her now.

During this massage, therefore, which I had innocently sought to remedy what I felt was mild muscle strain, Tema the medicine woman, with her intimate knowledge of the community, had used *edez* or touch as diagnostic massage to both comfort and warn me of negative gossip, thereby converting a "simple" massage into a very complex diagnostic/divination/psychotherapeutic session. I reflected upon some possible reasons for this alleged *togerchet* against me. Although never overt, I had noticed a slight coolness from a research assistant lately. Recently, I had hosted a smith/artisan at my home in the United States. His family, unbeknownst to me, became embroiled in a dispute with the family of my research assistant over crowded gardening plots, overgrazing, and access to funds. Thus unwittingly, I had entered the middle of political factionalism between parties who were equally my friends until their social divisions arose. They were no longer speaking to each other, and my host family for a while viewed my hospitality toward their enemy as somewhat disloyal. Economic jealousy also figured into that quarrel: many nobles, now impoverished, tend to resent some more successful smiths who profit from tourist art.

Distressed by this news, I retreated to my tent and sleeping bag for several hours and turned my head away from visitors. My host family became very upset, since a guest must never be unhappy in their home, and also, perhaps, because they feared I would become possessed by the Kel Essuf spirits. For as shown in Fatima's case, this condition is preceded by a kind of depression *(tamazai)*. The family sent several children to check on me and soon reverted to their usual openness; their coldness disappeared. The following morning, moreover, a marabout related to me a dream he had had the night before: in this dream, he reassured me, I had closed the mouth and jaws of a dog in the nearby dried riverbed. "This means," he interpreted, "that you have now vanquished your enemies."

More broadly, what was occurring here? As already shown, many medicine women combine nonverbal and verbal healing techniques of the body and mind, treat conditions that are difficult to classify as either "organic" or "inorganic," and to some extent, collaborate with other healers and participate in wider healing and social networks. This vignette suggests how they do this. At the forefront of their own techniques in this are touching and massage. These techniques, however, involve more than merely physical therapy. *Adana* in Tamajaq denotes a special type of massage *(arabaz)*, for *tarzak* illness in the back and shoulders. During this treatment, the medicine woman uses diagnostic touch and massaging treatment, contacting not only the woman patient's stomach but also the ground in order to take the disease out of both patient and healer. The medicine woman's obligation to throw the disease away (recall that the ground is believed to absorb the illness because the medicine woman is "heavy" from the patient's illness, and needs to have the ground take it off or away) has further significance. The ground, which opens up during childbirth, is associated with the Old Woman of the Earth (Waddawa), who threatens a woman giving birth. Many local patients came to medicine women for attention and resolution of personal difficulties, for example, to seek medicines to become fatter or to conceive a child.

Medico-Ritual Healing in Bodily Motions: Circling; Tapping the Earth; Rotating Alms; Diagnostic Touch and Therapeutic Massages

Massage does not occur in isolation; additional motions and pronouncements take place alongside touch and massage, all in a sequence of rituals. The medicine woman also rotates millet counterclockwise three times above the patient; this motion recurs in phases of rites of passage featuring pre-Islamic symbolism and women's participation. Many *ilaten* medicines are passed around almost casually, not only to the patient but also to other persons present, who are usually close kin, friends, and neighbors who accompany the patient, and they often taste or drink a bit of the medicine before administering it to the patient.

Emoud, a rare male bone-setter *(amadas)* who inherited this specialty from his father, offered insights into additional levels of significance of touch in healing, which focus upon but also transcend the body and extend into social, ritual, and cosmological domains. Like many elderly widowed or divorced men, he lived in the compound of a married daughter. In the past, Emoud was also a *wanzam* (derived from Hausa, literally denoting "barber," a circumciser of boys). The danger in that ritual is *anagar* (spreading illness, infection). He warned: "A woman with an illegitimate child looking at a circumcised boy can cause this affliction. After circumcision, applying rabbit dung prevents this.[5] I use a sharp knife for circumcision, but only my hands for bone-setting."

Emoud explained, "Male healers may use herbs, but they rarely touch the stomach, since that is the domain of Tagurmat and we men respect and avoid it. Marabouts don't touch the stomach or the bones. The *tanesmegel* (herbal medicine woman) touches the stomach; [whereas by contrast], I do not do this. I use my hands only; no tools. The *tamaswad* (diviner medicine woman) can see without touching: by imagination, memory, and speaking with spirits. The marabout does not use non-Qur'anic methods. The *(t)amadas* bone-setter does ablutions *(alwalla)* before she or he touches the bones and joints of a patient. There are Tamajaq terms for all the bones in the body; I know all of them. I advise a person with a broken bone not to work until after forty days. I set bones by realigning them in a normal position. The bones *(eghasen)* support intentional motion. The joints help motion. At memorial feasts, those balls made from millet, dates, and goat cheese [called alms, *takote,* in this solid form; in liquid form mixed with water, called *eghale* or *eghajira*] are like the joints of the dead. These are served and distributed among kin of the deceased in order to ensure that the deceased moves into the next world smoothly.[6] Curing is a skill, but ultimately the responsibility of God. I always think of God while treating patients."

Although male, Emoud's practice as juxtaposed against that of the more prevalent female practitioners illuminates some of the latter's distinctiveness. It should be noted that Emoud the male *amadas* uses his hands to set bones, but nonetheless, he does not touch the stomach, and touch as used by many medicine women is not limited to bone-setting. It involves much more complex therapeutic and ritual healing techniques. Also, despite the importance of massage in itself, medicine women's touching has medico-ritual, mythical, and cosmological significance surpassing the immediate therapeutic situation. This is evident in not solely the medicine women's comments but also in Emoud's acknowledgment that male bone-setters and marabouts avoid touching the stomach—the domain of Tagurmat, whom they respect.

Therefore local beliefs about the human body are vividly conveyed in therapeutic touch. Tanou, a medicine woman from Mount Bagzan, illuminated additional anatomical and spiritual beliefs concerning the body: "In the body, blood represents the person. When one lacks it, one becomes dry. The part of blood that contains the illness is what I know; (there is a swelling). In the body, blood is in the veins." This body is intimately connected to forces beyond it. Identities extend beyond bodily boundaries toward the earth and other dimensions of life, past and present—for example, to the earth *(amadal),* trees, and their spirits, which are the focus of bodily motions and ritual acts and prohibitions. A chief's drum cannot touch the ground. Medicine women touch the ground three times in healing, and babies should be born on the ground, on clean sand in the mother's tent. Certain foods and medicinal plants are believed to taste good or be healthy or effective only if used in Tuareg home regions where they grow; local residents insist "it is the earth here that is distinctive."

The centrality of the human body to cultural thought makes it a powerful mimetic referent that mediates all reflection and action upon the world (Lock 1993). This is clearly seen in indigenous medical systems throughout the world, for example, in locales where unseeable powers of nature are anthopomorphized in the form of two- and three-dimensional human figures used as ingredients in magical medicines, charms, and amulets (Wolff 2000:205). Usually, this is discussed in terms of sympathetic magic: figures act to direct or store these powers for a variety of positive and negative purposes. In the replication of human form as artifact, superhuman powers are encapsulated and controlled, to be brought into the cultural realm where they can be manipulated to benefit individuals or groups. Medicine figures are commonly used by practitioners in medical systems that have strong elements of what Foster (1976) has labeled "personalistic": illness and misfortune are believed caused by purposeful manipulation of superhuman powers, so that religious and medical systems are intermeshed. The medical practitioner in a "personalistic" system is an agent who is knowledgeable in those culturally determined rules of procedure that can be used to control superhuman powers to bring about predetermined effects for the self or client (Wolff 2000:205).

Yet these "personalistic" elements, as shown by Tema, Emoud, and Tanou, are not so separate from other elements: natural and organic, human and social. The assumption is that these forces act as part of a coherent, interconnected universe in which acts of "magic"—which I prefer to call alternative ritual power—can project specific forces along pathways between things to bring about desired human goals. Herbal medicine women do not practice what has been termed "sorcery" to interfere with the course of natural forces, causing them to act contrary to their natural program; rather, they attempt through their bodily touch and motions to act in concert with these forces and bring them into alignment with patients' well-being.

Somewhat like the Yoruba herbalist's *materia medica* (Maclean 1982), among Tuareg medicine women there is a division between simple medicines, which are prepared for imbibing or for applying to the body externally to relieve common physical symptoms, and those which are intended to operate at a distance. Maclean (1982:1650) refers to these latter as "really charms and countercharms" that "have nothing to do with modern science of pharmacology." Some are intended to produce a beneficial effect on patients or those close. Others may be necessary to counteract the suspected malevolence of enemies. Then there are amulets to promote good fortune and protect the wearer from general or specific dangers. All of these require that the user should have faith in their efficacy (Maclean 1982). Ideally the healer, too, should believe in his/her own medicines and should not be a charlatan. Tuareg medicine women are also somewhat like the Apache healers described by Perrone, Stockel, and Krueger (1989) as well as the Navajo ceremonial singers described by Trudelle-Schwartz (2003), who weave emotion, caring, and healing into a healing basket, in that they draw upon medicines from a special pot or calabash, in Tamajaq called *ten*. These objects constitute the universe in miniatured microcosm. Healing comes from these power objects and is infused with the energy of "wishing to heal" (Perrone, Stockel, and Krueger 1989:26).

In this, Tuareg herbal medicine women face three key problems: they must convince others that they do not harm; they must avoid being perceived as competing with Islamic scholars; and they cannot become associated with negative powers or destructive motives of sorcery *(ark echaghel)*. Thus their definitions and uses of power are always framed with these considerations. As the Apache healer's biochemistry degree links with the herbs she places in a medicine pouch (Perrone, Stockel, and Krueger 1989), so the Tuareg medicine woman's Islamic and bilineal/bilateral background merges with the matrilineally inherited plants she places in her own pouch, calabash, and pot and with the matrilineally inherited gestures and motions she enacts kinesthetically. In effect, these *ilaten* medicines involve an intricate interweaving of body, earth, past, present, and divergent sources of knowledge.

Tuareg herbal medicine women also capture and create power by "making imageful particularity" (Taussig 1993:16), albeit not exclusively in visual form. For their work is less anthropomorphic that of the Cuna described by Taussig and the Yoruba described by McClain and Wolff, reflecting the Tuareg religious (Islamic) traditions, but their work is nonetheless powerful in alternative ways. Rather than imitating the human body visually or representationally, medicine women enact it or embody it through their motions of touch and comment on it in their exegesis of illness etiology and treatment. Non-anthropomorphic figures used in medicines are equally powerful transformers that embody and channel the natural and spiritual materials from which they are fashioned.

In effect, Tuareg medicine women figuratively "carve" their power objects through touch and incantations but not through literally visual mimesis. As power objects, medicine figures (verbal, visual, and nonverbal and extra-visual) are differentiated from those used in other contexts by the labels applied. In this sense, their activities recall some, though not all characteristics of Yoruba healing (Wolff 2000). Yoruba medicine figures are not public objects and are not openly displayed on shrines. Rather, they are power objects used in *oogun*, a variety of techniques and materials that draw upon superhuman forces for healing as well as for sorcery. At the heart of the efficacy of *oogun* is a profound and pervasive belief in what some authors term "magic" (Wolff 2000:210), which I prefer to call alternative sources of power.

Physical contact with the hands and body also expresses Tuareg medicine women's knowledge of birth and other health-care treatments. Throughout European history and in widely varied cultures today, birth attendants have used touch in many different ways both to support the physiological birth process and to nurture others, in particular, a mother. Tuareg women assisting the woman in labor hold her by her shoulders. In many societies, any person who touches a childbearing woman has the implied or explicit authority to do so, including touch that is prohibited outside the birth situation (Jordan 1993).

Birth and herbal healing in Tuareg culture are women's work. They involve acquiring knowledge that is "in the hands" (Jordan 1993:192; E. Turner 1996). In this regard, Tuareg medicine women continue a long tradition found in many times and places. In medieval Europe, women formed the birthing circle and transmitted skills of nurturing a woman through childbirth; these were an extension of their own mothering skills (Kitzinger 1997:211). In many respects, this was a female process of bonding. In the nineteenth century, skill in diagnostic touch was a recognized element in esteem afforded an *accoucheur*. But each examination had to be negotiated with other women attending (Kitzinger 1997:214). There was much debate in Western biomedical journals as to how touch should be performed.

Among the Tuareg, as noted, the woman who bears a child remains for one week in strict seclusion and for forty days in a transitional ritual state, though in contrast to the case in medieval Europe, she is not considered polluting herself but is believed endangered by jealous spirits of the wild (Rasmussen 1991, 1997; Walentowitz 2002; Worley 1992). In other words, in addition to diagnosis, touch gives reassurance that all is well, and in cultures such as the Tuareg where touch is otherwise somewhat restricted, it also compensates for its absence in other contexts such as the reserve/avoidance one must practice toward parents-in-law, husbands in public, and firstborn children.

Like the elderly women curers in central Serbia described by Barbara Kerewsky-Halpern (in McClain 1989:115), Tuareg medicine women preserve, transmit, and practice a mode of healing based on imagery associations aroused by arrangements of motions, sounds, words, and utterances (Kerewsky-Halpern in McClain 1989:115). Their touch, motions, and words retain tropes and other elements carried over from ancient times. Among the Tuareg, human fertility is linked to more powerful forces that cause crops to grow and animals to be healthy. Here, the healer is not merely a birth attendant, however, but also has a spiritual function, and this finds expression in how she touches the woman, not solely during pregnancy and labor and following birth but at other times, as well. Physical contact is often accompanied by prayers, invocations, incantations, and ritual motions (e.g., circling). Tuareg medicine women often massage with oils that are believed to enhance beauty, and hence, fertility; they also sometimes use scented oils to diagnose illnesses and marital and other psychosocial problems. In touching the stomach of women and the earth, Tuareg herbalists sanctify the earth with *al baraka* blessing and convey this force like marabouts when they give items to people.

Senses and Body: The Total Sensorium

Relevant to touch, of course, is the bodily sensorium. In the foundations for an anthropology of the senses, a fundamental premise underlying the concept of an anthropology of the senses is that sensory perception is a cultural as well as a physical act (Classen 1997a:400). Classen and others (Classen 1997a; Rasmussen 1999; Olkes and Stoller 1987; Stoller 1989) have noted conceptual impediments in the anthropology of the senses: for example, the assumption until recently that the senses are transparent in nature and thus "precultural" and also that sight is the only or primary sense of importance (Classen 1997a:402). This attitude reflects a cultural bias (Olkes and Stoller 1987; Stoller 1989; Rasmussen 1999, 2001a; Classen 1997a). Sight came to distance itself from other senses in terms of cultural importance only in the eighteenth and nineteenth centuries, when vision became associated with the burgeoning field of science.

Tuareg medicine women continually emphasized to me that one difference between them and marabouts was their own healing by touch and marabouts' healing by writing. They also asserted that only a few among them use complex divination methods of "seeing in dreams," called *asawad*. Indeed, their own most widespread divination or diagnosis does appear, on first scrutiny, to be more based upon touch and tactile means, as in their feeling the stomach and their spinning the pot around. Other local residents, also, hold stereotypes associating marabouts with writing and more numerous and complex divination based on sight and text, but they are not necessarily considered more "scientific" than medicine women. However, as we shall learn, these typifications (of both medicine women themselves and other local residents) do not always hold up in practice.

Additional obstacles to fully understanding the total sensorium arose from the work of certain academics who suggested replacing or supplementing visual models of interpretations with models based on speech and aurality (Ong 1982). I agree with some theorists (Classen for example) that the oral/literate dichotomy tends to assume that the different senses will possess the same social values and have the same social effects across cultures. Tuareg herbal medicine women do more than simply challenge these assumptions; they break down the divisions between these senses. Taste and touch in particular, but also aurality, are important in herbalism and herbalists' divination/diagnoses as well.

In parts of Western Europe, women have been traditionally associated with the "lower" sensual realms of touch, taste, and smell, in bedroom, nursery and kitchen; men have been linked with the "higher" intellectual realms of sight and hearing (Classen 1997a:409). To what extent, and in what contexts, has sight become more culturally important among Tuareg? How does this affect herbalism, in which scent and touch and taste are so important in healing? How does this affect the perceived validation of authoritative knowledge or the bases of "truth," and what is the relation between scent in moral discourse (e.g., the odor of sanctity) and medicine women's practice?

In Tamajaq-speaking communities, scent is often associated with contagion. Somewhat like the Victorians, many Tuareg believe some illnesses can be spread by odor. Colds are believed to be transmitted through aroma, so persons with colds are advised not to wear strong perfume. Scent is also associated, in other contexts, with morality and other psychosocial states; for example, one must be clean and sweet-smelling to pray at the mosque, and many possessed women report they crave beautiful perfumes and incense scents (Rasmussen 1995, 1999). In a context particularly relevant to herbal healing, scent is also associated with pollution of fertility: marabouts say that one reason only elderly women ideally should become *tinesmegelen* is that "the scent of certain healing plants on Mt. Bagzan causes young women to become infertile." Yet this ideology, as shown presently, can become converted into positive connotations in the actual practice of medicine women's healing, in which these plants and the women who use them become imbued with their power to guard the force of reproduction in others.

Medicine Women's and Wider Cultural Concepts of the Body and Senses

Tuareg medicine women's view of the body in some respects corresponds to the Islamic Sufi scientific view described by Nasr (1993), as for example, in their widely held views of blood and in their important humoral, counteractive medicine. Some of medicine women's comments also revealed influences of Euro-American biomedical paradigms. Also expressed are local Tuareg cultural interpretations of gendered variations on these themes, as shown, for example, when medicine women and other women refer to the ovaries and uterus as *ehan n barar* (the child's tent or home), and in the association of the humoral balance with a local diagnostic category of depression and with altered states of consciousness and possession.

Also prominent in these medicine women's theories of wellness, illness, and healing are local cultural concepts of the body and soul. The head *(eghef)* is considered the place where spirits reside once they have entered the liver *(tessa)* and stomach *(tedis)*. While the stomach is also the symbol of the matriline, the back *(aghuru)* is the symbol of the patriline (Nicolaisen 1997). If herbal medicine women diagnose spirits "dancing" in a patient's stomach, they refer the patient to a marabout, who treats the patient in seclusion with counseling and the Qur'an, often also divining with the Qur'an and various cabalistic formulas. As noted, patients often see diverse healers in succession for the same ailment, for example, *bokaye* non-Qur'anic diviners who diagnose with scents and oils after seeing herbalists and marabouts The liver *(tessa)* is considered the seat of sentiments such as anger and love, and it is the place where non-Qur'anic spirits often enter; these require the *tende n goumaten* spirit possession ritual, whose public curing with music and a large, supportive audience who encourage the possessed person in trance in her dancing provide effective group therapy. The soul *(iman,* also denoting life and breath), is believed to leave the body during sleep and walk about. Upon death, the soul may be contacted through dreams or through offerings to graves. The heart *(ewel)* is connected to sentiments such as generosity and compassion and is closely associated with the soul and the liver in its psychosocial and nonorganic connotations; many nonorganic illnesses such as spirit possession are referred to as "illnesses of the heart and soul," and possessed persons complain of a burning liver (Rasmussen 1995).

As already noted, the body is perceived as tending toward the ideal of equilibrium between heat and cold states, and ideally balanced circulation of fluids (blood and mucus) that, in humoral medicine, is related to that of Greek and Arab medicine. This concept is similar to that in the related Moroccan Berber medical system (Greenwood 1981; Randall 1993). These are oriented toward interior and exterior of the body in relation to its interaction with the environment. Order and balance between hot and cold principles is organized like the universe; the human body is analogous to other things appearing in the universe (stars, vegetables, animals). There are also often interpretations of dysfunction and disequilibrium as a consequence of not respecting a religious role or social convention. Many medicine women expressed the belief that mental health is one basis of bodily well-being. Fundamental to the local paradigm is a continuum, rather than rigid opposition, between body and mind and between organic and nonorganic illnesses. Hadia, a very elderly and renowned medicine woman, expressed this clearly. She defined being in good health as

> being peaceful and doing your work. Bad health means having only illnesses, and aging also increases illnesses. Recently, there are more illnesses than before because food is more varied and people lack knowledge of how to prepare or eat it. The age of greater illness is after youth, which is from age of 25 upwards. To have a happy life, always care for the body, but do not undergo too many treatments. I believe there are dangerous places, for example, where people bury bad things. There are some bad marabouts who do this, and this also may cause illnesses. Also, there are places where there are spirits, for example, in the *idebni* ancestral tombs and near the tomb of a prominent marabout. If someone has a lot of misfortune, *goumaten* spirits are responsible because they cause worries and bad luck. A crazy person is often incurable, he/she has a bad fate from dangerous places above, or bad marabouts. There are people who are naturally lucky, or you can get luck from amulets of marabouts; also, there are lucky wives, identified by marabout divination. Wishes can be realized by good faith and good acts toward people. Medicine to ensure healthy baby and combat infertility is called *amagal n samodnen,* cool medicines, of leaves and bark.

Many Tuareg medicine women believe that the liver and intestines are located inside the stomach. Also, there are believed to be several types of blood *(azni),* and these change: blood is not the same from sunrise to sunset. Blood *(azni)* and water *(aman)* represent life. Blood establishes ties of fililations, kinship, and alliances. There can be pollution with blood; women in this regard constitute a link to the spirit world. Among some groups of Tuareg, women can become impure through shedding of blood and also by polluting conduct such as the breaking of sexual taboos. There is also a relation between the Kel Essuf spirits, blood, and the black color: certain women protect themselves with plant and antimony (kohl) applications on the face. Women are discreet concerning pregnancy. All blood must be taken out after birth. The new mother's body becomes cold, with its associated dangers, although it may also become hot, as shown earlier in Fatima's case. Transformations occur between states: for example, moonlight, considered cold and capable of absorbing vital energy, will be hot during the Ramadan fast period. Elements are not static but can change.

Nasr (1993:101) contrasts Sufi scientific views of the body to what he terms "rationalistic" systems: unlike "rationalistic" explanations, he argues, the symbolic and analogical language used to expound the inner relationships of nature is not limited within the boundary of "either-or" propositions. In this regard, Nasr tends to approximate Robin Horton's earlier (1967) views on "traditional" African thought and Western science and Levi-Strauss's (1962) views on the analogical thought of the *bricoleur*. In Sufism, there are poetic analogies, though many theorists now recognize that science also uses metaphor and analogy (Horton 1993). The same four principles of which minerals, plants, and animals are comprised constitute the human body (Nasr 1993:253) and in combination give rise to humors and qualities. The four elements—air (yellow bile), blood (fire), earth (black bile), and water (phlegm)—manifest in their admixture all the qualities of the human body. The interaction of these qualities determines the temperament of the human being. The temperament is equable when contrary qualities are in perfect equilibrium, and out of harmony and inequable when temperament tends toward a particular quality. Herein lies the basis of the humoral, counteractive ideal of "hot" and "cold" balance.

Implications

Medicine women in their theories of "hot" *(tuksi)* and "cold" *(tessmut)* therefore approximately articulate some variants of Islamic theory, such as Sufism, that much disease is believed due to destruction of this equilibrium by excess of some quality, and many cures attempt to reestablish harmony between opposites (Nasr 1993:254). The question now addressed is how these beliefs articulate with their other local Tuareg cultural theories of body and senses, and extend into gendered domains.

Growth and decay of the body of humans depend upon temperament. Growth depends on heat contained in the sperm, which is gradually used up. Moisture lessens in quantity and quality, thus preserving innate heat at a constant level up to the age of senescence. Among the Tuareg, similarly, childbearing women are considered "wet," and wetness is associated with fertility and life (Rasmussen 2000); whereas post-childbearing women are considered "dry," and dryness is believed to be opposed to fertility and childbearing, as in some other Islamic-influenced cultures (Boddy 1987). In Tuareg medicine women's theories as well as Islamic science, basic qualities combine together to generate humors.

Classen (1997b) describes how historically and culturally in Euro-American philosophies and cultures, theories are based in perceptions of the body and senses that are inflected with gender values. In Tuareg medicine women's and Islamic theories of counteractive medicine, it should be recalled, there are associations among hot vs. cold diseases, and "cold" women and "hot" men. However, Tuareg gender-coding of the senses is not as hierarchical as it is in classical European philosophies, despite the prevalent association of visual and written texts with predominantly male Islamic scholarship and Qur'anic healing. Most Tuareg do not denigrate or rank the senses in terms of gender.

While I do not seek to merely demonstrate Tuareg differences from Europe here (as this would be a tautological exercise—of course, this setting is distinctive!), nonetheless some comparison and contrast are instructive. Classen describes how in premodern Europe, women and men were allied with contrasting sensory qualities, which in turn embodied contrasting cultural values (Classen 1997b:2–3). In the visual domain, men were generally, in the Aristotelian tradition, associated with "rational" qualities of light and form, while women were associated with the "irrational" qualities of darkness and the sensual quality of color. Also most prominent in sensory differences associated with the sexes from antiquity to the late Renaissance in Europe, as among many Tuareg today, were the beliefs in the coldness of women and heat of men. Yet there are not evolutionary sequential correspondences in both cases: in contrast to females in Europe, Tuareg women are not deemed to be "half-baked males," thereby revealing interesting cultural alternatives to historic Euro-American ethnoscientific notions of the connections of sensory codes to gender and science and their implications.

While many Tuareg, as shown, also differentiate according to gender, and make gendered thermal/humoral associations in their counteractive medical system, there is a marked absence of a deficiency model here, and there is flexibility according to context. In the counteractive theories of balance and harmony, for example, "hot" vs. "cold" states of the body and diseases are caused for men and women alike by an imbalance of these forces. These states are indeed gender-linked: women should ideally be cool, and men should ideally be warm, but even these ideal gendered states should not become too pronounced or intensified; for example, a man can become too hot and fall ill. Too intense cold or heat, or conversely, an accumulation of the opposite of the ideally dominant quality brings illness and requires a cure. Thus there is symmetry, affecting both sexes.

In Tuareg gender typifications of the body and senses in social contexts, however, another sense of the terms hot and cold surfaces: when a woman has a hot character, she is vivacious and energetic, and "one advises her to find a partner with a cold character" (Figueiredo-Biton in Claudot-Hawad 2002:137). The goal is to find an equilibrium between hot and cold. My own and others' data suggest that one is therefore not better than the other; rather, one must avoid an excess of either. Nonetheless, the character of a woman should tend toward the cold, and that of man should tend toward hot. Hence the danger of either too great an exaggerated accumulation of the ideal or a sway toward the opposite quality (the latter represented in some "hot" illnesses of women, specifically, in Fatima's fever). Women and men cool off through washing the body and soul. This may be accomplished by several methods. Most require geographic mobility, as for example in pastoral nomadic work. Young men at puberty, when the blood mounts in their head and sexual energy is at its height, need to move, to accompany adults in their travels, in order to encounter other persons and expand their vision of the world (Figueiredo-Biton in Claudot-Hawad 2002:139). The expression for men's cooling off, however, metaphorically evokes women's menstruation process: *ashni* (or *azni*) *izgar taghasa*, "the blood leaves the body." Women also must do this in certain contexts.

Males' senses of sight and hearing in Europe were classified as distance senses, and female senses of smell, taste, and touch characterized as proximity senses. These were often interpreted to mean that men were suited for distance activities, such as traveling and governing, while women were made to stay at home (Classen 1997b:4). This is also true to some extent among Tuareg, but with very different implications. Predominantly men raid, trade, and travel on labor migration. Women own the tent and educate children. In this, however, there is overlap according to context. There is an association of sight with mental and smell, taste, and touch with bodily functions, yet women, as well as men, excel in the arts and sciences. In fact, Tuareg women traditionally were in charge of all early education of children inside the maternal tent, undertaken before Qur'anic or secular schooling.

But women also live in a process of transition and travel, albeit of a different kind, from the moment of their period. In some groups, they are sent to a medicine woman or another woman renowned for her knowledge of the human female body. This is the first educational trip and prepares the girl for her first menstruation. She learns that menstruation is a process of blood circulation and emotions that permits the body to cool off, preventing excessive heat that can have harmful consequences for the body, sentiments, and character (Figueiredo-Biton 2002:138). It is believed that during her period, a woman is in another dimension, that she travels in the beyond *(tasikal dagh elahaghat)*. This can be in the domain of the Kel Essuf or *goumaten* spirits of the wild, or that of God. In the Adagh region of Mali, Figueiredo-Biton (in Claudot-Hawad 2002:138) reports that seclusion is viewed not as a constraint, however, but as a means of finding peace and freedom, of permitting a woman's soul to travel peacefully by means of the blood in her body.

Several studies (Rasmussen 1991; Worley 1992; Figueiredo-Biton 2002) have argued that it is not because a woman is "impure" that she must not pray or touch Qur'an or amulets, but on the contrary, because her fertility needs to be protected from outside, impure, or hostile forces. In the Adagh region of Mali, the menstrual period is even called *tamesgida* (denoting "mosque") (Figueiredo-Biton in Claudot-Hawad 2002:138)!—whereas in other more maraboutique-influenced regions, it is called *iba n amud* (denoting absence of prayer) (Rasmussen 1991; Bouman 2003). On the eighth day following the onset of menstruation, the girl goes to the well, accompanied by young women already past puberty, and she learns ablutions necessary to reintegrate into society. People say she is washed, cleaned—but from excess of heat: *tesered.* Medicine women told me that menstrual periods "sweep the body like a broom" and that later in life, a woman who has borne many children is "rinsed clean." Excess is accumulated throughout the menstrual cycles over time. Thus the feminine cycle includes passage from a state of balance or equilibrium to a state of heat, then to a state of cold and finally a return to balance. Return to the state of equilibrium recovers vital energy, *asekhat,* denoting strength or good health. The goal of this interior journey is achieved by circulation of the blood and soul, in order to eliminate hot sentiments such as sadness *(turhena),* euphoria *(tadawit),* fear *(teksod),* and anger *(elham* or *atkar).* In these processes there are alternations between heat and cold, and wetness and dryness.

Other travels remedy an excess of the "cold" state and heat up the person. When a man remains for too long a time in the same place, in particular near his wife's tent, he risks cooling off (i.e., becoming feminized); he must maintain a rhythm of masculine daily life. He must avoid the tent by day when home from travel. Notwithstanding this ideal, I noticed some degree of flexibility, however: a few persons of ambiguous gender role are referred to as *"homme-femme"* in French, rumored to be in fact literally hermaphrodites; such persons display somewhat unusual conduct; for example, they excel at a particular task but never marry. I met one such person, a sex worker who resided on the outskirts of the town of Agadez, who cross-dressed and was rumored to be not only a bisexual prostitute but also literally a hermaphrodite. Local residents did not express any hostility or aggression toward him, but rather, regarded his status with some bemusement. The important implication here is symmetry and some flexibility between women and men, rather than hierarchy or rigidity, in local cultural gendered ideas of body and senses. Another point is that many women have the natural means to pass from one state to another without the need for travel; whereas by contrast, men must find their balance through geographic travel.

Yet a woman sometimes undertakes travel, for example, in order to give birth at her mother's home, where she also spends the first forty days following birth (this trip is called *tashegish*). If she is far, she goes back to her family (Rasmussen 1997; Bouman 2003). Women also may travel for economic reasons. A few herbal medicine women were described to me by other Tuareg as "hot," as "almost like men" (though never as *hommes-femmes*), in their wide-ranging travel to gather medicines and treat patients. Perhaps this underlies marabouts' allegations that some plants on Mount Bagzan make women infertile. Yet, as I show in subsequent sections, this association is not so simple; for medicine women must also be mothers, and they act, in many ways, as exaggerated or hyperbolic mothers and grandmothers.

In premodern Europe, the cold moistness of women was held to predispose them to putridity and inactivity. Heat supposedly made men intelligent, courageous, and forthright, and cold made women unintelligent, timid, and deceitful (Classen 1997b:3). Among the Tuareg, these are not such rigid binary oppositions. These states do not all line up neatly on one or another side; rather, they vary according to social context and time factors. Thus the Tuareg views suggest distinctions between the sexes, but also caution against assuming that differences inevitably add up to deficiency and hierarchy.

Among Tuareg of noble origins, as noted, there is some emphasis upon women restricting their motility, although this is variable over history and across regions, depending upon the importance of past slave labor. In some communities, this value of a woman seated inside her tent is important; in others, for example, in parts of Aïr, there is less stigma attached to physical labor of both women and men, and strength is admired in both sexes. In premodern Europe, women in vigorous physical activity were said to run the risk of burning up fat and menstrual blood and becoming "masculine" in nature (Classen 1997b:3). Some Tuareg theories suggest "androgynous" interpretations of highly mobile and successful women. There are stories of highly successful herbalist/diviners whose "doors were closed," i.e., their genitals closed up, in local belief. In contrast to the European belief, however, these stories rested on a belief that was not asymmetric; I heard no one state that nature always strives toward male perfection. Furthermore, Tuareg age and social stratum crosscut gender associations in the body and senses. For example, both sexes among smith/artisans are considered "hotter" than nobles of either sex; and both women and men of servile origin are stereotyped as harder and stronger than both women and men among nobles.

In Europe, men were deemed to use the sense of hearing to listen to weighty discourses and lectures, while women employed their hearing to attend to frivolous gossip and love talk. Among the Tuareg, male vanity is highly important, and clever speech is important for both men and women. Yet there is some hierarchy in the context of reading the Qur'an. Few women become professional marabouts. Yet even men who attempt to practice professional maraboutism may experience difficulty: some men are considered "not ready" to do this, and allegedly, they go insane or become possessed by spirits (Rasmussen 1995). There is in the Tuareg case no neat cultural uniformity or consensus, but rather, variation and inconsistency of evaluation in relation to the other senses and their relation to local concepts of body, rationality, and gender.

Tuareg medicine women do, however, tend to express their ideology of body and senses nonvisually and non-textually: through tactile and aural modes. They in effect enact or "embody" these ideas. Their communication of their knowledge is, in effect, "meta-tactile"; it is touch about touch, and "meta-aural," orality about orality. While they have much to say about such issues as how the "coolness" of women relates to rationality, they do so indirectly, recalling the noble value of *tangal* or indirect expression—both in their verbal and nonverbal narratives.

Oral Traditions and the Mythico-History of Herbal Medicine

It has been a long time since we learned [apprenticed] with our old woman [classificatory grandmother (aunt) or mother]. At that moment, I was not married. But I knew medicine (though I did not yet practice it professionally). She mentioned medicinal trees [to me]. She taught us how one makes medicines. I learned it with Lala, the older sister of my father. I learned it little by little, until I had children. I learned until I had my children, and then I began the [official, formal] practice. When one began, when one told the old woman "We wish medicine," she told us, "you also, you know how to make medicine." She gave us authorization to practice everything she told us [about]. Each time I brought my children, she told me, "You also, you know how to make medicine." She told us, "Some people steal medicine without obtaining authorization of elders. You have authorization to do medicine because our parents have inheritance. Everyone knows that."

When I received authorization, there was no elaborate ceremony, only alms, for example, dates and cheeses at my home for children . . . no need to assemble people. I offered my alms alone. Authorization occurred when she revealed to me all the medicines. She only spoke with her mouth. She gave me no rules, except not to do it without [alms *takote*] payment. She also said, "You must do it well, you must not be lazy." It is sufficient to recognize and distinguish products to be a good healer. But profound knowledge is found among persons who are old. From here to Aghaghagh on the Bagzan all [knowledge] is with old Lala, where one learns medicine. Among the very old herbalists, Lala only is living. Equals to her no longer exist. There exist those who are young, but Lala is the leader. I do not dream. I do not touch. The old woman does the work of touching. Each medicine that you wish, Lala can do it for you.

These words were spoken by Wasu, a medicine woman residing on top of Mount Bagzan. Wasu is a daughter of a local chief. She married a man from Mt. Bagzan, where she resided since her husband moved back there following the customary early marriage years of uxorilocal residence with groom-service and bridewealth payments. Wasu, her sister, Mina, and their mother and aunt all resided, gathered, and treated patients in their vicinity. Wasu took excellent care of me when I struck my head on the low doorframe of a stone house. She gave me cool water kept in a thermos in the shade and chunks of dried goat cheese. Many renowned old women healers resided nearby, but they were dying off. Some daughters and nieces gathered plants for them and learned from them, but others disliked the hard work of climbing mountains and gathering bark medicines.

Wasu's comments above revealed that, in addition to tactile and gustatory modalities, medicine women also employ verbal art in their mythology, incantations, and prayers, in both the transmission of healing knowledge and in their treatments; for example, they do this in their gathering of prayers, conferring of blessings, and healing incantations. For example, one must say "Bissmillahi" before entering water, showering, or eating; when finishing a prayer; and before putting on new clothes, because this pronouncement blesses and protects against spirits.

In learning herbalism, oral traditions are central: there are words going from older to younger persons. Apprenticeship of therapeutic knowedge is a long road: youths learn from elders; women of the same camp or village usually apprentice among themselves. If someone is ill, the women meet in council, and each tells what she knows concerning curing. This was shown in Fatima's difficult pregnancy, birth, and eventual spirit possession. It also became apparent to me on another occasion, when I was stricken with what appeared to me to be a case of strep throat, after, ironically, having emphasized washing as protection against "microbes" to local women.

On that occasion, when I fell ill, elderly women of my host family, their relatives, children, and neighbors crowded into my tent to express concern and offer healing advice, treatments, and medicines. One woman offered me spirits of camphor; another gave me cool leaves from the *ebisgin* tree; another offered a balm. I overheard one woman surmise that I had a "hot" illness. Another disagreed, stating, "The reason she is sick is because she goes out there among the rocks and bathes (thereby exposing bodily orifices to the wild and becoming vulnerable to spirits of the wild)." Hence the centrality of verbal consultations and dialogues in negotiations over diagnosis and treatment. Medicine women often debate and modify each other's knowledge in healing. In this regard, there are parallels to the performances of many other Tamajaq oral traditions. For example, women's riddles and some tales feature much interruption of tellers, continuation by other parties present, and continual revisions during performance.

Another means of learning is visual: one watches someone else prepare and administer medicines, as did the women's children on the occasion of my illness treatment. Some illnesses, as already noted, are shameful, but others are not, and the latter are relatively openly treated; no effort is made in these latter cases to seclude the patient. Thus children have the opportunity to observe, even outside formal apprenticeship. Yet the visual is never isolated, nor is it given absolute priority over other alternative senses. Rather, there are interactions between the visual, verbal, and tactile media. In local belief, the word *(awal)* is charged with weight: there is a time to speak, ways of speaking, different styles, gestures, and intonations appropriate to a given situation. Yet one must also carefully weigh words, for these are believed to have consequences in deeds (Casajus 2000). When herbal healers speak of illness and treatment, not only the content is important but also the aesthetics of their speech, which nearly becomes a storytelling event. Hence the importance of additional aspects of Tuareg herbalists' verbal language: their accounts of their mythico-historical origin, and images (verbal, visual, olfactory) in their healing paraphernalia and practice. These symbols are linked with each other and language in an interaction of verbal and nonverbal modalities in medicine women's healing.

Medicine women's profession in many regions is based upon oral traditions validating their heritage. Many local assumptions of competence and attitudes of trust are also based to a large extent upon medicine women's matrilineal genealogies within certain clans and their mythico-history of herbalism. Although some Tuareg men also see herbalists, nonetheless, choice of healers by sex is significant, and many people do make some distinctions in this according to gender. Most local residents claim that women, in particular older women, make good healers "because they are gentle and kind" and also because one can reveal personal, sometimes shameful information to them (except, notably, to those standing in a kinship relationship requiring reserve, such as the mother-in-law).

Somewhat though not exactly like a *curandera*'s power which comes from her religion and her deep belief that God has selected her to heal on earth (Perrone, Stockel, and Krueger 1989:9), many Tuareg herbal medicine women say they heal in order to compensate for their past sins *(ibakaden)*, to help others, and to act upon the mandate of their inheritance. These beliefs have their foundation in cultural mythology, or as I prefer to term it, "mythico-history," a body of stories and knowledge believed to explain how herbalism originated and how herbalists practice. The myth of "objectivity" and scientific credentials—for example, a degree from medical school—are founding principles of Euro-American science. Myth/histories are used as founding principles of herbalist healing, which, in the Aïr region, tends to be practiced in clusters of clans around the Bagzan Massif, namely, among descent groups called Kel Igurmadan and Kel Agatan. In the Aïr around Mt. Bagzan, these etiological accounts relating the founding of herbal medicine consist of several different variants on a single common theme or motif: of founding female twins and their murdered mother.

Here, I present several mythico-historical variants of accounts given to me about Tagurmat, the founder/ancestress of several healing clans within a major descent group All but one of the following variants were given me by herbal medicine women during conversations and interviews. One of them was related by a non-herbalist: an elderly woman, wife of a marabout, who refrained from pronouncing the name of Tagurmat—perhaps from respect, perhaps from some inhibition in the presence of her husband. Other similar variants, much briefer, were also recounted to me. I offer here six variants whose versions appear more complete and detailed.

These stories are very consistent with many other more general matrilineal origin myths in Tuareg descent groups outside the herbal medicine tradition, which relate more general origins of these descent groups in the different confederations.[1] These matrilineal motifs of herbal medicine therefore coexist with the wider mythico-history of Tamajaq-speaking peoples, and more broadly, with other Berber origin themes such as that of Tin Hinan and Kahena stories in North Africa.

Numerous anthropologists from at least the nineteenth century, for example, Morgan, into more recent times have analyzed so-called myths of matriarchy in different cultures in various times and places, from a variety of perspectives and from different analytical frameworks—evolutionary, feminist, and structural/symbolic and post-structural (Bamberger in Rosaldo and Lamphere 1974; Gottlieb 1992; Lepowsky in Goodenough and Sanday 1995). Tuareg herbal medicine women offer matrilineal motifs from a fresh perspective. Their stories validate their authoritative knowledge and skills in healing and beyond. They provide a charter to set wrongs "right," in particular, in social control of domestic violence toward women in gender relations, and remind others of wider concerns of descent, inheritance, and property preoccupations in Tuareg society. Their accounts should be considered pervasive and important, not necessarily because they are "true" or represent a consensus, but because most medicine women evoked this primary mythical theme or motif in explaining why they heal, and others took it very seriously, despite some competing alternative cultural themes and Islamic emphasis upon patriliny (Rasmussen 1995, 1997).

Most medicine women gave me their accounts in a highly formalized, nearly formulaic manner. Others related them more subtly and indirectly, on informal conversations and visits. On some visits, I was accompanied by a research assistant; on others, I was alone, though assistants helped transcribe and translate these accounts after I had tape-recorded them. Here are the various accounts:

1. *The tale according to Wasu:* "It was the Kel Igurmadan who obtained medicine. There was a man who had a wife, this man was very jealous. One day, he saw people passing and his wife said, 'I see men passing.' He killed this woman. He saw the stomach that moved, he tore it open, he took out two girls. These girls grew up. Then they began to play their little games of children, with little recipients of wood [cut cores of doum palms]. One held the small recipient, she made trees [medicines] in it, and the other made charcoal in it. Some people took the tree medicine, and they [i.e., herbal medicine women] practiced it. Others [i.e., marabouts] took the marabouage medicine from charcoal and vegetal ink and practiced it. That is how the people of the Kel Igurmadan received the wood and some among them have practiced Qur'anic charcoal and ink medicine. The twins had names, but I have forgotten them; maybe Fatima and Fatimata. . . . We learned that a long time ago because it was our elders who saw the era when they did that."

2. *The tale according to Tanou, Wasu's aunt,* a medicine woman related to Lala, the most senior medicine woman on top of Mt. Bagzan: "I practice medicine because it is our origin, inheritance from our parents (relatives). I inherited it from my father's side of the family. The grandmother *(kaka)* of our parents was pregnant with two twin girls. One day they were chatting. She mentioned that one day she saw a very handsome man. He [her husband] killed her with his knife. She died. He took out [of her stomach] the two little twin girls. When he took them out, their hands were holding tree woods [barks]. He took them out of their hands. He hid them until they grew. They buried the woman who died. When the girls grew older, he brought the wood and asked them, 'What is that?' They answered, 'That is the medicine.' Since they were [still] young, they began to gather barks. They played their games. [Later] they steeped them [the barks] in water and placed them on the fire [to cook] as practice. But for much information, you must go see Lala, the elderly senior medicine woman on Mt. Bagzan. I do not know the twin girls' names. I know [only] the name of the woman who was cut."

Tanou continued: "All the Kel Igurmadan, their origin is this [first practice of] medicine. The Igurmadan, there are several kinds. Not all of them inherited medicine. After that, some found the means of writing, others found ways of bringing medicine [i.e., according to Tanou, medicine is inherited, particularly within a specialized clan within the larger Igurmadan descent group]. Also, a person must learn [medicine] from someone who knows it. Also, a person obtains authorization. Children learn with their parents because there are many medicine trees. I learned from old Lala. It was she who taught me."

3. *The tale according to Tina,* who also divines by dreaming, from a village near Timia: "There was a woman whose husband killed his wife. She was pregnant. The day he killed her, there were two girls inside her stomach. He tore open her stomach, and took out the two little girls. It is jealousy *(tchismitene)* that led him to kill her. The parents of the woman left to see this husband to kill him. Arrived at his home, they saw him with the two twin girls. He gave them something to drink, and they left him without killing him. 'If one kills that person,' they said, 'one will be committing a sin. Among us, it is he who can find someone who will raise the twin girls. After that, one can kill him.' The parents did not succeed in finding anyone, and therefore, they left him [the husband] alone."

"When they [the twin girls] became big, one held medicine, and the other touched [to cure]. The two women of Tagurmat (their mother was named Tagurmat) and her descendants became a clan named Igurmadan, one girl was named Tanike, the other Tachida. Tachida was the older daughter, and the second one to be born was Tanike. They stayed on the Bagzan Massif."

"During the war years [with the Tubu, in the nineteenth century], another girl also was a healer.[2] The illnesses that she treated are serious illnesses, even evil mouth, she could cool it off. She cooled the spirits. The woman also treated *tuksi* (a "hot" illness), cooled it off. If it was a child, she dug a hole that resembled a tomb and she placed the child in this. This is the treatment for a child with many illnesses; next, one crushes *ebisgen* leaves and places them on the child's body."

4. *The tale according to Ana,* elderly woman married to an Islamic scholar; she did not mention Tagurmat but called this tale "Mohammed of Ibil" (collected in a village at the base of Mt. Bagzan—Ibil is a region at the gate of the Tenere, and to the east of Tamgak Mountains): "There was [at that time] a man named Mohammed of Ibil.[3] He had his wife. They were inside their house, and the woman saw some *meharis* (cameliers) who were passing, and she went outside to watch them. She looked at them to see them clearly. The husband slapped his wife, she died. He cut open her stomach, and he took [cut] out two little girls who were twins, whom they called 'those girls who were cut.' The two little twin girls, it was they who founded all the Igurmadan. One made the Igurmadan of the Kel Bagzan. All the Kel Igurmadan are from these two girl twins, who created them. Each made a part [of the descent group]."

5. *The tale according to Amina,* medicine woman on Mt. Bagzan: "Concerning the beginning of medicine, we were told, our parents told us that they obtained it from the twin girls, the Igurmadan twins *(tekanawene,* derived from the Hausa language). 'When they were little,' people told us, 'there was one girl who gathered barks and leaves. One day, their neighbor had the hiccoughs *(tazagat),* they gave him some barks *(teshawene),* he drank them, and he was cured. Another had a cold, and he drank, and was cured, also.'"

6. *The tale according to Lala* (at the time I collected this, she was the most senior medicine woman on Mt. Bagzan; she is now deceased): "I am seventy-five years old. I was born on Mt. Bagzan, in the Kel Igurmadan clan [descent group]. I touch and I make medicine. I have children, Akhmed Mohammed and others. When he was alive, my husband did caravan trading, and there were no gardens here. I do herbal medicine because it is the inheritance from my parents. From the time that I was born, I saw the old women making medicines. It is their inheritance, because there was once a very

jealous husband. He transferred [his wife] very far away. They lived [apart] so that men could not see her. One day, he saw people who were going to war on their camels, which were very decorated. People said, 'Look at the men who have left for war.' The woman looked and she told them, 'I see a very handsome man among those men. Someone who wore an indigo shirt *(alyale).*'

"As soon as he saw the woman [admiring the cameliers], he [the husband] killed her with a knife and she died. He placed her in the position of death.[4] But then, the stomach of the woman moved. He tore [open] her stomach and took out two twin girls. These two little girls each brought something hidden in their hands. He cut the umbilical cords *(taboutout,* umbilical cord). He arranged it [buried it beneath three stones], prepared [washed] these girls, and after that, he assembled the people in order to take the woman to the cemetery, and he said to the people nearby: 'Look at what is in the hands of the little girls.' People told him, 'These small objects held [in their hands], you must hide them until the little girls grow up, in order to find out [more] information about them. If they die, the news (information, *isalan*) dies also.' The small objects were of wood. He hid them until the girls grew. They [the other people] responded, 'That is the beginning of medicine.' They [the small twin girls] even had *icherifan* medicine [of the descendants of the Prophet], and *al hima* (denotes a sacred quality), and they taught how to practice medicine: one touched, they explained everything. Their names were Fatane and Fatoni. All the women on their side of the family taught those [women] who were interested how to practice medicine.

"So that was the beginning of medicine. Since they were taken out of the stomach of their mother, they held medicine. Before, other people, they used their hands [touch] in small massages and healed [that way]. At that time, they did not have many sins *(ibakadan)*, but now they have many sins [i.e., healers did not do harm before, whereas today, they are polluted or 'dirty' *(jergonen)]*. Nowadays also, for some others, it is not their inheritance [heritage, *tarek,* as this term is used here by Lala also denotes 'community,' family in Sufi sense, and 'history' or 'road'], but they [nonetheless] practice it. But even someone who has inherited medicine must obtain authorization, even in order to touch patients. It is not everyone who knows it equally. There must be someone who has received the knowledge from God, also."

Despite some differing details, basically these stories convey common themes. In these accounts, which describe an atrocity followed by death and regeneration, herbal medicine women validate their healing, as a special inheritance: an authoritative knowledge system. They trace its origins to the rescued twin daughters of Tagurmat, a female founding cultural heroine of the Kel Igurmadan, a local descent group fraction. According to these and many other medicine women and their patients in the Aïr region, herbal medicine began when Igurmadan twins (daughters of Tagurmat) were small. Many variants emphasize that one of the twins clutched barks and leaves at birth. Some relate that, one day their neighbor got the hiccoughs, and they gave him barks, he drank them, and he was cured. Another neighbor had a cold, he drank [their bark medicine] and was healed also. According to Rodd (1926), Tagurmat is the name of an old Igurmadan *tawsit* (descent group) who came from Ibil in the Tamgak Mountains; this is corroborated by the marabout's wife's variant, also an account of the origin of caravanning, which mentions Ibil. Ibil was the place where, according to some variants such as that of Ana, date and salt caravans to Fachi, an oasis in the eastern Niger

Sahara, also began. Other variants of the tale I collected were briefer: one, for example, stated only: "There was a man in the wild whose wife died. He took two twin girls from her stomach." In this latter, the motif of the wild—herbal medicine's origin outside civilization—is more explicit.

When I first heard these stories, I was puzzled. On the one hand, perhaps one must not take their verbal art imagery too literally (Evans-Pritchard 1950). Nuer twins, Evans-Pritchard observed, are not equivalent to birds, but rather share a triadic, analogical relationship with birds, humans, and Kwoth. On the other hand, the tellers of these tales do, in fact, take them literally, just as many adherents take the Christian Eucharist or communion ritual literally rather than as a metaphor. Yet the murder of a pregnant woman and the taking of twins from their dead mother's stomach is, unfortunately, all too possible, and has been known to occur. Another feature of these accounts, the twins' clutching of medicines as they emerge—may to some appear as more fantastic. Indeed, many such accounts blur the fantastic and the "real," myth and history. Perhaps, then, the solution is to move to the level of cultural memory and social practice, and ask: How can healing emerge from murder? How can a murderer also bring into the world healers and founders of a matriline? Interestingly, the jealous husband/murderer of the cultural heroine touched her stomach, but no man since has the right to do so. Here, what is crucial is a warning against domestic violence, and more abstractly, appropriation of women's descent and property interests. Medicine women attempt to protect from these dangers, as additional cases will show.

Suggested in these origin narratives is the idea that healing often includes empathy for others' suffering and confession, asking forgiveness and penance for sins—this resonates with medicine women's frequent emphasis upon healing as absolving them from sins. It also resonates with afflictions of the stomach—the predominant, though as shown, not exclusive, focus in many Tuareg herbal medicine treatments, particularly among women—these stomach and liver problems often metaphorically refer to marital and other social conflicts. Also suggested here is protection of not only the literal body and stomach (though these too are important) from harm (illness or antisocial actions), but also cultural transmission in reminding others of the "children of the stomach," i.e., the matriline and matrilineal *akh huderan* living milk property inheritance—these are ideally sacred—never supposed to be sold, only passed to sisters, daughters, and nieces. Domestic violence is a central event in this tale, however—and from the murder emerge rebirth and regeneration, with healing—ideally, alongside medicine, there is protection of women from natural illness and also social and physical violence. The healer, knowing the myth-given logic and ascertaining how individuals can violate the ideal in this logic, determines how to heal the ailment by bringing the person back into total harmony with society. In Tuareg culture, it is considered a great shame for a man to physically attack, or even argue with, a woman. Until recently, rape was unknown. Wife-beating in rural areas is rare and is condemned by both sexes.

More broadly, these myths contribute to a patient's trust, particularly a female patient's. Stories and myths one has been told and believes, and familiar, comforting rituals and symbols prompt patients to be more open to healing, whether in the form of an injection, a pill, or surgery, or among Tuareg, the *ten* or medicine pot, words, and the acts of touching the ground, circulating medicines three times around the patient's head, and ritually spitting on medicines. In other words, regardless of the viability of matrilineal identity and property today or the lack thereof (an issue examined in forth-coming sections), these myths establish a groundwork for symbols and ritual parapher-nalia of Tuareg herbalists and inculcate trust in their authoritative knowledge.

As Perrone, Stockel, and Krueger (1989) and others (Malinowski 1948; Levi-Strauss 1962) have pointed out, myths create trust. Stories extol the usefulness of given cure for other people. In the United States, for example, there is the strong belief that going to the Mayo Clinic will accomplish something favorable for the sojourner, like going to Lourdes as suggested by the myth of St. Bernadette in France for some others (Per-rone, Stockel, and Krueger 1989). Tuareg medicine women find and offer to others hope and trust. As shown, touching a patient's stomach—the nonverbal tactile anti-dote or structural inversion of the violence in the Tagurmat verbal art etiological myth—can be used to comfort, divine, or diagnose, and also, on occasion, serves as a natural human "polygraph" test, thereby opening up new possibilities for patient and healer of negotiating meanings of suffering.

Medicine women's work with wood, earth, and clay, rather than iron or other met-als worked by smith/artisans, or the paper written on by marabouts, in effect enacts and embodies the themes of this mythico-history. Herbalists primarily work with trees, plants, rocks, stone, and millet and other nonmeat cereal foods, rather than animals (with the marked exception of the goat's head); full animal sacrifices are more often of-fered by and to Islamic scholars and male diviners. Mountains, clay, and wood (barks and leaves) are resonant with symbolism in Tuareg cosmology, mythology, and ritual. The Saharan massifs (Bagzan and Tamgak) contain mountains described in myths as related to one another in kinship, "like people." Babies should be born inside the mother's tent, on the ground. A possessed person is believed to be cured of spirits upon falling, exhausted, to the ground (Rasmussen 1995).

As in some other African cultures, for example, the Yoruba, the Tuareg medicine woman learns about a very large number of herbal preparations since being appren-ticed as an adolescent into the service of a senior healer. Herbalists not only recognize the pharmacological properties of different plants and their uses in day-to-day medical and ethnobotanical practice, but are concerned with their origins and inheritance. Some of the medicines in common use do, of course, have a direct biochemical action within the body when absorbed, but in many other cases the effectiveness of a remedy de-pends on more nonorganic principles, deriving from a symbolic resemblance—whether "sympathetic magic" or "mimesis" (Taussig 1987, 1993), between one or other of the in-gredients and the condition for which they are prescribed. This mimesis need not, how-ever, be solely or predominantly visual. During Tuareg medicine women's collection of plants from the wild, they murmur blessings and benedictions (both Qur'anic and non-Qur'anic) and sometimes write prayers in the sand. These actions recall the special praise songs sung by Yoruba herbalists, which make explicit their desired medicinal power; an incantation is necessary to incorporate the influence of the spoken human word, "without which matter alone is neutral and negligible" (Maclean 1982:165).

This evoking of Tagurmat, in effect, places the ailment or problem in a wider per-spective and serves as a mnemonic reminding patients of the great sacrifice Tagurmat made, of her death, but also of her regeneration through the survival of her children—those twin girls—who passed on her medicine despite her murder at the hands of a violently jealous husband. Even in cases of male patients, evoking Tagurmat verbally and nonverbally also has the effect of at least foregrounding the matrilineal mythology in healing rituals whose aim is wellness, and perhaps, by extension, reminding men of the importance of respect and protection of women when men are tempted to forget these cultural ideals. Medicine women therefore in effect remind many of their patients of the significance of their past heritage and certain gendered arrangements, which are often under threat or—perhaps more distressingly—half-forgotten. These memories, while not all-determining, still matter because they are enacted—sometimes verbally, sometimes nonverbally through touch, the sound of words, and bodily postures and motions—by medicine women in their healing actions and in their evocation of wider cultural memory.

The None Too Distant Past: Herbalists, Ancestors, and Cultural Memory

The question arises here, is the past present, and how? The environment in which many medicine women work is resonant with chronotopes which refer to spirits and humans in the past—both recent and remote, located on the borderlands between myth and history. Place-names evoke tropes connecting this environment and experience with it to past events impinging on it. People originally went up to settle on Mt. Bagzan to escape from wars: from Kel Geres and Tubu raids, and later, from French massacres. During French massacres, some fled to the top of the Bagzan; others fled to Hausaland.

Some Igurmadan elders say they are descended from the people of the Bagzan, known collectively as Kel Bagzan ("People of the Bagzan"), who came down from that mountain massif, but gradually, over time, rather than from any single event in living memory. The Kel Bagzan constitute a larger category, including Kel Agatan, Kel Igurmadan, and other closely related descent groups in the Aïr region of Niger near the Bagzan massif. There, medicine women climb into the high mountain areas to collect their tree medicines.

When I went to see one herbal medicine woman in that region, Anta, in an old section of a seminomadic camp, I noticed many historic landmarks along the route. She lived in a beautiful area with rock art said to be painted by Aligouran (Adigouran), another prominent culture hero, who is believed to have also invented the Tifinagh alphabetic script. Nearby there are many stone ruins called *ibedni*, left by untraced ancestors, called variously the People of the Past or the People of the Night (Kel Arou or Kel Nad).[5]

As I arrived at Anta's home on foot with a pack camel, the sun was just setting, and women were baking *tenderu*, a dish of flat wheat bread. Her village had experienced some violence several years before during the Tuareg separatist rebellion, and I was uncertain how local residents would regard me.[6] Nonetheless, Anta greeted me warmly and willingly discussed her work and heritage with me:

> I believe I am sixty years old, I was born here. My father is Kel Azanghaydan, my mother is both Kel Igurmadan and Kel Agatan also. I am married and have nine children. I touch and I do herbal medicines. But I do not do the large pot of medicines. I know it, but I do not do it now. I particularly treat children. I work with trees of the Aïr and Hausa country *(Agala)*. I do the work to treat my children, and sometimes other patients, when other healers are not available.

Also, it is our inheritance (or heritage, *gado nena*) and our origin *(arasal nena)*. I [also] treat unrelated patients, if they come to me. I inherited the healing from my mother's side. I do not know a story or myth explaining how the Kel Agatan began practicing medicine, I was only told that we inherited this medicine from a woman who inherited that from her father, the first ancestral healer. To my knowledge, our ancestors did medicine. When I became a woman, I learned medicine. My parents died when I was young. I practiced it, I learned well like that. It originated from my parents. I apprenticed only for a year. I began to treat people when I had my family [i.e., upon marriage and having children]. At that moment, I was in the wild *(essuf)*, in the wilderness and crazy, I had not been interested in it. And then, I followed my older sister who practiced it. I have practiced it a long time now, because I obeyed [her]. Among all people, the best curers are from the Kel Agatan clan, who are related to the Kel Igurmadan clan, and also preferably, those who have inherited this. Also, [the best] is someone who is nice.

I find the illness with the aid of my fingers *(adade)*, I touch the patient. I do not dream. I am not a specialist, I am a generalist. But all who come to me, I can treat them. I treat hot illnesses or *tuksi*, and stomach illness *(tezoufnine)*. I know the medicine of the pot. It is from Hausa country that one brings [medicines] to me. Those from the South. My children, who are caravanners, bring them to me. I follow some rules. The days I do not place medicines on the fire are Thursday and Friday, since my parents did not. Also, if someone takes medicines on those "great" Islamic holy days of prayer *(emud)*, he/she will not be cured. Also, if the medicine is not well cooked, one cannot drink it. The medicine must remain on the fire for three days. If a woman comes and she wants medicine to drink, I must touch her in order to verify that she is not pregnant. If she takes [some] medicines, she will miscarry. A pregnant woman's medicine is distinct, especially in cases of *tuksi* illness. The goat's head plays a role in the stomach; it purges it of everything inside it. At that moment, one vomits it. I touch the earth in order to not catch the illness.

First, I must encircle millet around the patient. I encircle the millet around the patient three times. That is what our ancestors did. As one holds millet, one retracts the fingers because the fingers not retracted signify hostility or fighting. Because even if you harm someone by bad words, you must not extend the finger [that is a grave insult]. . . . Women, men, children—everyone comes to me, but their medicines are not the same. I only treat women for reproductive problems in the case of a fetus with problems in the mother's stomach. If the woman falls, there will be problems. In the past two weeks, I have treated about five [adult] people, and a girl: one woman, others men. The girl had a blood problem and a dislocated liver. They paid me. For *tezoufnin* I am paid 1500 CFA (about US$3). The girl paid 500 CFA (about US$1). But they pay me anything according to capacity. The herbalists and bone-setter/masseuses are often the same healers, though their skills are distinct.

At several points in their narratives, Anta and others alluded to relatives, parents, and ancestors. Anta identified herself as of both Kel Igurmadan and Kel

Agatan descent on her mother's side. The Kel Agatan came originally from a dried riverbed near Timia. Although as noted, the Kel Agatan descent group is also represented by many hereditary herbalists on Mount Bagzan and also farther northwest, near Mount Tamgak, their precise origin myth and founding ancestress name were not available. In beliefs concerning death and ancestors, local cultural, pre-Islamic, popular, and "official" Islamic cosmoligies and rituals interweave. Dead souls are believed to wander in the vicinity of graves, and some communication with them is possible through dreams and divination. The name of the deceased is not mentioned by immediate descendants, and many persons are even reticent about the more distant and remote ancestral names. Tagurmat, for example, was not mentioned to me until late in my field research. Graves are not individually marked, although stones are piled higher on tombs of prominent marabouts and chiefs, and offerings such as dates are made to them. While ancestor "cults" among Tuareg appear less elaborated than in some other African societies, as there are no domestic altars or regular libations, nonetheless, there are some important mortuary commemorative rituals; for example, rituals *(takote)* consisting of animal sacrifices, mortuary feasts, and prayers led by marabouts for the deceased held at intervals following death, which feature almsgiving and reading from the Qur'an (Rasmussen 1997). Medicine women often gather their medicines in the vicinity of ancestral ruins and tombs. They describe the alms they offer to children and trees by the same term, *takote*.

In keeping with many "official" Islamic beliefs as interpreted by Tuareg Islamic scholars, local residents emphasize judgment day following death, when angels measure the relative weights of bad and good deeds of the deceased in life. Many herbalists undoubtedly reflect upon this when they indicate that one reason they practice medicine is to compensate for their earlier sins.

How exactly is the herbal medicine mythico-history used today? Medicine women's voices indicate that there is room for ambiguity and alternative interpretations of cultural memory. Indeed, these narratives and their associated practices reveal modifications and mutual reconstructions of knowledge. Some elderly persons, such as Ana, identified Tagurmat as both an old Igurmadan clan who came from Ibil in the Tamgak Mountains, around the same time that caravan trading to Fachi and Bilma also began, and also the name of the two female twins. These contradictions are not necessarily problematic, but rather they constitute an important characteristic of multiple voices in post-Bakhtinian perspectives; there may indeed be internal contradictions within a single narrative, not merely dialogic between narratives, and these all may be accommodated or drawn upon as needed.

The mythic and historical past are blurred. Many ancestors important in herbal medicine are not recent or precisely genealogical (or at least, their links cannot be exactly calculated) or historical but are more merged with distant "mythical" time. These include the Kel Nad or Kel Arou "People of the Past or Night," Aligouran the Saharan culture hero, and various matrilineal tree spirits. According to a local primary school director, Tagurmat was an ancient woman chief who led Tuareg ancestors in a battle near Mount Bagzan, on a horse. She had sons, twins, whom this man called by male names: Alhassane and Alhosseini. By contrast, his female relatives provided me with additional female names of girl twin founders/cultural heroines: they were called Aaneghale and Chite.

To this day, there is an *oeud* (dried riverbed or *cori*) in the Tamgak Mountains called Igurmadan. Elders from whom I collected genealogies and histories indicate that the origins of Kel Igurmadan before they arrived in their present-day village at the base of Mount Bagzan were in a nearby village just a mile down the dried riverbed, and before that on top of Mt. Bagzan. Before the Bagzan, they were in Hausaland where they had fled at various times, around 1917 to escape from the fighting of the Tuareg Senoussi revolt led by Kaoussan and the French punitive repression and famines in the 1920s following its suppression. The genealogy of the current Kel Igurmadan chief's family that I collected goes farther back to a marabout leader named Boulkhou, approximately the great-great-grandfather of the current chief of the Kel Igurmadan, whose mystical power in resistance against the Tubu has been recorded elsewhere (Rasmussen 1997). The current chief's father died this past year, and his grandfather, who died in 1985, was born in Ajirou, east of Bagzan, and was Kel Igurmadan. He was a caravanner and herder. He went to Hausaland and returned to the Aïr later, where he built the first mosque and sank the first well in the village where the current chief of the Kel Igurmadan resides. During my early field residence, he still lived, but was retired and confined to bed because of a foot malady and so no longer took an active part in politics. All men in these chiefly families have been caravanners and marabouts. The younger generations continue these occupations, though caravanning is on the decline. Many younger men today supplement these traditional occupations with oasis gardening and labor migration in the increasingly monetarized economy.

The point here is that alternative mythico-history remains powerful in medicine women's authoritative knowledge claims. While I show presently that they are not always successful in its social enactment—in protecting women from all dangers—nonetheless, they are respected by both women and men for reasons having to do partly with this heritage and partly with their own actions and character. Many women patients indicated to me that "although there are many trees on Mt. Bagzan they are not the sole reason herbalists there do medicine. Rather, they do medicine because of their inheritance of their medicine knowledge and their character."

On the other hand, the experiences and perspectives of two other medicine women show that heritage and inheritance are desirable yet insufficient conditions in themselves for respect and the successful transmission of herbal medicinal knowledge. According to Rahma, a medicine woman who did not know her age but had several grown adult married children, "a *tanesmegel* is someone who brings medicines from trees to patients. I have been a *tanesmegel* since becoming older. I learned myself, by experience. Not just anyone can become an herbal medicine woman, however, since it is difficult. My mother was one, also, although my daughter is not apprenticing."

Thus Rahma admitted some informality in her learning to heal, although she also inherited this profession; she described it as her *gado marawan* (literally, "parents' bed," from *gado,* the Hausa term for bed, and *marawan,* the Tamajaq term for parents or relatives). Although Rahma, like others, emphasized this importance of clan inheritance. she also indicated that she practiced this career because people asked her to. Rahma was born near Azel, a village near Agadez now famous for its artisan soapstone tourist art. She was a widow with four adult children. Her husband was not a curer; he went on caravans.

Rahma's family genealogy included many noble herders and caravanners, but they were not wealthy and also stood outside the circle of influential chiefly families. Rahma's late husband left nothing to his widow. Her bride-wealth *(taggalt)* camel also had died, and so she was poor, despite her herbal medicinal practice. Rahma's brother, a herder and marabout, lived outside villages in pastures, and he sometimes visited her.

Given that inheritance is so important in many medicine women's professional credibility, I wondered why her daughter Asalo was not apprenticing with Rahma. In her comments, Rahma emphasized a combination of independent learning and inheritance. Events in Asalo's life, however, suggested that even these criteria are not sufficient to win over a clientele if the medicine woman's family is not respected in the community, if she is very poor and socially marginal, and/or if her kin violate important social and sexual taboos. Asalo did not continue her mother's herbal medicine profession because of her own problematic social status in the community. She was a young divorcee, and although divorce does not bring social stigma among most Tuareg, it is the conduct between divorces that determines a woman's reputation: Asalo had allegedly given birth to several children out of wedlock, considered shameful in that community where Islamic scholars are influential and respected. Also, rather than hiding her illegitimate children, or leaving the community herself, Asalo remained, and her behavior was considered unstable; for example, she was rumored to run naked through the desert.

The point here is that, in learning and establishing an herbal medicine profession, what is important is not solely technical knowledge per se (although that too is a criterion) or inheritance (although this, according to many healers and patients, makes for even better skill) but also exemplary gender-based social conduct. Central concerns here are gendered and aged experience.

My experiences with medicine women drew my attention to this importance of age, as well as gender-based social mores. First, successful medicine women must be well integrated into the community themselves. While their relatives may violate social norms, they themselves must be reasonably well-integrated into the community. While there is a great deal of free social interaction between women and men in Tuareg society, illegitimate births are shameful and the mother (though not necessarily the grandmother) of such a child is stigmatized. Additional factors explained why Rahma's daughter did not apprentice and both women were relatively marginal. Rahma rarely participated in communal work parties or rites of passage. She was prevented from doing so, not solely because of her daughter's conduct but because of her poverty; for such participation requires substantial contributions in alms and other offerings. She also lacked kinship connections to the influential chiefly families.

In fact, another medicine woman—Hadia—also had a daughter who had given birth out of wedlock, but her own career by contrast was not adversely affected by that, for several reasons. First, Hadia was better off in herds, and this enabled her to take a much more active role in community events, particularly rites of passage, which are crucial to elders' status. Also, Hadia came from an old oasis, caravanning, and herding village where the shrine of an important marabout-founder was located. Finally, while Rahma's daughter remained in the area, Hadia's daughter (whose story is told later) left the community immediately following her out-of-wedlock birth, and Hadia hid the child for a while, raising him outside in pastures.

I have known Hadia for nearly twenty-five years. I first met her in a neighboring village at the home of one of her daughters. She was constructing a conical grass building in her daughter's compound, where we were both participating in a communal women's work project. Hadia was also a frequent guest at the local rites of passage and contributed many alms offerings to ceremonies at the mosque. Thus a number of factors in addition to inheritance in clans and technical expertise emerge as important in the relative degree of influence and respect of medicine women: age-related appropriate conduct, minimal economic security sufficient to enable sociability and generosity, and if not "scandal-free" family history, at least discreetness in handling scandals. Participating in rites of passage—name days, weddings, and mortuary condolences—are activities all elders must do, but herbal medicine women must be even more exemplary in fulfilling these obligations. Hence the cultural significance of age, as well as gender and inheritance, in herbal medicine.

In another study of the more general significance of age in Tuareg culture and its impact upon ethnographic field research, Rasmussen (1997) has observed that Tuareg elders in effect become pre-ancestral. This leads to another important point: since youths and elders in Tuareg society are usually very distant in public sociability contexts (except for close kin such as maternal grandparents and grandchildren, who practice joking relationships), medicine women, on one level, therefore counterbalance and relieve this reserve relation between most elders and most youths. Local residents confirmed this when they told me they could confide in medicine women, in particular very elderly ones, about sexual matters and other delicate topics otherwise kept hidden, during private healing sessions. Only in more intimate family settings, including the curing of illness, can such reserve be dropped. In order to serve others in this way, as trusted confidante, the medicine woman must be exemplary in her conduct, ideally at least, above reproach in local concepts of proper gendered and aged conduct.

Ethnographically, such conditions offered challenges but also insights for me. Reserve and respect run counter to the close proximity required for an ethnographer's apprenticeship, which is valued in some recent "experimental" ethnographic narratives in order to become nearly merged with the healer in practice and ideology (Peters 1981; Olkes and Stoller 1987; Stoller 1989). Reserved distance was necessary for me at first, in the earlier years of my field research, due to my age and social status as a married woman of childbearing age, but one without children. Years later, upon my returning several times to their communities, my relationship with some (though not all) of these women changed considerably: many whom I had known longer opened up more to me, and our interactions became considerably less stiff and formal. While closer friendships and increasing trust clearly were also important reasons for this, my advancing age probably also accounted for their openness. Thus Hadia only gradually related her life to me, and primarily on my later visits. I present one selection from her narrative here and another one later.

Hadia indicated that she was born at the time Kaoussan (leader of the 1917 Tuareg Senoussi revolt against the French in the Aïr) escaped. This suggests that she was approximately 85 years old in 2002, when she still herded goats and donkeys, and healed, though kin gathered for her.

She continued her story:

Me, I saw Kaousan of the Ikazkazan [leader of Tuareg Semoussi Revolt against the French in 1917].[7] Before, we lived in Ajirou. When raiders *(izingan)* came, we ran. When the raiders came, at that moment my family was celebrating my name day [held for a baby one week following birth]. People ran, they left the meat on the fire, one fleeing parent even dropped their child, whom we later adopted. I have four living children. I had a husband, but he died. He was a caravanner. I inherited the work of herbal medicine from my parents. We were children when we began gathering the medicines. It is not an obligation. But people prevented me from resting; they sought medicines [from me], as they knew that it was inheritance from my parents. My parents did it, after their death, I inherited that. I do medicine for the stomach, I treat everyone. I go up the mountain, I bring the bark medicines from the trees. I was eighteen years old when I began to learn, to gather. At that time, I learned it, but I did not practice it. I apprenticed with my mother, I waited until her death and I myself was old before I began practicing full-time, around 1980 [three years before we met]. One must have a "complete head." And a person can even be jealous of relatives. Like that, it is like obedience. I refused to practice full time independently when I was very young, although I already knew some techniques and medicines. This skill was inherited and learned [down] through my mother from my grandmother. But even a few men in my family do this. Being a *tanesmegel* is specialized; one must be of a certain family. It is in the blood.

The grandparent *(kaka)* of medicine is the Kel Agatan (clan). It is they who make good medicine. We received medicine from our grandparents who lived among the Kel Agatan. It is in the same *tawsit* that is the origin of medicine [i.e., it is related to the descent group Kel Igurmadan]. I am Kel Agatan. I touch to know the illness. Sometimes I touch something hard, sometimes something soft, sometimes something like grains.

Illnesses Hadia cured include the following: cold illnesses or *tessmut* (which she and an accompanying marabout described to me as including gonorrhea; also cold in general); hot illnesses or *tuksi,* which she and the marabout described as stomach-related, and other conditions caused by heat in general. "*Tessmut* ('cold' illness) makes the bladder become hard. If there is *tuksi,* the body is torn and soft on the interior. These are the roots of other illnesses. With *tessmut,* one has difficulty urinating, also vomiting can be *tessmut. Tuksi* ('hot' illness) disperses in the body; the entire body becomes hot." She explained that there are many sorts of *tuksi:* examples are conditions from too much sugar in the diet or salt. Hadia's treatment for *tuksi* from heat in general is to rest at sunset on a mat. Hadia also treated infertility of women and men. She believed that the causes of this are too many illnesses, especially of the stomach. *Takokiat* is one bark she used as a stomach remedy; this is a grayish-black when pounded.

She said, "All sorts of persons come to me, but usually, when they are first attacked (afflicted). I prefer 'new' illnesses [i.e., in their early phases]. I think women have more illnesses. Women suffer more from food, sun, and wind. The treatment for food-related illnesses consists of plants, barks, wood from Hausa country, and incense *(tafarchit),* which is also a spirit medicine. For illness from the sun *(ezziz* illness), I use plants called *chamin* and *akkamum*. I touch the stomach to verify and diagnose the illness. I touch the earth to cure, as part of my medicine. I also attach a cloth to a tree in order to leave the illness behind. I pronounce *'Bissmillah'* not only while touching a patient but also while pulling up or picking medicinal plants."

Therefore among female patients, in particular, those whom medicine women diagnose and treat for stomach and liver afflictions, there is far more at stake than organic illness. In the next chapter, in narratives and in several case studies, I examine more closely medicine women's roles in relation to gender, age, and sexual and social reproduction.

5—Medicine Women, Gender, and Physical and Social Reproduction over the Life Course

Some medicines are the same for people with the same ailment; others are not the same. The medicines of men and women are not the same. One uses different parts of plants for men's and women's medicines in some illnesses. For example, men's and women's *tuksi* (hot) illnesses are the same; their *tessmut* (cold) illness is not the same. Men's medicine for one type of *tessmut* uses only the roots of the *afazo* plant; whereas women's medicine from *afazo* uses the entire plant (grass). Another type of *tessmut* (cold illness) of men needs the root of the doum palm and wild millet because the illness is not the same as it is for women. Women's barks are usually of a red color. The man goes [sexually] to many women. Women do not go [sexually] to as many men. A tree called the "donkey's date," this entire tree treats the woman's cold *(tessmut)*, except the leaves. Women do not take millet as medicine for this, because for men, some illnesses are not the same. Medicine for woman's *tessmut* caught from the husband consists of *toberas* tree leaves. But not many women here have caught this from their husbands. I have heard of SIDA (AIDS), but it is still rare here. No medicines cure SIDA.

Tana, whom we met earlier, is speaking again here. She also described a medicine for *ezziz* (predominantly a women's illness, from sitting on hot mats or sand, a type of "hot" affliction): this consists of incense *(tefarchit n aman)*, the urinary tract of a jackal, dried elephant droppings or rabbit droppings, and crow's eggs, crushed and mixed together. The patient washes the genital organs, puts this medicine in the fire, and then approaches the fire.

The foregoing comments suggest that in some medicines and treatments, the gender and age of patient and herbal healer are important considerations. Some medicines are believed to be more effective for women (for example, red clay from a natural hot spring at Tafadek), others more effective for men.

According to Tata, the medicine woman who treated Fatima, "Pregnant women should avoid some tree medicines, but take others, preferably fresh rather than dried. After periods cease, women have less strength. Sometimes there are problems with anger *(tourgoum)* caused by the husband. Women's problems [also] stem from lack of instruction about the body. [For example], when I first got my period, I hoped it did not last; I was afraid. I had no instruction. Menstruation is like a broom *(afarat)*; a sweeping of body. As we get older, there is greater respect. Also, children are helpful in providing support in later years."

Hadia, whom we also met in the previous chapter, also commented on these topics: "Women can catch the cold illnesses of *tessmut*, but it is more widespread among men.

The food women eat is not the same as the food men eat. Also, women take raw *eghale* [the millet, date, goat cheese, and water drink], that is what can give women the cold illnesses of *tessmut*."

One day while I was visiting, Hadia examined and treated a woman, whom I shall call Mariama, wife of a local chief, who had walked to her residence from a village about five miles away. This consultation illustrated the importance of gender-specific treatment and psychosocial marital counseling in medicine women's treatments of many married women.

The Unhappy Co-Wife

Hadia explained, "Mariama has a very high body temperature. Sometimes women only want to modify their body, that is the reason they seek medicine [for cosmetic reasons, for example, to get fat]. Mariama is not only ill, sometimes it is because of her husband that she seeks medicine. For a long time, Mariama tried maraboutage (Qur'anic verses). She has had this illness for a long time, and I believe the separation from her husband provoked that. For several years, Mariama had moved her tent off to the distance [from her husband's adobe mud house]. People later helped them reconcile. She returned to their home [inside the compound], but she became ill. She took many pots of my medicine and did maraboutage often. When she came to me once recently, and returned a second time, she had hot illnesses of *tuksi*, so I prepared the pot of medicine for that. I calmed her down. She feels better now."

I had known Mariama since early in my research. As I sat in on her consultation and healing session with Hadia, Mariama assured me that she was now cured of the spirits that had afflicted her in the past, but she complained that she now suffered from another illness "of the stomach and liver." During Mariama's examination and treatment, Hadia used massage *(arabaz)* and touch *(edes)*, contacting not only the patient's stomach, but also the ground, in order to take the disease out of both patient and healer and throw the disease away (the ground absorbs the illness). "The medicine woman is 'heavy' from the patient's illness and needs to have the ground take it off or away," she explained. Upon the conclusion of Mariama's treatment, when she was not present, Hadia commented to me that "Mariama was not really that ill. She came to me primarily for attention and also because of some continuing difficulties with her husband. She sought medicines to become fatter. Many women do this in seeking my treatments. There are certain herbal medicines that make women fat, more attractive to their husbands. They drink them, and then should supplement the medicines by remaining at home and eating lots of meat."

When I first met her, Mariama was a frequently possessed woman, about thirty-five years old. Her first possession attack had occurred just after her marriage, before she had children. Her immediate possession symptoms were extreme weakness and respiratory problems. Her more general health problems were fevers, headaches, and nosebleeds. A maternal aunt, also, was frequently possessed, and a female cousin was rumored to have gone insane. During my early visits, Mariama was hospitable, but she seemed to suffer from extreme mood changes and frequent "depression" *(tamazai)*. She indicated she was prone to colds as well as stomach ailments, though she added that spirits "circulate like colds." I often found her resting alone in her tent while her oldest daughter did the housework.

Later, I learned that at that time, she was separated, though not divorced, from her husband. As Hadia recounted, Mariama had moved her tent off slightly to one side of the main compound. Her husband, the chief of a local descent group, was a caravanner and an Islamic scholar who often traveled on trading expeditions and pilgrimages. The couple were of noble origins and were close relatives in an arranged marriage: his father was a cousin of her mother. Both owned livestock, and the husband also had a small store inside their compound. Since he was a chief, however, their property was jointly owned, contrary to the usual pattern of independent women's property ownership, so if this couple divorced, the property would revert to the husband.

The couple did not divorce after all but reconciled. Eventually they had seven children, though two died. By the early 1990s, however, the husband had contracted a polygynous marriage with a woman who resided in a village about fifteen miles away.

Over the many years I have known her, therefore, Mariama has been plagued by not solely those possessing Kel Essuf Spirits of the Wild who attacked her liver (the seat of strong sentiments, especially love) and head, requiring the *tende n goumaten* exorcism, but also by afflictions of the stomach (the symbol of the matriline) more usually cured by herbalists, unless diagnosed as spirits. She medicated these problems eclectically, by undergoing a number of *tende n goumaten* rites and by taking the medicines of both Islamic scholar/healers and herbal medicine women. Verses performed at Mariama's possession rituals conveyed concerns of mother/child ties and orphanhood; they alluded to an uneasy "truce" between the possession songs and orthodox Qur'anic verses and the ambiguous relationship of their respective knowledge systems. The songs also referred to natural resources that are alternately nurturing and threatened. For example, in one verse, the soloist sang: "The word of the mouth (in this song)/This is not the science of the Qur'an that marabouts study/let them study and finish/I have been orphaned from my mother." Another sang: "One milks (a goat or camel) for the child/He drinks it/One pounds doum/palm pits burned in the fire/he eats all"[1] (Rasmussen 2001c).

Following her extended massaging of Mariama, Hadia administered a purgative medicine to her. She explained that it is preferable to administer this in the morning rather than the evening. She added that "even 'hot' illness *(tuksi)* [i.e., not just spirits] can sometimes make a person crazy." Just as Tata did in Fatima's case, Hadia, in her treatment of Mariama, alluded to marital problems. Many herbal medicine women treat those problems of women—particularly pregnant women—whose husbands make them angry, as in that special kind of anger of pregnant women called *tourgoum*. This latter condition is especially dangerous: it is feared to cause birth defects if it is not treated. This is exemplified in the following related case, of the next patients to arrive at Hadia's on the same morning.

Takhia, from Mariama's village, arrived by truck at Hadia's village. She complained of liver problems. Takhia had in addition sought treatment by another herbalist, Tina, also a diviner specialist who related one of the variants of the Tagurmat motif to me. Takhia was accompanied by another woman from her village, her sister-in-law. During Takhia's consultation, Hadia made complex kneading motions in a lengthy stomach massage, pulling the flesh to the side. Hadia's more specialized touching *(edez)* treatment for Takhia here was called *kulan tessa* (characterized by kneading or massaging and pulling of the skin over the stomach so as to manipulate the liver and reset it). The precise illness, *aratak (azenkes)*, denotes in local translation into French a *foie tombée* or "fallen liver," but Takhia also appeared to have more general problems of "hot" illnesses. Hadia did this action for about five minutes. There was also a lot of casual, pleasant conversation, joking, and visiting among women before Hadia made her actual diagnosis and began the treatment. Neighbors dropped by. Thus not all phases in all consultations are private or secluded. The degree of seclusion depends upon the needs of each case and each phase of treatment. Takhia later indicated that she felt better and said she would walk back to her village that same day, after resting.

When Hadia later brought over cooked *ilaten* medicines for Takhia to drink standing up, she indicated that Takhia would perhaps be treated again, in her home. "Sometimes," Hadia surmised, "women see herbalists for problems the clinic can't heal, or problems they view as too personal, for example, to get *ten* for conceiving a child, or to get fat. But as women age, there is no more need for adornment because prayer becomes important." The rumor among local residents was that Takhia had a "hidden" illness (i.e., another underlying problem or a shameful illness). Her two-year-old son was staying at her mother's.

The next patient of Hadia's later that day was the baby of Takhia's sister-in-law, who suffered from *tenede* (fever) and stomachache, diagnosed as a hot illness or *tuksi*. Hadia administered the counteractive cold medicines as the baby slept. The mother of the baby indicated that she preferred herbalists to the clinic, saying, "the clinic is only good for shots, and the mobile medical unit visits only occasionally." Then Hadia was called to a village about five miles away to treat a small girl's stomach problems, diarrhea and vomiting. She took *ilaten* medicine of the large *ten*, containing a combination of many more powerful medicines. Her mother did not want to take the child to the clinic about twenty miles away in a large oasis, she said, because it was too far to travel with the child so ill. The girl improved after Hadia's visit but was still not cured.

Another medicine woman, Amina, further illuminated the age- and gender-related aspects of herbal medicine in relating her life and apprenticeship to me:

> I was born here on Mt. Bagzan. I have seven children. I touch, I use barks. I practice medicine because of the illnesses I feel [touch] and I treat them. Our medicine is our tradition, among our elderly women, it is among these elders that we learned it. For practicing medicine, the person must be [at least] forty years old, you must attain this in order to practice it. I apprenticed when my mother did medicine, I followed her, it was I who gathered barks for her at the time I was learning. I spent five years learning. When my mother died, I began to do it as she had authorized me already. While she was living even if I could do it, she had not yet authorized it. Also [I waited] because of respectful obedience *(adeleb)*. The persons preferred for making bark medicine are those of the Kel Igurmadan. Especially, those who are on the mountain. Also much preferred are women who have ceased giving birth; after that, one can begin to do medicine. Also, one prefers medicine women who are no longer interested in men.

Most Tuareg medicine women study with an older relative—usually a mother or aunt (and occasionally a father) and need their authorization to become herbalists themselves. Upon authorization, there is a small ritual of almsgiving in which the new healer offers dates and goat cheese to children at home. Many patients insisted that "An old woman heals best. To be qualified, it is sufficient for the healer to recognize and distinguish different medicines; but for really deep knowledge and competence, the healer should be elderly." Several reasons were given for this. Male patients are reserved toward most young women, and women patients also prefer to confide in elderly women. Additional reasons were given. One elderly herbalist commented, "One must be clean or pure to practice herbalism [i.e., a woman of post-menopausal status]." As observed, some marabouts stated: "Some trees on Mount Bagzan give off a scent that causes infertility; thus young, childbearing-age women are vulnerable to them, because they can be made infertile [by these trees]."

An herbalist in Agadez stated, "A young woman plays the *anzad* (a one-stringed, bowed lute associated with courtship); [whereas] an old woman practices medicine and prayer." In local cultural values, secular music and festivals often feature courtship and freedom of association among men and women of diverse social origins, who are forbidden to marry. These events are considered "anti-Islamic," held far from the mosque, and avoided by older persons in general, as well as marabouts.

But one must not jump to facile conclusions! I argue that medicine women are not simply "androgynous" figures (Fitz Poole in Ortner and Whitehead 1981; Wood 1999). For the most important qualification for being a medicine woman is having been a mother. The Agadez herbalist also insisted: "A childless woman cannot become a medicine woman." Ideally, then, the herbalist begins healing after having had all her children, and she waits until the senior female relative who taught her has died or retired, out of respectful obedience *(adeleb)* for that person. The criterion of having had children is crucial, albeit with a preference for being post-childbearing in order to practice fully as a professional, to "have a complete head," and to inspire more trust and respect from patients. Additional qualifications for herbal practice mentioned were physical strength, willingness to forego comforts, and desire to assist others. These qualifications suggest that herbalists ideally manage the "coming and going" between the deceased and the living, past and present, youth and age, and human settlements and the wild—though these pairs are not always rigid binaries but are realigned or repositioned in different contexts.

Here we encounter paradoxes and contradictions. Marriage is not forbidden, but encouraged, since legitimate children are essential for everyone. But many (though not all) medicine women are single for lengthy time periods—either widowed or divorced. Reasons are complex. There were hints of marital problems during their professional practice from competing obligations and, perhaps, some husbands' jealousy. Indeed, a husband's jealousy is one theme in their founding mythico-history. The essential qualities of herbal medical practice—physical and spiritual mother, commemorative figure, and social mediator—are particularly evident in the ambivalent attitudes toward a few medicine women's more specialized divination by dreaming, in addition to the more widely practiced and less controversial touching of the stomach and spinning of the pot (the latter's form is rather like a stomach, in fact). The implications here are interesting. Perhaps medicine women cannot become too powerful in domains beyond, first, their "hypo-maternal" status, and secondly, their mediating, boundary-straddling role as negotiator. If they do, they risk social censure, marginality, and rivalry, or at least, domestic conflict, as detailed later.

Although herbal medicine women do indeed treat patients suffering from head as well as stomach and liver ailments, nonetheless, they cannot venture too far into more powerful forms of divination with spirits or risk intruding upon marabouts' domain too openly. In principle, they are supposed to deal with head and mind problems, as noted, by referring them to marabouts—however, as shown, many medicine women actually treat these problems, as well, albeit covertly and unobtrusively. Thus in their ideology and public discourse, medicine women are modest; they emphasize their dealings with problems of the stomach and fertility. In practice, they handle both domains. Moreover, actual cases I collected of medicine women's treatments—for example, Tata's of Fatima, Hadia's of Mariama, and Tema's of me—revealed the boundaries among these domains as very porous and overlapping.

Recent works on Tuareg and other cultures' gender cosmologies (Buckley and Gottlieb 1988; Gottlieb 1992; Rasmussen 1987, 1991, 2000; Worley 1991; Figueiredo in Claudot-Hawad 1996; Figueiredo-Biton in Claudot-Hawad 2002) suggest critical refinements of earlier observations concerning female "purity" and "pollution."[2] Although Tuareg women of childbearing age practice restrictions against participating in some specific Islamic rituals during menstruation, and some regional variation exists in attitudes regarding, terms for, and connotations of menstruation, this condition also confers adult status and introduces responsibilities to observe Islam more strictly in prayers and fasting. Nevertheless older, post-childbearing-aged Tuareg women do appear to more closely approach male ritual roles in one way: their greater public participation in Islam (more closely approaching men and boys in the mosque and prayer-ground spaces). In this respect, their roles resemble the roles of post-childbearing women in some other cultures (Fitz Poole 1981; Brown and Kerns 1992; Lamb 2000; Rasmussen 1997, 2000, 2001b). Yet younger childbearing-age Tuareg women are generally not restricted (not secluded or fully veiled, may travel and visit and receive male visitors after marriage).

Thus there is no linear "progression" from impure to pure, or from restriction to greater "liberty" over time. Yet some distancing from "secular" courtship and sexuality occur as women and men age, and a closer engagement with more "sacred" religious devotion is often the ideal, particularly in those groups more influenced by marabouts (Rasmussen 1997). Why is it better for an elderly woman to practice herbal healing once she has ceased to bear children and is no longer interested in men, is "clean" and "free of sin"—and yet she has more *al baraka,* which is also associated with fertility and life?

Local beliefs surrounding reproduction include the idea, expressed in local slang, that during menstruation, a woman's eggs (pl. *chikikaten*) are "broken"; at other times, they are whole. Some beliefs and practices vary according to gender. For example, men describe women as being like "containers" or "leather sacks" during pregnancy, whereas women describe female reproductive physiology as centered on the stomach *(tedis)* and womb, called *ehan n barar* ("the child's tent"), and also tend to place greater emphasis upon love as important in conception. The male is believed to transmit "heat" *(tarraf)* during conception. Iblis, the Devil, is considered to be the ultimate source of reproductive force. Some men are alleged to possess more sperm than others (also a finding in biomedicine); but among Tuareg, this condition is believed to be the force driving some men to monopolize women in polygynous marriages.

Women must protect themselves from malevolent spirits believed to cause birth defects and infant mortality. During menstruation, there are ritual restrictions against praying, touching Islamic amulets, handling animal hides, planting crops, and dressing hair. These measures are believed to protect *al baraka* in living things, and by extension, the yet-to-be-born child. In the past, noble purity was also protected by these taboos, in that they were most strictly practiced by noble women and, as such, also tended to discourage noble women from coming into contact with men of ambiguous or low status (Rasmussen 1991). Certain ritual measures seem to encourage legitimacy, and formerly, perhaps the underlying idea was to discourage liaisons that were not within officially endogamous marriage arranged by parents.[3] This is why conception should not occur outside the tent under the moonlight, nor before the end of the weeklong wedding. In rural communities, babies are born within the mother's tent, in her own mother's compound, with elderly female relatives attending.

There are also many pregnancy-related precautions. Hadia observed: "During pregnancy, women should avoid bitter medicine [from tree bark] and potatoes and coffee, which cause *tuksi*. Mountain plants are good to eat; and acacia bark and leaves, as well. Many women have problems during pregnancy here because of *tessmut*, cold, which attacks the bladder." On her own first pregnancy, she felt fear. Her first birth was easy, however.

Many believe that women are most vulnerable and fragile when they have just given birth and also during childbirth itself, when the ground is believed to open up and form a grave. In the countryside, infant mortality is approximately 60 percent. Spirits are believed to sometimes mistake babies for goat-hide water bags and try to pull them back into the spirit world. Efforts therefore must be made to protect mothers and keep newborns in the world of humans. When a woman goes into labor, she and the unborn child enter a dangerous threshold state. The earth remains wide open until the birth of the child. The Old Woman, Waddawa, the elder among the spirits of the wild, rises from the earth and sits nearby, threatening serious illness or death to the mother and child. During childbirth and for six days that follow until the name day, mother and baby are therefore in a liminal state (Worley 1992).

Dynamics of Menstrual and Post-Menstrual Cosmology in Relation to Herbal Medicinal Practice

Local concepts of the life course are, nonetheless, not strictly linear, chronological, or biological. Rather, these phases are socially and ritually defined in ways not always in accordance with Euro-American chronological notions (Rasmussen 1997). For example, females are considered to "become women" at marriage, rather than upon menstruation; and males are considered in need of being made men and then become marriageable upon taking up the men's face-veil, at approximately eighteen to twenty years of age. Adolescents of either sex, but particularly women, are believed to be vulnerable to the jealousy of spirits and humans at life transitions.

Thus women and men are considered full jural and social adults only upon marrying and, more importantly, becoming parents. Informal adoption is often practiced in cases of childlessness, but rituals promoting fertility convey the importance of having children, and eventually, children-in-law (Rasmussen, 1997), who are important to old-age security. Sons-in-law contribute economic resources to their affinal household through bride-wealth and groom service. There is an extreme respect/reserve relationship between a man and his parents-in-law, particularly the mother-in-law.

"Menstruating" vs. "no longer menstruating" women are nonetheless recognized as socially salient categories, though primarily defined as social and ritual statuses that do not always correspond to literal biological processes. Local residents describe these age categories and transitions in terms of social and ritual roles as well as physiological processes. Hadia observed: "A woman's illness after she is unable to become pregnant was called *akarambarza*, or turning of the stomach. On getting old, there is no more need for adornment, due to the importance of prayer. The age menstruation stops depends on the number of children and the woman's own limits, and her health in general. When menstruation stops, this is not good; there is a lack; one has less strength than before."

She added, "during menstruation, a woman should not wash; if she does, she gets sick, has no sexual relations. She wears old clothes. She cannot pray or wear amulets or henna. While menstruating, a woman tends to get fat. On first menstruation, I told a good woman friend, but not my own mother because it is shameful. I was afraid, because I did not know what this was. . . . After she stops having children, a woman is free from these restrictions but is also less strong." Hadia also believed that the most important change from menstruation to no menstruation is increased respect.

Tina, a mediumistic medicine women with specialized divining powers, added insights here: "We seek an old woman healer because she is free and clean (*tazdag,* her periods have stopped). That is what our relatives (parents) do, one after the other. When menstruation stops, women are not sick. A few are, but not many. I treat all illnesses: cold *tessmat, alafaz* (sour blood, from a fall or a burden). I treat everyone. There are some illnesses that attack women and not men. Some women have problems with hemorrhaging. During childbirth there is sometimes much blood."

The Tamajaq term, *tamghart,* denoting "old woman," refers to women who have ceased to menstruate, as well as women who, while literally still of childbearing age, are classified as post-childbearing in their ritual and social roles (Rasmussen 2000). Transition from menstruating to non-menstruating status, while subtle and gradual due to frequent childbearing and breastfeeding, is nonetheless marked by tropes with both cultural and biological referents. Metaphorical post-childbearing roles therefore do not always coincide exactly with literal cessation of fertility. Nor, for that matter, it should be recalled, are childbearing roles exclusively organized in terms of "menstrual pollution." Yet there are clear expectations about the meaning of entering the post-childbearing phase of a woman's life. Two key local concepts serve as points of departure for this. The first is the local notion of "prayer," culturally opposed to "lack of prayer": the former describes post-childbearing status, while the latter describes menstruating, though not necessarily general childbearing, status.

As already noted, in several dialects of Tamajaq, terms for menstruation vary: *iban emud,* denoting "lack of prayer" (Rasmussen 1991; Bouman 2003); and *tamesgida,* denoting "mosque" (Figueiredo-Biton 2002:138). Some Tamajaq-speaking women also referred to menstruation to me as "woman's friend." Yet the issue here is whether the connotations are also different. Perhaps many researchers, including myself, have overlooked that these slang terms for menstruation may well be used, as in many cultures, as a kind of shorthand or even women's in-joke, among women used to refer to their condition, as for example, such English language terms as "George," "visitor," etc. In retrospect, these additional and contrasting slang terms for menstruation pose intriguing analytical challenges to interpreting the meanings of medicine women's and others' stated ideals of the "best healers as preferably no longer menstruating women." More revealing, perhaps, is that among themselves, I noticed women used a variety of these terms, even *ta jerga,* denoting "she is dirty"—suggesting that yes, indeed, there may be some degree of pollution perceived here, and by women themselves. Several medicine women, in fact, used this latter phrase to me. They also, as already noted, spoke of the need to be free of sin. Hence the complexity and ambiguity of meanings of these associated ritual restrictions, and the difficulty of positing either the absence or presence of clear-cut "pollution and purity" beliefs in Tuareg menstrual and post-menstrual cosmology.

For many herbal medicine women with whom I conferred, however, "prayer" clearly evokes the absence of menstruation—at least metaphorically if not literally. Since many women are defined as socially and ritually post-childbearing even if they are still menstruating, once their children are of marriageable age or married, the physiology of menstruation or its cessation is less important than its metaphoric elaboration in the experience surrounding a woman's social and ritual status as "elderly" or "post-childbearing"—in particular, in herbal medicine practice. As shown, older women in general are integral to performing many rites of passage, and medicine women are important in managing fertility, birth, and wellness in life. At any rate, the point here is that "mosque," "full of prayer"/"lack of prayer," and "dirty" all refer to a combination of ambiguous, situational physiological processes and social/ritual roles. These concepts and terms implicitly convey ideas about, not just childbearing and menstruation, but more crucially in the case of medicine women who are ideally older, what it means to become symbolically defined as old or "no longer menstruating," even if one is not literally so. Many women are culturally defined as post-childbearing by virtue of their position as actual or potential mothers-in-law upon the marriage of their children (or adopted children). Medicine women in effect act as icons or paragons of these statuses: as quintessential mothers, grandmothers, ancestors, and mothers-in-law.

These ideas are further illuminated by another phrase used to describe women who no longer bear children. Medicine women explained that physically, women are "rinsed clean" after having their last child. Men and women alike linked the folk exegesis of the term for last-born children, *iliuwaten (alilui,* sing.), with the verb "to rinse." Women friends indicated explicitly that upon cessation of menstruation, they felt "diminished" or "lessened" in physical strength, depleted by childbearing. Children "use up" the mother's menstrual blood, from which they are formed. However, the women also recognized increased social status and respect, in their view derived from post-childbearing women's greater participation in religious (pre-Islamic as well as Islamic) rituals and from the marriage of their children (Rasmussen 2000).

Local cultural definition and elaboration of becoming "old" in older women's public conduct, and of the physiological processes underlying the end of fertility, are interrelated. However, these definitions and interconnections entail more complex associations than a structuralist analogy such as "prayer" is to "menstruating" as "lack of prayer" or "mosque" is to "no longer (culturally) menstruating." Yet ritual restrictions are important, and medicine women play key roles in guarding them.

Some medicine women, for example, observed that their medicines will not be effective if given to a woman who has sexual relations with her husband; during many treatments, then, there must be abstinence from sexual relationships. Medicine women did not reveal to me (perhaps from reserve) whether or not they, too, needed to abstain from sex themselves during their treatment of others, an additional restriction noted among Navajo female ceremonial healers by Trudelle-Schwartz (2003). There is no strict taboo against Tuareg medicine women being married. I found that smith women (who tend to be less reserved on sexual matters) revealed to me that they should not dress a noble woman's hair or manufacture leather amulet cases for clients during the client's or the smith's menstrual period. This and the foregoing restrictions suggest that there may be some sexual restrictions surrounding medicine women's healing that were not always explicitly articulated. It was also unclear whether all medicine women had literally ceased to menstruate; for they stated, in more social terms, the ideal for them to wait until they were "older" and their mentor had authorized them or had died, for full professional practice independent from their mentor. Since literal chronology and physiology are not the sole yardsticks of age, and since many women who still menstruate are defined as social or ritual "old women" when their status changes upon their children's marriage, menstruation itself may not be the central criterion but rather may be mentioned as a kind of metonym for wide processes.

Medicine women's practice, while metaphorically associated with transformations over the life course, is not dependent upon literal physiology or precise, linear transitions or chronological age. This idea conforms to more general local cultural concepts of the life course and aging. Many older women's increasing participation in religious rituals—pre-Islamic as well as Islamic—does not stem solely or simplistically from their literally non-menstruating state, but rather from metaphorical extensions of this state, from their more generally increased social status with advancing age and experience. Participation in religious rituals, in particular rites of passage, becomes much more important for women later in the domestic household cycle, when children reach marriage, than during their childbearing years. Researchers have reported a similar occurrence among other Islamic peoples (Abu-Lughod 1986; Delaney 1988; Mernissi 1987). In this light, medicine women appear to be expected to inspire other women with their exemplary conduct in their own life transitions. Tuareg women in effect become exaggerated social and ritual mothers upon their assumption of culturally defined post-childbearing status. Herbal medicine women model or embody these roles and guide other women through these transitions. They and the ancestresses lead the way, so to speak.

Upon their children's marriage, women are culturally "old," to convey their increased authority (Rasmussen 1997). While sexual relations and pregnancy are not exactly taboo after this event, it is nonetheless considered shameful to have more than about ten children. Hadia indicated that it is acceptable for mother and daughter to both be pregnant at the same time if it is the daughter's first child; if it is later, however, this is considered shameful because "the mother has a son-in-law with children, and these two persons would be ashamed at a name day to see each other." These situations are shameful because they reveal an excessive sexuality and lack of reserve; older women should ideally minimize sexuality and maximize reserve in public.

Medicine women's theories about the effect of childbearing upon women in later life show further how the physiological and the cultural are intertwined. Many explicitly connect ailments of some post-childbearing women to the effect of having given birth to several children, which they warn gradually causes increased vulnerability to illness. Here, medicine women are clearly advocates for women's health interests to men who, increasingly, pressure women to bear more children and earlier in life than considered healthy. Also recurrent in herbalists' explanations was the belief that menstrual periods maintain health. Several told me that, "Since menstrual periods give strength, one is less strong after they cease." Hadia commented that, "When menstruation stops, the health it brings also stops; for menstruation sweeps the body like a broom." Several other women who were healers as well commented, "Menstruation brings health and preserves strength, and once it ceases, the body weakens." Another stated, "Without menstrual periods, old age arrives and bends or folds the body, leading to additional problems. The strength and health that menstruation represents, and the resistance that it confers to such problems, cease upon menstruation's permanent ceasing." This seems connected to a local medical theory that menstrual periods anthropomorphically become children. Yet on another level, women are relieved of their "lack of prayer" status and in some respects, though not all, grow closer to men in their potential official religious participation. Yet, as Crapanzano (1980, 1992) notes regarding Moroccan circumcision, this transition varies according to context. Thus elderly medicine women become archetypal women: in effect, although they are now "dry" and "rinsed clean," they are also grandmothers, namers of babies, and potential ancestresses—protected from spirits threatening young women (who are "wet" and "open") and thus able to be closer to spirits and tame them. Women told me that children nonetheless are valuable, for "once they become adults and marry, while you diminish, your children grow and help through economic and emotional support."

Thus medicine women work to keep a delicate balance (though not an equilibrium) between sometimes opposed forces. They act at the nexus of male-female power struggles. In compromise solutions to tensions, they facilitate transformation of natural and cultural forces in ways that transfer powers between men and women, but they also sometimes appropriate or co-opt women's viewpoints and may threaten their long-term interests. In effect, despite the criterion of having in the past borne children themselves, herbal medicine women should ideally be distanced from their own biological childbearing in order to culturally help manage it in others. But they must be sufficiently close to childbearing in order to interpret it in ways constructive to the social order: they must translate and comment upon the wider social concerns of men and older women.

In other words, medicine women must strike a balance, somewhat like anthropologists, between objectivity and subjectivity. The injunctions by marabouts against young women gathering from trees on Mount Bagzan, which allegedly could render them infertile, emerges in this light as enjoining younger, non-herbalist women to preserve and transmit another kind of fertility and identity: of paternally traced kinship. As among the Beng (Gottlieb 1992:27), Tuareg in their cultural ideology do not perceive these spheres to be necessarily mutually exclusive or contradictory. However, in social and legal practice, these spheres sometimes can become the battleground for different agendas, of men's and women's conflicting viewpoints and interests in biological and social reproduction. This idea was corroborated in a somewhat different context by a (non-herbalist) woman working for a health agency, who commented during a discussion of family planning in Niger: "Islam does not necessarily restrict women's [reproductive] rights. But some men interpret it that way . . . as anti-women's [reproductive] rights." Medicine women, while perhaps aware of these contradictions, do not speak openly about them. Rather, one must look to the details of their practice and its wider constraints to illuminate their roles here, as in the next case.

A Long-Married, Childless Couple

These processes are clearly shown in the following story, of efforts to treat one couple's childlessness. Although as noted, Tuareg recognize that childlessness may sometimes result from the man's sterility, and men also seek treatment for it, nonetheless, childless women feel pressure, since some husbands respond to childlessness by contracting polygynous marriages. Men and women alike see herbal medicine women and marabouts when they are childless. But many women find marabouts intimidating and hesitate to see them unless medicine women refer them to marabouts, or husbands pressure them to do so. Women prefer to consult medicine women first when they have reproductive/gynecological problems. In efforts to conceive a child by a childless couple I have known since the early 1980s, both outside and local healers played a role, but herbalists and marabouts were more prominent over the long term:

One married couple, both friends and assistants of mine whom I'll call Amoumoun and Hadijiatou, graciously hosted me in a rural community during several research projects.[4] They married around 1986. He was from a noble and chiefly family; she was of mixed descent, with some Tubu ancestry. Although oasis gardens have been in the Aïr region for several centuries, and Amoumoun's father had formerly owned a garden where clients had worked in the past, the families were nomadic herders before the late 1970s, when drought in the region had compelled many to settle down and mix subsistence patterns. Like many in that region, Amoumoun came to practice a combination of herding, gardening, and labor migration. As a young man before his marriage, Amoumoun worked in Nigeria as a security guard at an embassy in Lagos. Later, he became active in local aid programs and cooperatives, and he also assisted me with many transcriptions and translations of oral art texts.

Hadjiatou had been among the first local girls to be educated in the *École Nomade* in the neighboring village. She recalled: "When I was about twelve, soldiers came to our small nomadic camp, announced, 'not enough girls are enrolled in school,' swept me up onto a camel, and led me to the *École Nomade* (Nomadic School).[5] I boarded nearby with an elderly woman, the maternal grandmother of my future husband. At first, I resisted and detested classes, but later, I started to enjoy school." A very bright student, she became proficient at French. Amoumoun was also one of the first Tuareg children to attend secular school, in another primary school established in the early 1970s in the area, and was also bright: he graduated first in his class and also attended Qur'anic school. His father was a prominent marabout related to local chiefly families.

By the early 1990s, Hadjiatou and Amoumoun had been married for about ten years, and the couple remained childless. During the first years of their marriage, there had been little concern, and many couples in such circumstances remain married and monogamous. Later, however, the couple became worried. In 1991, Amoumoun did not blame his wife directly for infertility, visited herbalists, and conceded that he himself might be at fault. But he began joking, in front of his cousins, that he would soon have to contract another, polygynous marriage to solve this problem. Another woman cousin joked back, referring to me, thus far also married but childless, and warned: "If you (Susan) eat with this man, you too, will remain childless!" This joke implied that childlessness may be contagious, through eating: an allusion to the central symbol of the stomach. It also expressed the local symbolic analogy between eating and sexual relations (for example, at weddings, smiths sing of "eating the meat of a fat cow," a positive allusion to a beautiful, healthy bride). Negative powers such as sorcery and spirit attacks causing childlessness may be transmitted through food and sex. But positive powers may be as well: Islamic *al baraka* blessing, for example, is believed to be conducted through saliva and semen.

Soon after these incidents, one evening as we prepared dinner, Hadijiatou worriedly inquired whether I had any medicine for conceiving a child. She also saw herbalists, although their treatment produced no effect. In 1992, Hadijiatou and Amoumoun traveled to the hospital in the town of Agadez, where she underwent a gynecological examination by Western-trained medical staff. Since Hadijiatou had some primary school education and spoke French, and her husband had previously worked for an international NGO livestock aid program, she had experienced somewhat greater contact with outsiders than most women in her rural community. Perhaps for these reasons, Hadijiatou submitted to an exam at the hospital, which many other rural women shunned. But she complained to me that the nurses and doctors there "were not nice to Tuareg from the countryside" and that "their medicines (prescribed) were too expensive." The hospital at Arlit, a mining town to the northwest, was reputed to be a better place. But the couple did not go there, since this was farther away and the route was at the time dangerous, due to banditry and fighting in the region. The Agadez Hospital examination did not reveal anything conclusive.

During the rainy season of 1995, Amoumoun saw several herbalist medicine women, and several diagnosed him as having a "cold" illness called *tessmut*. One treated him with herbal remedies, steeped into tea she instructed him to drink at home, adding that he should not bathe for ten days during the treatment. Amoumoun also saw another, more elderly herbalist, Hadia, with whom he had a lengthy discussion in private, during which she questioned him closely about his state of health and his relationship with his wife. Afterward, Amoumoun again expressed concern about the couple's childlessness and now indicated that he himself was "in good condition."

About ten days after Amoumoun's consultations with the herbalists, he arranged for a marabout, Eliman, to visit their home and conduct an examination diagnosing the cause of the couple's childlessness, followed by a ritual cure. Eliman arrived in the morning to perform the Qur'anic divination techniques *itran* (literally denoting "the stars," similar to the horoscope) and *alekhustara*, involving taking measurements of the patient and consulting Qur'anic verses, and to sacrifice a goat of Hadjiatou's as alms. Amoumoun gave an advance payment of 20,000 CFA (about US$80) to the marabout. First, Eliman calculated numbers based on Hadjiatou's and Amoumoun's names. He spat three times on the measuring cord. He then measured Hadjiatou's forearm length and also her waist with the cord. Then he calculated in the sand. He felt her ankle. The cord measure became longer. The marabout explained, "This means that the woman is less than fertile. This (infertility) is caused by a blocking from pills and also from spirits who are against children. Because of them, her condition is diminished and lacking."

The marabout then sacrificed the animal. This had to be a young, white male goat of Hadjiatou's, and its meat had to be eaten by the family and marabout at once. The meat must not dry, or this undoes the treatment. In three days hence, the patient would drink Qur'anic verses written in vegetal ink by the marabout. This writing must be on a tablet never before used. Later, the couple would eat three soft-boiled, shelled eggs (one and a half each) with the same writing on these eggs as on the tablet. This would have to be repeated three more times at intervals afterward. If the treatment was successful, the couple would give the marabout 1,200 CFA (about $6) more later.

The marabout butchered the kid goat with the assistance of Amo and a third party, a male friend of Amoumoun's, distantly related on the paternal side. The marabout took part of the meat home. The intestines and liver were cooked with a little fat in a pot over the fire; these were eaten first. They discarded the bladder, large intestine, and stomach contents. Hadjiatou would eat the lungs of the sacrificed kid goat. The women of the immediate household grilled the rest of the meat in the compound. These women were Hadjiatou's sisters-in-law, Amoumoun's sisters. The couple now resided next door to them and Amoumoun's parents, for they had moved away from her parents after the obligatory first few years of postmarital residence there.

As he was leaving, Eliman explained, "Childlessness or having few children runs through women in certain families; this is inherited. We (marabouts) must do a calculation *(lisafe)* to find out which ones." He also looked at me and briefly remarked that, "in the future, I would like to 'measure' you, Suzanne, as well, and perform some calculations to discern your own state of health." This remark, like the joking of Amoumoun's cousin, perhaps expressed a fear of contagion and underlined the need for mediators and facilitators to control ambiguous agents and powers, within and outside the maternal tent. Hence the blending of social, physical, and spiritual levels of treatment here.

Years passed. Still, Hadjiatou did not conceive a child. Although we both enjoyed friendship and respect in the community, women continued to sometimes tease both of us concerning our common childless condition: they warned us again to not eat with childless men. During a name day celebration, one woman regarded me gravely as we ate from the same bowl and slowly stated: "Amoumoun and Hadjiatou have not had a child. You have not had a child, either," and she solemnly reflected upon this. Thus local residents worried about all of us, unsure of the causal direction or precise etiology of our common affliction of childlessness.

Upon subsequent visits to the family in 1998 and 2002, I felt some tension between the husband and wife, though they remained married. Amoumoun continued to consult marabouts and herbal medicine women. Hadjiatou, likewise, saw a variety of healers. Adding to their preoccupations with individual childlessness were more collective concerns, in new dangers to the entire community. In 1997, there was an outbreak of post–Peace Accords fighting in Amoumoun's village between some former rebel factions and government militia when the latter accused local residents of sympathizing with rebels. The militia attacks forced many to flee into the mountains. The couple moved back to the small nomadic camp of Hadjiatou's own parents, on the foothills of the Bagzan Massif, where Amoumoun started a new oasis garden and occasionally guided tourists up nearby Mt. Bagzan on camel rides. For a while, Hadjiatou informally adopted a baby of a sister. Their compound was now much smaller, however, and their garden was flooded by unusually heavy rains in 1998. Subsequently, peace negotiations in Algiers settled the political conflict, though residents remained traumatized by the violence. Some children mistook my camera case for a gun holster. Others inquired anxiously, as I unloaded a suitcase from a truck, whether there were guns inside it. Amoumoun and Hadjiatou remained in their home in her village, although he frequently traveled to his own family's village to see relatives. His elderly father, now very ill, resided in their abandoned compound, pillaged in 1997 but now repaired—where he was cared for by his daughters and grandchildren next door.

Around 2000, after several years of alternating drought and floods in the Sahara but also relative political calm, international NGO aid agencies had returned to the region to start cooperatives in gardening, herding, and artisan work. Hadjiatou had lost some of her livestock and now owned only a few goats. She became responsible for distributing beans to local women in exchange for work around the village, including building fences. This program, funded by a German bank, also gave some money to the women. Hadjiatou also displayed some talent for tailoring; occasionally, she borrowed a relative's sewing machine, but this item was either stolen or broken during the 1997 militia attack. Later, I purchased a sewing machine for her as a present upon my departure in February 2002.

Despite her success and responsibilities, however, motherhood remained important, and Hadjiatou grew more and more distressed concerning her childlessness. Whether this resulted from her own wish for children, from her husband's pressure, or both, was not clear. During my most recent visit, Amoumoun indicated to me that he was now thinking of contracting a second, polygynous marriage. He said that he would install the second co-wife in his former compound in the other village, which was now at peace, nextdoor to his own relatives. Hadjiatou indirectly expressed concern about this tentative plan one evening, as she and I prepared wheat pancakes over the fire: she remarked, sadly, "You know, some women's husbands want to become polygynous." As I sliced onions, my eyes tearing a little (from the onions or perhaps the news!), I tried to comfort and encourage her, asking rhetorically, "but isn't it true that many Tuareg women oppose this and even divorce husbands who do this?" She replied, with some resignation, "Yes, but you know, after a while, they are so sad, that they take them back, even with another wife."

Discussion

Details of this couple's history reveal the complementary and mediating roles of healers but also show how their actions during consultations, diagnosis, and treatment marginalized the wife. Hadia's role here is a bit ambiguous, but there are suggestions that ultimately, she deferred to the men's definition off the situation, particularly during the later stages of this treatment (around the time of the marabout's consultation/treatment/ritual), which she did not contest. Initially, the cause of the couple's childlessness and responsibility for curing it (particularly by women in their popular "lay" or "folk" theories) had emphasized pollution/contagion, perhaps emanating from males, or even from another female, perhaps an outsider such as myself. Some women considered childlessness to be the husband Amoumoun's responsibility, but this burden later became transferred to the wife, Hadjiatou. Here, I interpret this as double-edged: on the one hand, the positive element was recognition of this woman's empowering responsibility for fertility; but on the other hand, the negative element was the assignment to this woman of blame for lack of fertility. Indeed, Hadjiatou was diagnosed by Eliman as "less than," implying lacking, short of something. The important question here concerns the consequences of these processes, still unresolved; as of this writing, in letters from the field, I have not yet learned news of either the birth of a child, or the contracting of a polygynous marriage, in this family.

Therefore interpreting this case in terms of "loss" or "gain" for women such as Hadjiatou, and women in general, remains partially open-ended, and it is difficult to predict future relations between this couple. However, herbalists' roles in this process are striking, and several patterns can be discerned. During one stage of this treatment for childlessness, Hadia the herbal medicine woman in her referral, in effect, enabled a redefinition of this problem and a redirecting of attention onto another causal agent: the wife. Hadijiatou, in effect, was placed "on the hot seat." Recall how Amoumoun had earlier been diagnosed by one medicine woman with a "cold" illness, a urinary tract infection, the suspected cause of the couple's childlessness. He had been dissatisfied with the earlier diagnosis, and also reluctant to follow her treatment, not wishing to refrain from bathing. He then sought a "second opinion" from the second elderly medicine woman, who clearly facilitated transfer of the cause of childlessness to his wife, by referring him to the marabout.

In effect, the final divination/diagnosis stage of this treatment with Eliman the marabout provided a kind of closure, at least for the time being, for Amoumoun. It articulated men's interpretations of childlessness and their interests in reproduction, in their own "rewriting," mirror-image version of matriliny: fertility, but also infertility, are women's responsibility. It did not denigrate women, but did give their reproductive powers a possible negative face in attributing the withholding of children to them. This interpretation opened the path to possible displacement of Hadjiatou as sole wife, tent owner, and head of a single household, in possible future polygyny. This interpretation recognized women's bodies as the ultimate controlling agent, in granting or denying men children through the body as container. This is further expressed in Tuareg men's comparing the uterus to a leather sack. Women, it should be recalled, use different tropes for this: some equate it with the stomach *(tedis)*, also the symbol of the matriline, and others refer to it as "the child's tent (or place)" *(ehan n barar)*. Spirits "who do not like children," it is true, were also mentioned by Eliman in this causation; but these non-Qur'anic spirits are believed to be inherited through women and, as he added, "they run in women's families [i.e., the matriline]." This bodily imagery therefore expresses, in microcosmic form, wider tensions and struggles surrounding the maternal tent. In this universe, a variety of agents conduct either positive or negative powers. Some are on the periphery—forces outside the maternal tent—others are more central. These forces are contagious and inherited in different ways. They are not rigidly opposed but are part of a system of powers that is multicentered (Arens and Karp 1989). These powers are manipulated, reversed, and redefined in specified contexts to suit the interests of various parties, when identity and relatedness are in dispute.

"Children of the Stomach" and "Children of Men"

Many authors now agree that kinship among many Tuareg has been bilaterally traced for centuries, with vestiges of ancient matriliny combined with patrilineal institutions from Islam (Nicolaisen 1961; Murphy 1964, 1967; Bernus 1981; Spittler 1993). These systems are now being rearranged, redefined, and disputed. Many leaders of cultural revitalization and NGO aid programs in Tuareg regions often invoke the importance of women and matrilineal institutions in their speeches and even sometimes attempt to model some policies on this heritage. In some groups, for example among the Ifoghas and Kel Geres, there are more marked matrilineal traits, such as succession of maternal nephew to traditional office and stronger alternative inheritance forms for women. Among many maraboutique and *icherifan* clans, by contrast, there are stronger patrilineal institutions from the influence of Qur'anic law (Oxby 1990; Walentowitz in Claudot-Hawad 2002).

In general, inheritance occurs mostly before death. On marriage, women receive jewelry, blankets, a bed, other household items, and sometimes cloth and sandals. Women's personal property is passed down mainly from mother to daughter; men's, from father to son. The tent remains, in all but the most sedentarized and urban, and the most destitute and disenfranchised cases, important property and the residence of the married woman. Nowadays, in more sedentarized communities, increasingly one finds an adobe mud house, built and owned by men, alongside a woman's tent in the same compound. Upon a man's death, his house is not destroyed as is a deceased woman's tent, but is inherited, usually by a son. Although a woman has the right to eject the husband from her tent upon divorce, if he has a house in the same compound, there are often disputes over who remains there and who leaves (Rasmussen 1997).

The most valuable asset of the descent group has traditionally been livestock, although in some regions, gardens are also important, particularly since the 1984 drought, which decimated many herds (these latter are more difficult to replace than gardens). Most gardens are owned and worked by men, whereas herds are independently owned and managed by both men and women. Women have lost out in this decimation of livestock, with its consequent pressures toward sedentarization and more intensive gardening and migrant labor, since these remunerative activities involve predominantly men. There is increasing monetarization of bride-wealth; whereas in the past, bulls and camels rather than cash constituted bride-wealth. In this, women are at a distinct disadvantage because, with animals held in trust for them in the past, herds usually increased; whereas nowadays money is often spent by relatives and thus no longer provides older women with security.

Some Tuareg say, "It is the stomach that colors the child." Another source of shared maternal identity is breast milk. Possession by spirits not curable by Qur'anic verses is believed inherited matrilineally, from mother to daughter in breast milk. Many Tuareg believe that the maternal nephew inherits intelligence from the maternal uncle. But some others, such as the Kel Ewey in Aïr near Mt. Bagzan, do not use separate kinship terms for maternal vs. paternal nephew; they refer to both as *tegazay.* Brother-sister ties, prominent in myth, are also important in social life and sometimes benefit women legally. Brothers accompany sisters on distant or dangerous trips and sometimes defend their sister in disputes: one brother successfully assisted his sister, an older woman, in preventing her adult son from selling her bride-wealth camel.

However, over the long term, this concept of maternal kinship identity tends to be submerged and disputed in most legal practice. Qur'anic and patrilineal influences often extend to naming, ideas about children's affiliation and identity, and marriage. Most men refer to the offspring of a polygynous man and one of his co-wives as the "children of men." They tend to disparage an older form of naming of a girl as "daughter of *(oult* or *welet)*" as "only done with an illegitimate child," considered shameful, antisocial, and greatly stigmatizing to the mother. In most Tuareg groups, a child belongs to the descent group or clan of his/her father. Many men insist that the secret, Tamacheq name that older female relatives bestow on the child in the unofficial naming ritual is "not important; it means nothing," whereas many women argue that the latter is as important as the Arabic name from the Qur'an in the child's identity.

Women's "living milk" property, as noted, still viable but under considerable threat in the wake of droughts and war, on one level retains power because, as shown, this property is continually evoked throughout medicine women's healing. Recall how medicine women used this term *(akh huderan)* to describe their inheritance of herbal medicine as a profession and associated it with "women's property and secrets." In this association, therefore, medicine women preserve and transmit knowledge, material objects of the herbalist trade, and cultural and intellectual property, in the face of men's more Qur'anic-based legal property interests.

Yet the hard reality is that children of the stomach, from the time of Tagurmat's twin daughters, are sometimes pulled away by men, as embodied and enacted in the myth of the husband's murder of his pregnant wife. Upon divorce, young children go with the mother, but later, their father may claim them. In the matrilineal imagery of Tagurmat, there are oblique references to disputes over bride-wealth. A woman's bride-wealth camel is held in trust for her by male kin. Upon divorce, the marabout grants bride-wealth reimbursement to whoever he rules is not at fault, and most consider the woman at fault if she requests divorce on her husband's polygyny. For this reason, many women are reluctant to see marabouts about marital problems. Since property and inheritance issues are so closely connected to fertility and descent issues, this reluctance may also extend into seeing healers: it is likely that Hadjiatou was pressured by Amoumoun to see the marabout concerning this couple's childlessness.

Certain rites of passage over the household cycle—for example, the *taneqait* ritual (held when a married woman disengages her herds and kitchen from those of her mother)—in some regions are no longer done, because of fewer herds and greater sedentarization. An older woman now has less power to decide if her daughter's marriage is stable and whether the couple may choose to remain near her or leave and establish virilocal residence.

Therefore women's property of tent and herds has greater leverage in some situations than others: namely, in nomadism and during husbands' travel on caravan trade and migrant labor, and during years of sufficient rain and good pasture. In more sedentarized gardening oases, households become more patrifocal. Men at home stand as economic middlemen between women and the marketplace and tie women more to the home. Women may send their camels with male relatives on caravan, but unlike some other African women, Tuareg women did not until recently usually sell food snacks or conduct market trade directly.[6] Relevant here is Schlegel's insight (1972:5–6) that, in examining matrilineal societies, anthropologists need to address the allocation of authority and property in the domestic group. Factors such as sedentarization and postmarital residence affect attitudes about authority and power relations in the household. Men in positions of strength—in more sedentarized gardening households, and in residence next door to the husband's kin, such as Amoumoun—tend to give orders to their wives, and these wives also have more domestic work in processing grain.

In these conditions, medicine women's roles are contradictory, however. In some respects, they provide comforting continuity with the past legacy and represent a continuing viable force counterbalancing challenges to women's interests. In other respects, however, as shown in forthcoming sections, some medicine women's roles are being co-opted by wider authorities. Medicine women serve, in both their ritually commemorative and socially mediating roles during their healing, to move the physiological closer to the social and cosmological concerns. They seek to align the physical, the social, and the mythico-historical—and their medico-ritual work facilitates this process. While many older women tend to retreat from their roles as literal childbearers and take up roles as culture bearers (Rasmussen 2000), medicine women most prominently orchestrate this process as hyperbolic mother and grandmother figures. Over the long term, medicine women's treatments, while of course aimed to relieve very real physical suffering, also merge the ancestral and living experience.

On the other hand, in more immediate social and healing contexts, medicine women also depart from the roles of elders more generally: medicine women also provide a contrastive relief from the usual elders' reserved conduct toward youths, as shown in the earlier observations about their touching therapy. In the curing context, despite their more general reserve toward many youths, medicine women's touch of patients makes them more accessible emotionally. But they also must be somewhat distant in public contexts, since they also address a wider dilemma: guarding women's physical health seems to compete with the desire for many children to assist with adult work and provide affinal connections later. This problem constitutes the "subtext" recurrent throughout medicine women's treatments of women's gynecological problems and marital conflicts. But there is more at play as well. Conflicts—between matrilineal and patrilineal rituals and institutions, cognates and affines, spirits and humans, and illegitimate and legitimate—need mediators. Medicine women mediate between domains— they are close to Islam but also to the spirits of the wild; they are close to official marriage negotiations and weddings and naming, but also able to handle others' illegitimate children without risk of ritual pollution or social shame. Hadia, for example, raised one daughter's illegitimate child in the wild outside village centers. In much herbal medical healing, therefore, medicine women aid in reminiscence, evoking ideals in their cures, associating wellness with more general coping with problems of the life course. This mnemonic or commemorative role is of central importance in their work.

Implications

Many anthropologists now agree that female images are neither static nor universally uniform: they can be equated with rubbish (Strathern 1981), with nature in the sense of being outside and below culture (Ortner 1974, 1996), with evil (Hoch-Smith and Spring 1978), or with mystical beings that threaten men (Ortner and Whitehead 1981). In some cultures, women's qualities, substances, or essences are widely perceived as harmful to men

(Douglas 1966, 1996). On the other hand, men or their substances can also pollute, as among Kafe and Hageners of Papua New Guinea highlands (Reiter 1975). Thus it is not that women pollute men, but that all reproductive secretions are potentially polluting. Yet even this view can be, and has been, disputed (Buckley and Gottlieb 1988; Di Leonardo 1990; Gottlieb 1992; Goodenough and Sanday 1995; Brown and Kerns 1992; Rasmussen 1991, 2000) in post-structural studies recognizing that cultural gender symbols change with social and historical contexts. Both males and females in some contexts may become associated with good and evil, healing on some occasions and harming on others. In the Tuareg case, ritual extensions of the mythico-historical matrilineal ancestresses defend against the challenges to women from outside social, economic, and political forces but also remind others of the potential for violence between the sexes in the killing motif.

I am well aware of the problem of romanticism or essentialism of "women's healing" or "women's science," as in some feminist standpoint theory (Harding 1987), which implies that there are uniquely "female" approaches to problem-solving and the science of healing. I also seek to avoid reiterating classical anthropological structuralist oppositions—for example, between public and domestic or nature and culture. Hence my caution here in assigning Tuareg medicine women to an exclusively "women's science." I agree with Jane Flax and Michaela Di Leonardo that gender relations have no fixed essence; they vary both within cultures and over time (Flax 1990; DiLeonardo 1990). Yet there is some salience to gendered aspects of Tuareg herbal medicine since, as noted, although some Tuareg men also see herbalists, local choice of healers by sex is nonetheless significant, and local people do make some distinctions in healing according to gender. And mostly women see them, in actual practice. Thus I have attempted in this section of the book to identify the gendered and age-related assumptions on which herbal medicine women's healing is based. Tuareg women's healing power comes through negotiating contradictions, not fixed oppositions, in wider Tuareg society. As such, they have much to teach anthropology concerning ways to revise, yet also salvage, the best of structuralist and post-structural worlds of meaning. Medicine women, in effect, cross over between tent, village, camp, and wild; and for many more nomadic women, the "domestic" household has always been very elastic, extending into the pastures and mountains well beyond the tent, camp, and village. Also, medicine women treat organic and nonorganic illnesses, and their administration of herbal infusions involves much more than solely pharmacopoeia; it also includes advice on lifestyle, diet, and interpersonal relationships.

Herbal medicine women therefore facilitate communication and transformations, and they address and negotiate conflicts and contradictions. Like their herbal recipes, their actions combine, reinterpret, and negotiate important cultural themes. Their science is not, in other words, merely "a science of the concrete" (Levi-Strauss 1962), but neither is it neatly or unambiguously "our science." It occupies a unique space in between these categories: neither "African" nor "Western," neither quite male nor quite female "science" or problem-solving. This positioning may not completely resolve, but still, it hopefully remedies the problem, noted recently in African studies and African philosophical study (Karp and Masolo 2002), of tendencies toward either allocating African modes of thought to an exaggeratedly "exotic" contrast to our own, or, in the other extreme, implying there is nothing distinctive about them at all.

Thus medicine women are simultaneously mothers and professionals. Some literature in feminist anthropology has tended to assume these are mutually exclusive roles, reflecting a cultural bias toward compartmentalizing these roles and a view that motherhood is somehow limiting (Chodorow 1974). Other literature tends to assume that female healers' success depends solely upon their extension of maternal roles (McClain 1989). The question here thus becomes, would Tuareg medicine women be equally successful if not surrounded by maternal imagery? In the past, many women in Euro-American culture cooked at home, but most famous chefs tended to be men; in the Tuareg case, by analogy, the problem is, to what degree is medicine women's professionalism detached in come contexts from their literal mothering roles? Here it is necessary to distinguish between medicine women's ritual and mythico-historic symbolic roles and their technical healing roles in actual process and practice. Even their symbolism is not unitary or one-dimensional, as Wood (1999) observes concerning older males who ritually "become women" among the Gabra. On the one hand, herbal medicine women express the female model in symbolism of ancient matriliny; on the other, this symbolism is not always consistently isolated or opposed to other models in contemporary Tuareg culture but rather is intertwined with them. For example, some herbal medicine women enact Islamic symbols and rituals, and some also work closely with state and NGO–sponsored biomedical personnel. Yet there are also some tensions between these roles and systems, explored later. In the countryside, at least, medicine women's position does not suffer diminished status from treating predominantly women and children, and furthermore, as noted, they treat some men as well. Men, too, express confidence in them, though their treatments more explicitly address women's problems. In a later chapter exploring medicine women's relation to wider authorities such as staffs trained in Western established biomedicine in the towns, there is some evidence that their authoritative knowledge faces greater challenges.

Medicine women's commemorative or mnemonic role is further illuminated in the substances and spaces of their work, which are imbued with great powers in local cosmology, the subject of the next two chapters (6 and 7). Their socially mediating role is further illuminated in the subsequent three chapters (8, 9, and 10).

6—Natural Imagery (Arboreal Tropes) in Herbalism

Plant Uses in Nature and Culture

I did four years of apprenticeship. In apprenticing, first I offered alms *(takote)*, and afterward I went on to practice. I gathered, also. Some trees, you must arrive by them and pour the offering on them. Sometimes, one circles the alms around the sick person that one treats with the trees' medicines. Me, I practice medicine that is steeped in water *(adir-adir)*; I do not cook it. I treat *lama* [an illness when the body is heavy], I make small cuts and prepare barks, which I have the patient steep in water like a tea and then drink. I do not practice the entire medicine "pot," though I know it. I do not touch, except I do sometimes give a special massage, the type that pulls the body *(arakab*, a special massage to reset a dislocated liver). I also do some standard massage *(arabaz)*.

I received authorization four years ago. I obtained authorization from my father's older sister, Lala. When she gave it, there was no need of a test. She only increased my understanding and prevented me from doing something wrong. She pronounced all the names of the trees. Now we [Tuareg] have multiplied. Before, people of the past did not live as long. Now some persons do development. We have an old grandmother (the Tamajaq term that Tanou used here was a kinship term, *aya*). We are her children. She was named Aya. I have no news of her now. A good herbalist knows what Aya taught. She who does good medicines is healthy and certain, she does not always need to be elderly. As soon as I see someone, I know he is ill. But I am not a diviner. I bring my children to see old Lala, or all those who come to be touched [i.e., Tanou refers patients needing touch to Lala, who knows this skill better]. . . . After Lala touches to diagnose, she refers some patients to me. I treat, for example, for illness from a fall, *alafas,* I use *mananad* (leaves and seeds from Hausa regions). I treat a dislocated liver, hot illness *tuksi,* I also use barks that I find.

I am about forty years old. I do not touch in order to set bones [i.e., am not a *tamadas*]; I only make [tree] medicines. I do not do divination. I am Kel Igurmadan. I was born here on the Bagzan. In addition to herbal medicine work, I also do some harvesting work in the oasis garden and help with preparations of grains. I have five children. I have been divorced for six years. Those children who are grown, all are men. The girl is little.

Ten [Eng. pot, translated into French as *la marmite* (French)] is a generic term: there are different combinations and proportions of *ilaten* medicines in each *ten* used for different purposes. For example, one pot makes women fat. Women consume certain *ilaten* mixed with meat and stay home for several days in order to get fat. If a woman has the means, sometimes she even slaughters and eats an entire animal for this purpose.

Tanou, an herbal medicine woman on top of Mt. Bagzan, thus explained her work with herbal tree medicines. I did not attempt to elicit all ingredients or combinations used because some medicine women regarded these "recipes" as secret, esoteric knowledge. I only recorded those specific plants and combinations given me by those who permitted me to write about them. Also, I wished to reassure a few medicine women who were concerned that I did not seek to steal or sell their medicines.[1] Besides, Latin terms were not available for all these tree species. Trees and other medico-ritual paraphernalia of Tuareg herbalists certainly have botanical properties; they are not solely cultural objects. Yet they are not solely instrumental in healing either, but also operate expressively as well as botanically and pharmacologically, to powerfully symbolize concerns of living and deceased, past history, and contemporary society. The total *ten* repertoire consists of approximately one hundred trees.

Each herbal medicine is often a combination of different plants or parts of plants; and herbalist healers mix their own recipes and pass them down in their family, camp, or village. This pharmacopoeia has significance extending into myth, history, cosmology, and ritual in ways that validate medicine women's authoritative knowledge. Moreover, the prevalence of medicine women in certain clans in areas with mountains and trees is not completely explained by ecology alone; for as observed, many women emphasized to me that, "although there are many trees on Mt. Bagzan, they are not the sole reason *tinesmegelen* do medicine; rather, they do medicine because of their inheritance and their character. . . . Also, Mount Bagzan is believed to be 'blessed' with medicines; it has a special benediction on its land."

Medicine Trees as Symbols of Life and Herbal Medicine Women as Protectors of Life

Although the Sahara is a different world altogether from another part of the world where there is an abundance of herbal medicine—the Amazonian rain forest—nonetheless, trees, though rare and sparse, exist in parts of the Sahara and are central to local concerns. Their shade and coolness are sought after. They provide shelter from the harsh sun and medicines for a variety of illnesses of humans and livestock. Some livestock, in particular, goats, are fed with tree products. Some women's Tamajaq names derive from plants: for example, Rinkidan is plural for a large bush with lots of branches. Tabaidot denotes an herb species. In more nomadic groups, men, upon being ejected from a woman's tent in a quarrel, sometimes temporarily "camp" beneath trees.

Tuareg herbal medicine directed my attention to another relevant issue: to which symbolic ends have trees been used? As Rival observes, trees and wood are widely deployed as social symbols (Rival 1998:xiii). In Tuareg herbal medicine, trees are deployed as symbols of transgenerational continuity. Tuareg medicine women offer a local cultural variation on a widespread human theme: the vitality and power of self-regeneration of trees, central in rituals, medicines, folk tales, myths, and poems. They are tropes of semiotics of space and time. In this chapter, therefore, I explore the symbolic significance of trees. I draw on, and hopefully constructively critique, anthropogical studies of ways in which natural processes are conceptualized and the natural world is classified, and ways in which humans interact with their natural environments and use natural resources (Rival 1998:1).

Long debated in anthropology is the broader issue of how cultures as symbolic systems derive meanings largely from natural elements (Rival 1998:1; Durkheim and Mauss 1963[1903]). Anthropologists have pondered the social origin of human representations of natural categories, as well as the emergence of accepted "objective" natural history. Herbal medicine women's practices contribute to theorizing interactions between human societies and their natural environments. While much anthropological writing deals with animals, landscapes, and domesticated crops, there is less attention to trees per se. Tree symbols open up perspectives, not solely on herbal medicine, but more broadly on the interconnections among cultural constructions of nature, gender, and modes of thought. Trees provide some of the most visible and potent symbols of social process and collective identity. Medicine women reproduce, but not solely naturally or literally; they bring together natural and cultural elements. Like smiths, who convert nature into culture (McNaughton 1988; Rasmussen 1992, 1998b, 2001a), medicine women bring together disparate elements. Tuareg notions of nature and culture are not, however, diametrically opposed or discrete (Ortner 1974; MacCormack and Strathern 1980).

Tree symbolism reflects the more general human urge to express ideas through external and material signs, no matter what these signs might be (Durkheim 1976[1915]:127; Rival 1998:1). Durkheim described how Australian Aborigines carve, tatoo, and paint their totems. This desire "to translate thought into matter" led him to reflect on the relevance of externalization, materialization, and physicality in social theory and to conclude that "a collective sentiment can become conscious of itself only by being fixed on some material object" (Durkheim 1976[1915]:236). Material forms have social effects in their physical manifestation (Rival 1998:2). However, while material cultural studies tend to treat anything material as if it were object-like, as this chapter illustrates, the physical presence of a tree is not that of an artifact; a tree is to many medicine women and other Tuareg a living organism, albeit a superhuman, spiritual one.

As Rival (1998:2) points out, trees offer escape from such a dualistic frame. Trees and plants have social and metaphysical significance that does not seem to reside in drawing an absolute distinction between nature and culture, but on the contrary, in reaffirming the continuity of biological species within the living world.

Despite the persisting general importance of livestock herding, Tuareg medicine women are firmly situated in this "vegetal" world. Although they occasionally conduct animal sacrifice, the latter is done much more frequently by Islamic scholars and male household heads. Herbalists and their tree medicines break down the distinction between nature and culture. Trees are much more than mere background settings or functional means to herbal medicine women's work. They are intimately connected with their heritage, both in the bilineal social system of healing knowledge transmission and in the cosmological system of spirits and ancestors. Trees, moreover, in much local folklore stand metonymically for particular historical events and cultural values, act as witnesses to deeds, and serve as points of orientation—not solely in literal geographic travel, but also in psychological and symbolic internal quests. Trees are therefore part of the literal and imagined landscape.

The tree in Tuareg communities represents humidity and moisture, a symbol of life (Ag Solimane 1999:67). Yet trees do much more than form a natural category, background, or life-form. Trees are used symbolically to make concrete and material the abstract meanings in life. Trees are ideal supports for such symbolic purposes precisely because their status as living organisms is ambiguous. Among Tuareg, they have superhuman, spiritual attributes and powers; specifically, trees are the locus of matrilineal ancestral spirits and some Kel Essuf spirits of the wild. As Rival observes, tree symbols revolve around two essential qualities, vitality and self-regenerative power (Rival 1998:3). They are life-affirming and death-denying cultural representations. Here I explore how medicine women work with trees, beyond the obvious fact that they yield herbal plant medicines. While clearly, their medicines are significant, there is more at play here than their leaves, bark, and roots as *ilaten*. Trees have ritual value for additional reasons. I argue that trees are not merely artifacts or even merely "props" or paraphernalia; they are essentially cultural and historical.

The ritual focus upon tree spirits and "enchanted" *(al hima)* land among the Tuareg also evokes the sacred and *al baraka;* I pursue these latter concepts in connection to herbalism in another chapter. Here, I explore ways in which trees illuminate herbal medicine women's work. Trees in myth and ritual in effect commemorate important cultural values and aspects of historical and social life. As among the Uduk (James 1988:303; Boyer in Rival 1998:90, there is among the Tuareg the anthropomorphic idea (most likely from pre-Islamic cosmology and mythology) that certain trees can participate in conversations. Indeed, part of wood's property is to absorb sounds and other signals. The point here is that tree symbolism shows not so much a transfer of intentionality onto nonhuman living organisms, but, rather, "a need to find within the natural environment a material manifestation of organic processes that can be recognized as similar to those characterizing the human life cycle, or continued existence of social groups" (Rival 1998:7). Life cycle rituals make extensive use of trees. Among the peoples of Nusa Penida and Bali (Giambelli in Rival 1998), coconut palm is the central ingredient of birth, marriage, and death rites.

How do Tuareg conceptualize growth and life in their very different environment of desert and mountains with few, but nonetheless very important trees, dominated by the acacia and various palm species? Not surprisingly, water is a more pervasive natural image. For example, a Tamajaq proverb states: *Aman iman* ("Water is life"). Yet trees also receive much ritual and mythical focus. Until recently, a widowed or divorced woman who was obliged to undergo three months of *ida* (sometimes called *al ladat*) or seclusion from men could circumvent this rule by making an offering to a tree, begging it to release her from this restriction and allow her to remarry sooner. Medicine women suspend the clothing of sick patients in trees in order to metaphorically take away their illnesses. Many herbal medicines are supposed to be administered beneath or in the shadow of certain trees in order to be effective. Herders often suspend a goat carcass from a tree to ward off jackals from herds.

Date symbolism is also prominent: dates act as amulets, tomb offerings, and a source of blessing. Women sometimes inherit date palms as living milk property. In regions where trees and palms are more numerous, fibers from palms and wood from trees are used in everyday implements and buildings; smiths, for example, manufacture axes, spoons, and ladles from wood; women and elderly men make basketry from palm fibers; and women build wooden frames for tents and in some regions, mats from doum-palm fibers for tents. Their central posts, alluded to in women's songs, support the female-owned tent and by extension, the matrifocal household during men's absence on caravan trade, labor migration, and battle. The wood for tent frames is obtained by the bridegroom from smiths attached to the marrying family. Over the life course, there is imagery comparing an aging human to a wooden canopy frame, with its supports gradually giving way (Rasmussen 1997). Even in the Sahara, therefore, trees have symbolism as resonant as the symbolism of water, wells, grasses, pastures, rocks, and earth. Many healers indicate they communicate with and receive instructions from tree spirits while gathering leaves, roots, and barks.

In Tuareg rituals of gestation, birth, and growth, there are both animal and vegetal substances used. Uses of vegetal substances (for example, millet and dates) have feminine connotations, whereas uses of meat (animal sacrifice and grilling of meat)—despite herding by both sexes—have masculine connotations. In rites of passage, these elements are complementary: at the baby's name day, for example, during the women's naming of the child, the dates, millet, and goat cheese that elderly female relatives carry are said to confer *al baraka* upon the child. Animal and plant substances are also offered as alms to guests at memorial feasts for the dead. Hence the complex symbolic uses of trees and other natural materials and places in the landscape in Tuareg society, structured as it is by hierarchical ranking, but cross-cut by relative gender equality in the contemporary bilateral system.

There are analogies between the human body and trees, as well as other natural phenomena such as mountains, which are anthropomorphized in local folklore. Some mountains are referred to in myths as kin to each other, for example, brothers and sisters. Trees are not seen as hermaphrodite, but rather, tend to be more often feminized with matrilineal spirits: many bush and tree names in Tamajaq are in the feminine form. Trees in mythology and poetry stand for families and other social groups, namely descent groups, clans, and various occupational strata. Tree spirits in myth and ritual evoke mother-daughter and brother-sister ties. For example, trees in some tales give directions to brothers searching for a lost sister or vice versa, to a sister searching for lost brothers.

Trees are ritually opposed to metals (for example, iron and weapons). Medicine women say that trees "do not like" iron (hence their taboo against gathering medicine with an ax) but "prefer" rocks or clay (hence the preference for cooking herbal medicines, by stricter adherents at least, in a clay pot). Yet in contrast to other more sedentary African farmers, many Tuareg tend to shun NGO efforts to plant trees and erect fences, and trees are not a central feature of Tuareg villages or camps, in the same sense as, for example, the Kapok tree is among the Beng people described by Gottlieb (1992). Some Tuareg, moreover, are suspicious of efforts by such agencies as *Eaux et Forets* (Waters and Forests) to restrict and demarcate certain forested areas. By contrast, they pay more heed to local marabouts' proclamations designating small forests or groves as "sacred" lands because these are associated with prominent past holy persons, such as founding marabouts.

Fernandez (in Rival 1998) argues that in many societies and cultures, trees express health and vitality. The empirical world gets symbolically elaborated and is used in the creation of moral orders and moral communities. Tree symbolism helps give meaning to social life and "facilitates the imagining of corporate bodies full of vitality" (Rival 1998:25). More broadly, "common sense" is intrinsically symbolic because it is rooted in experience, in perceptions that are both phenomenal and sensible (Rival 1998:25). Hence the blurring of distinctions between everyday knowledge and specialist ritual knowledge and representations. Tuareg herbalism ritual and myth construct moral communities through the personification of tree tropes.

Levi-Strauss (1962) has pointed out that animals are good as tools with which to think about human society. This applies to plants, as well. Yet these classifications are not arbitrary differences but depend on the recognition of what is known and shared between animals, plants, and humans (Bloch in Rival 1998:40). Tuareg culture, like many others, greatly dwells on kinship and mutual dependence between animals, plants, and humans. Among the Tuareg, despite or perhaps because of their desert environment, the role of sheltering trees in ritual and symbolism is prominent in healing both organic and nonorganic illnesses, above all in spirit possession songs and in herbal medicine women's healing. It is also prominent in traditional and modern Tamajaq and other Berber poetry.

Sheltering tree images are centrally relevant to medicine women's commemorative role, for they embody so much about the way many Tuareg identify with their desert and mountain home, and so much concerning their feelings about gender and healing realms. As Rasmussen (1995) observes concerning Tuareg spirit possession, natural features in possession songs embody Tuareg feelings and sentiments because of their intimate connection with the transitions from tent to wild and natural world and spirit world, and back again to the social/cultural world, in exorcism processes. Like birds for the Kaluli (Feld 1982), trees for the Tuareg are ideal mediators because they embody the existence of spirits as well as expressions of protection and sheltering so central to ritual and healing concerns. Thus they evoke a profoundly emotional response. Most prominent poetic images derive from pervasive (though not consensual or monolithic) cultural values that remain meaningful to many Tuareg. These include idealized brother-sister ties, beliefs concerning twins, and enduring mother-daughter ties. These values are expressed in themes of searching for sheltering trees in the desert and for lost kinspersons, focused on the desired state of emotional support from the maternal tent and fear of abandonment or lack of support. Social relations are also expressed in themes of lost kin and trees used as markings of territory and guidance in orientation. Natural arboreal features and places in the terrain appear in sung poetry, acting as models of balance and social mediation for men and women alike. For example, there are widespread aesthetic themes of searching for shelter, and the tree branch trope, *azel* or *fage,* is a metaphor for song.

These arboreal themes, found throughout folklore and other expressive domains of Tuareg culture, are paralleled in medicine women's practices. Hence the complementarity between medicine women's ideology and practice and other domains of culture, which, though submerged in some contexts of everyday life, become highlighted in medico-rituals and mythology. There is a continuum in medicine women's herbalism between art, science, religion, and "magic" forms of power. Therein resides the continuing power of medicine women's art/science work, which breaks down some Euro-American cultural notions of the art/science split. Medicine women are artists, ritual specialists, and scientists all at once. They face the challenging task of protecting women's interests in communities where these are increasingly subject to debate.

Tree Symbols in Ritual and Song

Many songs performed at the ritual spirit possession exorcism ceremonies, to which medicine women frequently refer patients, make connections between geographic spaces and the sheltering tree symbolism of herbalism and pre-Islamic spirits, relationships between women, and relationships between women and children. A drum pattern and title called *talawankan* was described metaphorically by my assistant as "swaying gently back and forth, like a tree branch moved by the wind" and characterized by a "sad, slow" pace. The women adepts confirmed this and connected it to their head dance of swaying back and forth.

In one *talawankan* song, the soloist encourages chorus and audience to support her in her singing performance: "I am alone / I am like a mother's orphan / This piece is *talawankan* / that Aujem dances / I am alone / I miss the young girls." Here, singers praise a renowned male dancer. Appeal is also made to maternal kinship ties in an image of being orphaned from a mother and missing the young girls of one's neighborhood. These images encapsulate the contradiction between courtship and mixed-sex festivals, on one hand, and parental ties and official marriage obligations, on the other, as well as problems many women face when they must choose between following their husband to remote work sites and leaving their female kin, or remaining behind; in either case, one misses distant loved ones, and this is another prominent theme in Tuareg poetry more generally.

In the verses of another *talawankan* song, natural arboreal images evoke the solidarity of uxorilocal residence in early marriage, as opposed to later virilocal residence and its obligation, for women, to leave close female kin. Recall that virilocality is now becoming more frequent earlier in marriage, upon sedentarization and men's planting of oasis gardens located farther from their home due to land shortages: "Oh, my self (being) says the Hausa / in his field / located alongside the well / My women 'twins' (whose husbands are brothers) / They have all left on travel / Some have gone to Emdigra / Others to Telwa / She (a camel) eats branches of the *atanin* tree / the *atanin* tree of Alawa region." Emdigra refers to an *oeud* (dried riverbed) with many trees where there is herding of livestock and gathering of herbs for sauce, plentiful in the Aïr region except during drought. The fruit of the *atanin* tree in the Alawa region is used in leatherwork tanning/dying. These images of place, particularly the arboreal tropes, provide the listener with an escape from recent ecological and economic problems of drought, experienced by men and women alike.

The reference to twins here refers to women married to the same brothers. *Anemelu* denotes both a literal twin and, in its plural form, can refer to pairs of brothers married to pairs of sisters. *Tanemelout* or *tanemilet* is the feminine term for a sister-in-law in these unions of two brothers married to two related women (sometimes cousins, but referred to as classificatory sisters). This is a marriage encouraged by many older women, particularly female cousins and sisters, in order to keep property in the family and provide women with greater support and companionship. Several brothers, drummers at the ritual where these songs were sung, were married to pairs of sisters. Here, this trope is connected to women's marriage, kinship, and residence, and also their nomadic and gathering activities.

In another song of this *talawankan* drum pattern, images refer explicitly to female kinship and relationships in connection with natural features and place names, marked by trees to orient and shelter: "Tomorrow / I shall leave in the evening / for a faraway country / My friends [female neighbors in adjacent compounds, traditionally also matrilineally related] / Repeat what I say / The *atanin* tree of Assadek / Under them repose / Four twins / Moussa and Assadek, Ata and Anourra / You, the girls / For the sake of God / Speak / Speak and applaud / My sister-in-law / Where is my Habsu? / I call my Chimo / Where is my Chimo?" Here the chorus and soloist address the solo singer's cousin, who is present, and appeal to women's mutual support networks. The phrase "twins in the shelter of trees" among Tuareg, as elsewhere in Africa (Arens and Karp 1989), has cosmological significance. In local belief, one must never hurt or offend a twin. In one Tamajaq tale, one twin snatches food away from the other twin sibling and is blinded, although the wronged twin later restores his sight through mystical powers. In this context, the possessed is compared to a twin who must be protected and sheltered from pain.

Songs with another drum pattern, called *idougdougan,* are preferred by many possessed persons because the rapid rhythm makes them dance vigorously and become tired soon. Exhaustion and falling to the ground are the objectives, indicating being cured of spirits. In pre-Islamic Tuareg cosmology, the ground is a place highly charged with significance: it is associated with Waddawa, the Old Woman (of the Earth) present during childbirth as the earth opens up and threatens the woman giving birth. People seldom pronounce her name directly, however, from fear this would activate her powers.

Verses from one *idoudougan* song are as follows: "Clap your hands and make the t-hum-a-hum (men's rasping sound in the throat said to imitate spirits) sound / and accompany me / (Refrain) / I am beneath an *agar* tree / of the village of Assaqamor." The *agar* tree is said to shelter spirits. Its wood is useful for implements made by smiths, its ashes and smoke protect from spirits, and its leaves are used by medicine women to cure that illness of the brain and respiratory system called *okouf.*

In another (untitled) song, there is allusion to a *techkout,* denoting a female slave and confidante of noble women in the precolonial social system, and to Amougai, the name of a nearly broken-in riding camel, very young and still slightly wild: "By God, I cannot be a slave of my village / She to whom one said to take the cord of the camel bridle / to lead the riding camel to meet the herd / Toward Abadayan, with the trappings especially attached to the camel from Arabs / Sadik, solid as a trunk of the *tegar* tree / The word of Sadik / is worth more than the fertile yellow female camel in value / By God, I cannot be the tree in the oeud / where Alhou and Maghrak rest / Two young people who resemble twins in their features." The camel praised here was taken from the Arabs in a victorious raid in the Algerian Hoggar. Here is a sense of nostalgia for past triumph and prosperity, defended against outside intruders and enemies. The Tuareg and the Chamba Arabs were traditionally enemies. The French colonial administrators manumitted slaves in the early twentieth century, and Tuareg subsequently forfeited their rights and resources from the trans-Saharan trade. The *tegar* tree yields very hard wood; here, the singer praises a man, Sadik, by comparing him to this tree's toughness. Implied here is endurance in the face of historic challenges to precolonial Tuareg social and economic bases of power, but more as well. *Tasakay* is a highly valued camel. The singer is also defending her own value, to be worthy of Sadik. And, as already observed, injuring a twin has dangerous consequences, for twins bridge natural and cultural domains. In this song, humans are given attributes from nature to convey physical and moral strength and to prevent loss.

Another untitled song continues these themes of solidarity in times of duress, through arboreal imagery: "My women friends, pray for me / So that my soul (life) does not leave on Wednesday / For the sake of God / I cannot become *atadan* or *ebizguin* tree / where two men Alghou and Amghak rest / these two twins / whose voices resemble each other / Last night when you were sleeping, me, I was not sleeping / Cares (worries) prevented me from this / Cares for young men." A transcriber assistant explained that many Tuareg believe that *iman,* soul or life, leaves the body and wanders in sleep as in death and during travel. Here the soul is in a sheltering place, protected from outside dangers and hardships. Medicine women explained that the *tadan* tree is feared; it is believed to shelter spirits, but its fruits are eaten. The *ebizguin* tree's cool leaves are chewed or inhaled as medicine for those *azni* blood illnesses, colds, and sore throats. Its fruits are a rich source of vitamins, often given to children. The soloist fears becoming a slave to men, using the metaphoric image of trees giving women shelter as they rest, and potentially, also, offering women remedies for illness or vitamins as sources of strength.

Similar themes appear in selections from a lengthy song called *Taraye Tetrema,* denoting "Road That Leads Toward the West": "I pray to God who brought me into the world / He who made the sun / (Refrain) / God who brought me into the world, and who will take me back to my country (village) / Takriaz, Agalal, Anou-migrin / (Refrain) / · Young girls of the Kel Tates group, may you protect me may you keep for me a life that is for everyone / (Refrain) / Have pity on someone in love / When it attacks, even the science of marabouts does not take it away / (Refrain) / Even the sorcerers of Kano do not take it away / Nor the Tubus of Kawar / (Refrain) / Nor those of Bilma, the Sougou people / The switches of love are numbered nineteen / The *aza* tree [with thorns and inedible fruit] and the *abaka* tree [with thorns and which bears fruit] which scratch the liver / (Refrain) / Like a burn from fire of straw mats / My soul / (Refrain) / Young girls with me, some have been reclaimed / Others have been sold for billfolds / Others have been sold for tobacco / (Refrain) / Others have said that I am not beautiful, that I am not pretty / (Refrain) / But I do not care about the regards of day and night / (Refrain) / Adoula who is of a pretty pale complexion and who made pretty anklets."

The *anage* tree is considered very beautiful. Sand dunes are sometimes said to be the abode of the Devil, Iblis. The song also refers to villages near Iferouan in northern Aïr, the Kel Tates, a group of Tuareg within the Kel Igurmadan descent group, and to neighboring ethnic groups: the Hausa of Kano and Tubu of Kawar, the latter said to be skilled at curing and sorcery. In local belief, love has nineteen switches that beat the one in love. The *aza* is a tree with thorns and inedible fruit; the *abaka* tree, also, has thorns, but yields good fruit, yet one cannot remove the thorns easily. Here is allusion to pain that wounds over the long term, despite more immediate pleasures.

Context of Time and Place; Trees as Shelter and Medicine and Tree Symbols in Mythology

The *agar, afagag,* and *tiboraq* trees have an extensive mythology. They are significant in pastoral nomadism, herbal healing, and divination practices. Medicine women sometimes treat a child's fever with a mixture of charcoal from the *agar (Maerua crassifolia)* tree, which shelters spirits, and onion pounded into a black powder mixed with water, and then smoothed over the body and face. Many Tuareg refuse to rest in its shadow or sleep at its base unless they have given its trunk a few ax blows to make the spirits harmless. Smoke from its wood is believed to cause blindness. But its powers may be focused in a positive direction also. A person who has been bitten by a rabid animal should climb the *agar* tree, which must then be chopped down, causing the spirit to leave (Nicolaisen 1961). The *afagag (Acacia raddiana)* tree forms large, nest-like clumps believed to hide spirits, and again, people should avoid sleeping beneath it. The *tiboraq (Balanites aegyptiaca)* is also believed at times to shelter spirits. Many fear its ashes and smoke but also use them as protection against spirits. Smith/artisans, to whom many nobles attribute demonic powers, manufacture ladles and axes from its wood.

All three trees described above have certain features in common. Their interiors are difficult to penetrate, and they have a tufted, hirsute appearance, suggesting dangerous powers hiding in their thickness. They are associated with spirits, madness, and danger, but also with creativity and natural/cultural transformations by medicine women and other specialists, such as smith/artisans, with pre-Islamic spirits, and matrilineal ancestresses. The possession song verses, drum patterns, and dance motions associate the solitary soul of the afflicted with spirits: the soul is said to be in the "wild," outside human habitation (Rasmussen 2001c). These natural environmental images pervade Tuareg verbal art; for example, they appear in a widespread folktale motif of lost siblings looking for each other.

Consider, for example, the following tale I collected from a group of women cousins as we sat inside one night huddling near a fire, weaving palm-fiber matting for tents, during the cold, windy harmattan season. This tale is entitled *Tellilen* (the name of a bird and also a woman's name, from *teylall*, denoting guinea hen, translated by local assistants into French as *la pintade)*. This tale contains prominent tree images which are personified:

A woman had seven children, one of whom was different (he had two tufts of hair). This woman was told: "When you have a daughter, you must beat the drum and give a great cry." When she had a daughter, she beat the *acanzam* (drums played by smiths to announce a birth) and gave the women's (ululating) cry. The other children left, they went to make camp. She, the daughter, was there, at her mother's, but they left. She asked her mother: "Well, mother, am I the only child that you have?" The mother replied, "No, you have your brothers seven, among whom there is one different from the others, with two tufts of hair. They went to pasture a long time ago." She (the daughter) went to follow them. She walked, walked, until she came to a tree called *tichghar*. She asked the *tichghar*, "Haven't you seen seven other youths, among whom there was one different from the others (with two tufts of hair, one on top and the other below?" She (the tree, fem.) told her: "Oh, it has been a long time, they passed by here nine months ago today." She walked, and walked, until she arrived at a tree called *abizgine*. She asked the *ebizgin*, "Have you, in the name of God, if you believe in God, seen seven children among whom one has two tufts of hair?" "They passed by here eight months ago." She walked and walked, until she arrived at the tree called *ezin*. She said, "For the sake of God, if you believe in God, haven't you seen seven other children, among whom there was one with two tufts of hair?" It told her, "They passed by here seven months ago today." She walked, walked, until she arrived at the *agar* tree. She asked, "For the sake of God, if you believe in God, haven't you seen seven other youths, among whom one has two tufts of hair?" It told her, "They passed by here six months ago." She walked, walked, until she arrived at the *aza* tree. She asked, "For the sake of God, if you believe in God, haven't you seen seven other children, one of whom has two tufts of hair?" It told her, "they passed by here five months ago." She walked, and walked, until she came to the *atise* tree. She asked the *atise:* "For the sake of God, if you believe in God, haven't you seen seven other youths, one of whom has two tufts of hair?" It said, "They passed by here from today, four months ago." She walked and walked, until she came to one *tagaye* tree (doum palm). She said to this tree (the doum palm): "Haven't you seen seven other youths, among whom, one has two tufts?" It replied, "They passed by here yesterday."

She walked and walked, until she arrived at their camp. No one was there. She prepared the meal and she ate, and then she hid herself. When they arrived, the meal was prepared. They said, "Well, who has prepared the meal for us?" The next day they went on another trip. She was once again hidden, came out, and prepared the meal. When they arrived (returned), they said, "Who has prepared the meal?" The next day, they told the one with two tufts of hair, "Hide. See who is preparing our meals." He hid himself. She came out, she prepared her meal. Then she was on the point of hiding again, when the son with two tufts of hair came out and caught her, and seized her. The others arrived, they embraced her, crying.

They placed her on a riding camel. They wandered until they came to a well. They prepared her decorated camel harness. They went until they arrived at a well. They put their bucket down into the well. Someone caught it, a devil (spirit) with a single fingernail. One of the brothers told him, "This thing, leave us [let us have] our bucket; we will give you a young cow." He said, "What do I want with a young cow?" "With a young bull, my father has one already and my mother has one already and I have one [already]." "You thing there, that catches us, leave us our bucket, and we'll give you a female camel with a dromedary." He said, "What am I to do with a female camel and a dromedary? My father has one, and I, myself, have one." "This thing, let us have our bucket. We will give you a fiancée who is on a pretty harnessed camel." He (the devil, spirit, *aljen*) let them have their bucket.

When he left them, they pulled and pulled, and drew up the bucket, until they had finished watering their animals. The spirit dug his fingernail into the knee of Telilan's camel on which their sister was seated, and they (the brothers) pulled at the camel, trying to raise the camel. They pulled, and pulled. The camel cried, he refused to get up. When they seized Telilan, she said to her brothers, "Leave me, leave me, I am torn, I am torn." They were there, until they became exhausted, they ran, and they came back. She said to them, "Kyaydara, Majila, you went, you abandoned me, woe unto you!" Once more, they returned, and tried to make the camel get up (from the well). She said, "I am torn, I am torn." They left her.

The spirit was there, he was there, he left, and he seized the girl. He told her: "What will you become for me, my daughter or my wife?" She told him to make her his daughter. Then he put her under the bed, he was a hunter. He came, he killed their meat. The spirit and the girl cooked their meat and ate it.

One day, a brother arrived (at the spirit's), and he hid himself under the bed. The spirit came (home) and put their meat on the fire. The pot said, "*Bidille, bidille* (vocables), there are two strangers under the bed." She said, "That is none of your business." The spirit asked, "That pot, what does it want?" She told him, "It wants us to take it off the fire." They took it (the meat), she ate it. He asked her, "Have you eaten well?" She replied, "No, I haven't eaten enough. Give me some more." She then passed some meat to the brother beneath the bed. Then she said that she had eaten well (she had given some meat to the brother under the bed). Then she asked the spirit, "My father, where are your souls, so that I may place mine with them?" He told her, "My soul is inside the horn of a moufflon that has a single horn."

The gazelles came to the well. They drank until the arrival of the moufflon with only a single horn. She took a little water, she looked here and there. They (the brothers) went to hide, the gazelles came to the well to drink. The brothers went and hid themselves, the gazelles came to the well to drink. Finally the moufflon with one horn came to drink. It drank a drop of water and looked here and there. He (the brother with two tufts of hair) hit it with a stick, the horn broke, the little box fell. He opened it, the spirit ran, saying "For the sake of God, you must leave me my soul, I will leave your girl, for God and his prophet." He caught at the hair and tore it, and the spirit fell.

They took their girl and left, until they arrived at a place where they made their camp. Finally they left, then they went off, they left her alone. She was in the camp. The crow came, she was taken away by some crows who placed her in their nest. When the brothers came back, Telilan was not there. He with the two tufts of hair, he walked, he gathered together his camels, until he arrived at a nest. He said, "My white camels are for Telilan, My red camels are for Telilan." She replied, "What is wrong with her, poor Telilan? She is in the crows' nest who just defecated on her and flew away." He arrived at the camp. He said, "I have seen Telilan today." They said, "That is a lie, a lie." He told them, "We will go, I am going to show you, if I have lied, you must sharpen your knives and cut my throat." He sang that refrain three times. Some of them said they must cut his throat. Others said they should let him continue to sing one more time. "If she does not answer that time, cut my throat." She answered: "What is wrong with poor Telilan? She is in the crows' nest who just defecated on her, and flew away."

In this tale, a sister, named Telilan, has been separated from her brothers, including the one with two tufts of hair, a style associated traditionally with a firstborn noble male. She wanders, encountering trees that, personified as spirits, lead her to them. Upon arriving at her brothers' nomadic camp, she prepares their meals. Following their reunion, the sister has been kidnapped by a spirit or devil (here the term is from the Arabic, indicating a Qur'anic spirit). In some other versions of this tale, when her brothers depart in search of her, en route, they also appeal to trees for clues to her disappearance and directions for finding her (Rasmussen 2001c). The tale ends with a lamentation, performed in "sing-song" style, conveying the sister's ambiguous fate and sadness.

Upon asking for the siblings' whereabouts, one by one, each tree indicates when the lost siblings passed by earlier—namely: the *tichghar* (a tree eaten by camels), *abizgine* (a tree whose fruits are eaten, whose wood is used for enclosures for houses and gardens, whose leaves are cold medicine and whose roots are used as stomach medicine—they are pounded and placed on a bloated stomach), the *ezin* (a tree with bent thorns, very difficult to remove; its bark is a medicine women's preparation drunk for "hot" ailments, believed caused by too much salt, and its fruits are eaten), the *agar* (mentioned earlier, the tree whose leaves and fruit called *ebalaqan* are eaten during drought, and which is believed to shelter spirits and the devil), the *aza* (the tree with thorns, whose gum is eaten; it is located not in a village or camp but on the mountains; it makes a noise in the wind, associated with spirits), and, finally, the *atise (acacia epinee)*, with which the mortar is made, also the mortar drum in the possession exorcism ritual.

The crow steals eggs from other animals and brings them back to his nest; many Tuareg believe that when the stolen eggs from other birds hatch, crows nonetheless emerge. White and red camels are considered prettier than camels of white and black coloring. Red camels are less preferred than white ones, but more preferred than black camels, and they are, accordingly, intermediately priced. The *akatar* is a very decorative harness placed on camels and donkeys ridden by women to marriages.

Hence the marriage imagery between the siblings, which is opposed by the intrusion of the Qur'anic spirit. This theme—of lost siblings who search for each other and prepare for marriage—is a widespread motif in Tuareg folklore, suggesting the struggles between matrilineal and patrilineal forces upon conversion to Islam. As chronotopes, these trees orient and, more abstractly, situate and evoke matrilineal ties and nomadism in jeopardy. This imagery also has broader significance, in that it enhances anthropological understandings of nature and culture, in both symbolic and historical contexts of herbal medicine.

A binary opposition, nature/culture, once claimed a large constituency in anthropology (Levi-Strauss 1962; MacCormack and Strathern 1980; Ortner 1974). More recent work has shown that nature and culture contrasts differ from society to society and that different societies juxtapose gender symbols with those of nature and culture in distinctive ways. Thus Euro-American definitions of nature and culture may have little to do with contrasts that other cultures use to order the world. Yet there is an interesting idea here that can nonetheless be salvaged: perhaps women healers are marginal, albeit positioned not between culture and nature, but between different contexts or planes within social and cultural worlds. For example, Tuareg herbal medicine women mediate between the tent and the wild, and between the living human world and that of the deceased ancestors, in particular, matrilineal founding ancestresses, and these domains are not locally viewed as necessarily always opposed, but rather dynamic and shifting in meanings according to context. The foregoing imagery suggests that much ritual healing by medicine women addresses contradictions and struggles over how these domains are converted into social and legal policies under the impact of contemporary patrilineal, Islamic, central state, and increasingly, sedentarizing forces, some of which threaten women's traditionally high social prestige, economic independence, and relatively free social interaction with men. In their view of their work, classification of the world, and medico-ritual roles, medicine women therefore offer to anthropologists a means to escape binary oppositions with Euro-American cultural baggage, namely, science and *bricolage,* nature and culture, and religion and magic.

On another level, in other contexts, these images must be placed in their sociopolitical and historical context, as well. In more recent times, the historical grounding of these images widens their gendered specificity, expands their meaning, and resonates with how many Tuareg men and women experienced colonial and postcolonial state policies with important consequences. Many Tuareg still rely upon herbal medicines—barks, leaves, and other bushes and plants—since Western biomedicines are of difficult access. Many tree medicines are locally grown, purchased in markets, or imported by caravans from the South. French colonial and independent state policies have combined with natural ecological droughts to force many Tuareg to sedentarize, and there have been restrictions on nomadism, herding, gathering, and caravans, which were formerly relatively freer to roam across borders. Early in the twentieth century, many children were marched forcibly at military gunpoint to nomadic boarding schools (Dayak 1992; Rasmussen 1997). More recently, aid programs have tended to favor oasis gardening over pastoral production (Childs and Chelala 1993; Decalo 1996). Livestock herds are more difficult to replenish than gardens after drought, and while both men and women own and inherit livestock, men own most gardens. Droughts have also threatened many valuable medicinal plants. In this light, the arboreal imagery contains a paradox, reflecting wider contradictions, but also unities, in Tuareg society: these natural images of trees refer to the wild and natural as both threatening and sheltering, for men and women alike.

Herbal medicine women work in both the home space of nomadic camps and sedentarized villages—they usually cure inside the tent—and the wild, where they gather. They gather many tree medicines in the vicinity of ancestral ruins. Herbalists pray before pulling leaves or bark off trees and bushes. One herbalist I accompanied on gathering expeditions, Mina, told me, "For each tree, one offers a different prayer because some are big, important medicines and others are small." While gathering medicines, before pulling leaves and/or bark off each tree or plant, Mina prayed. She knelt before each tree—here the *obdeg, tadeine,* and *gamji* trees—and said a different prayer. She carried Islamic prayer beads along with her. Mina said she would dry the plant medicines after gathering them. She stopped and explained names and uses of plants to me. As she pulled them up or picked them, she softly murmured "Bissmillallah" and other prayers/benedictions. "For these medicines to work," Mina explained, "one must respect the tree and also give food to children." She said "Bissmillallah" before some trees, touched the ground three times and did Islamic ablution motions before others. She also did full Islamic prayers; wrote Qur'anic verses in the sand; and spat to convey *al baraka* on some leaves and barks before placing them in her medicine bag. She was accompanied by three young nephews, sons of her older sister. She explained that grown men don't come on these expeditions because "only women know trees." Also, in order to make their tree medicines effective, medicine women believe they must give millet and sugar to children before embarking on medicine-gathering expeditions and offer millet to the tree before taking its products.

The spaces where herbal medicine women work are both "cultural" and "natural": they include both the home space of villages and camps—where they heal—and the wild of dried riverbeds, mountains, and deserts—where they gather. The latter are all distant from homes and the maternal tent, male-dominated mosque, and houses. Herbalists alternate between the wild and these points of habitation. Thus they cure in domestic spaces but gather medicines in the wild near stone ruins of ancestral spirits. Before they leave to gather, they circle millet and sugar three times over the heads of maternal nieces and nephews. They pray before pulling leaves or bark off each tree and bush; for each tree, one offers a different prayer, because some are big, important medicines and others are small. In local cosmology and ritual, these trees are associated with matrilineal spirits. Medicine women are obliged to remove bark from trees with a rock or stone, but not an ax or any tool made of metal, particularly iron, which is believed to make the medicine ineffective because iron repels spirits, and in this gathering context, medicine women seek to attract rather than repel these spirits. Yet herbalist/diviners also display devotion to Islam. Thus they stand on a boundary or borderlands.

The gathering of herbal medicines from tree spirits has moral and political implications. The arboreal tropes in local aesthetics—poetry, song, and folktales—also strongly evoke these concerns: female-female and mother-child ties. Feeding children and giving to trees in effect perpetuate matrilineal ties, many of these now becoming threatened, in the uprooting of matrifocal uxorilocal households in the wake of drought, sedentarization, and patriliny imposed by Qur'anic and central state influences. As trees are uprooted, so are humans and their ties. The founding ancestress of herbal medicines and her twin daughters who emerged from their murdered mother's stomach holding tree barks and charcoal, symbols of herbalism and maraboutism professions, respectively, are commemorated in these tropes, as well as in medicine women's actions in healing.

Therefore trees have ecological and ethnobotanical significance, but their significance transcends this, extending metaphorically into myth, ritual, nomadic, and matrilineal concerns, though these concerns are by no means irrelevant to men. Yet more gender-specific meanings also emerge. In many verses' reference to the traditionally important role of women in nomadic communities as cultural educators and facilitators, they also echo the voice of a mother warning daughters and of brothers warning sisters to be cautious in love. Many married women nowadays are pulled away from matrilineal kin and property (Rasmussen 1997).[2] The outside stranger, fascinating and feared, is a frequent motif in local verbal art generally—there are hazy boundaries between the suitor, husband, and raider. Nowadays this latter includes marauding militia and bandits. Even after the peace accords negotiated between rebels and government, there have been sporadic armed conflicts in some regions between former rebel factions who have splintered off and some militia. Some Tuareg women have been raped by, or have married, soldiers and left their local communities.

In the wake of this violence, women and men face considerable turmoil. While some former rebels are honored in poetry and song for their battle exploits—as were warriors in former eras—others have become uprooted from their community, unemployed, and alienated, even "bandits." Moreover, strange male outsiders have entered the region in post-Rebellion regional aid programs, and these men do not always respect local customs. For example, some soldiers and functionaries, new to the region, have misinterpreted Tuareg emphasis upon free sociability between the sexes as implying prostitution (Gast in Yacine 1992:168); whereas by contrast, Tuareg courtship traditionally emphasizes music, poetry, and conversation, but not necessarily sexual intercourse.

Against mythical images of gender, therefore, are juxtaposed tropes of natural environmental features and geographic spaces: many references to women and female social ties are interspersed with sheltering and medicinal trees. Tuareg state that "only women know trees." They also state that the person performing the head dance in possession trance is "like a tree swaying in the wind," and many songs allude to the sheltering shadows of great trees, or in a verbal pun, of great songs (Rasmussen 2001c). These aesthetic themes are rooted in the powers of trees to heal, to witness altered personal states in social and emotional life, and to restore a sense of a unified self. Indeed, trees are personified in the natural terrain, as social witnesses of beliefs and practices that are important, yet disputed.

Medicine women's healing therefore evokes a more general cultural preoccupation with inner experience and altered personal states, oriented to external position in the

natural and social terrains. These are all interrelated in their common symbolic repertoire: of local cultural constructions of natural terrains and states of human rootedness
and wandering in interior and exterior spaces. These terrains give a kind of sensual per-
suasion (that is, aesthetically creative appeals to memory, emotion, and creativity) that
is crucial to the tactics through which the sick patient regains control over the self,
through shared memory. These natural tropes in herbal healing, rituals, songs, and
myths orient the person toward returning to society, not solely in physical health but
also in social community, and stand as moral witnesses. These expressive domains,
therefore, deploy similar tropes to convey a wandering of the soul. Herbal medicinal
imagery and pharmacopia refer to important activities in everyday and sacred spaces.
Many of these sacred spaces are imbued with *al baraka* blessing.

Part Three / Medicine Women and Wider Systems of Power

7–Medicine Women, Sacred Places, and *Al Baraka* Ritual Benediction

Although very elderly and becoming somewhat fragile, Lala was nonetheless still respected as the most senior among the herbalists on her mountain plateau. She was well cared for; her tent was clean, and she was surrounded by her daughters and grandchildren. During one exam, she felt her patient's spleen *(aousa)* by touching the patient's stomach; she said that blood flowed from it. She murmured *"Bissmillah"* as she touched to diagnose.

Lala stated: "If an herbal medicine woman gives anything to someone, even earth, this contains *al baraka*." She gave some to her patient and to me. She also explained that rotating medicine constitutes giving alms. She elaborated on additional protective measures during treatments to safeguard the patient's wellness:

> All patients should be far from moonlight because that provokes shivering. I cook and mix my mixtures of plants overnight; while cooking, no one else takes ashes or wood from my fire. We medicine women cannot work during the healer's menstrual period. . . . I apprenticed with my mother. Me, since I have had my memory, I have understood it [medicine].
>
> Nowadays, for some people, medicine does not require inheritance. Knowledge of it is too widespread [dispersed; i.e., what was in the past secret has become more open and subject to distortion or appropriation]. Me, I learned with my old mother and by studying with my other elderly female relatives; I watched until I learned. In order to study, you must receive the medicine from someone who knows it. I cannot tell you how old I was (when I began practicing), but I began when I understood everything. I touch (in order to know the patient's illness). I treat hot illnesses of *tuksi*, cold illnesses of *tessmut*, spirits also *(eljenan)*, and all irritations, as well.

Medicine women, in particular elderly ones, are believed like marabouts to conduct *al baraka* blessing/benediction. Many medicine women also reside near areas designated by marabouts as sacred *(al hima)* spaces (though they tend to gather on the boundaries of these areas, and to examine patients inside tents). These *al hima* spaces are believed to be filled with *al baraka*. Medicine women also gather many of their medicines in outlying areas near ancestral tombs imbued with *al baraka*. In this section, I explore medicine women's long-standing and changing uses of this Islamic ritual power in relation to those sacred spaces. There are contradictions facing those who activate *al baraka* and protect places endowed with *al hima*; for as shown presently, *al baraka* ritual protection of the sacred is increasingly challenged by contemporary leaders and new organizations who appeal to ties extending beyond descent, kinship, and social stratum origins. Local and outside authorities attempt to manipulate and benefit from evoking *al baraka* and its sacred aura. The central paradox, I argue, is the following: those vary forces that endanger *al baraka* and its sacred *al hima* spaces are now also needed to restore *al baraka* to land and people. Thus two forces—benediction and the sacred— hitherto united, have become detached and in mutual battle. This paradox affects medicine women's work. How do herbal medicine women cope with this predicament?

Certain groups and lands are associated with water and wells in local mythico-history. For example, many founders of villages and/or culture heroes are credited with sinking the first well, as well as building the first mosque. In the medicine woman Hadia's village, an Islamic scholar from a prominent family, descendants of the village's marabout-founder, gave his account of its origins and reasons for its status as protected, consecrated *(al hima)* land filled with *al baraka* benediction. The marabout, whom I'll call Aghaly, gave the following account of the origin of his and Hadia's village:

> In the beginning, this village was inhabited by the Itesen (ancestors). At that time, then the marabout [named] Atkaki came and lived here. This region is named Atkaki [after him]. Three hundred years ago last year, he was here. He passed by Tewar. Sidi Mohammed [who was a companion of Atkaki] was the first after him. Arabane [another marabout from the East—either present-day Iraq or Turkey] arrived. After them, Atkaki arrived in the Aïr. Once arrived, he stayed in the mosques of Aïr [Atkaki was the first to arrive in this place named for him, Atkaki, but the third to arrive in the Aïr region generally]. Three hundred years ago, Atkaki arrived in the Aïr. Sidi Mohamed stayed in the mosque at Teffess [region next to Tchighozerine, at the entrance to Tenere]; the other [Arabane] stayed in the mosque of Tchighozerine. That which pushed them to leave their natal region, it was that there was too much wealth there. They said that they did not like that, they wanted a region neither too rich nor too poor, so they could practice religion [better]. They [i.e., the family] stayed in Tewar a hundred years. Four hundred years ago, Atkaki the marabout arrived in Tewar; 300 years ago, Atkaki the marabout [or his descendants] arrived here [in this place, named after him, Atkaki]. As soon as he saw our spirituality [religiosity], he stayed to live here. My family is responsible as ritual caretakers for Atkaki's tomb; we are relatives and descendants of Atkaki.

Aghaly gave another reason, as well, for the sacred status of his and Hadia's village:

> The first marabout who came to choose Atkaki to live in, while walking, he saw *al baraka* blessing, while walking in the night, he saw the place becoming very light, like daytime, and he said, "Me, I have seen the region where I am going to live." The marabout Atkaki kept a forest here, guarded by slaves, in order to conserve the grass and regulate gathering there. During that era, there was no millet grown here, the marabout Atkaki had that forest guarded by slaves on each side of it, in order to prevent people and animals from depleting it. One had to wait until the wild herbs and grasses were ripe and after the marabout authorized people to gather there for their food. As soon as the rains came, the slaves guarded it. People then had ears [i.e., they listened to authorities] and were afraid. Now they only have eyes and do not listen to or fear anyone. Also, if the

slaves saw an animal wandering without its owner, they seized it, and they guarded these animals to prevent damage [to the forest crops]. That forest *(efaye)* was considered like Hausaland [where caravans go], as a source of food [i.e., a granary or "breadbasket"].

Then, after a time, people began to go to Hausaland (on caravans) and also traveled throughout the Aïr. Now, before Atkaki had been a region where there was plentiful food: *adoua* trees, *jujubier* trees, *arounkoud, anizame, anzenan, tezagh,* and *yadia* trees, all bearing fruits and leaves.

Aghaly continued and gave another reason Atkaki had decided to remain in that village:

Before, the marabout Atkaki wanted to go to Hausa country. When he faced toward the south, he saw darkness like night, he looked toward the north, he saw brightness and light like day, so he decided to stay and live in the Aïr [i.e., in the middle of the two]. All the mountains became white [color of happiness, purity, and good luck] at the beginning, when the marabouts arrived, with their Qur'anic students and small birds that they caught alongside the water sources. At night, they refrained from lighting fires in order to protect from enemies, [and] their homes were partially in the sand [subterranean]. When the marabouts first came, they passed through Fez, Morocco. They had their books and other supplies transported [here] on an elephant.

At that time, one did not cut down trees or sink wells [here at Atkaki] because anyone who does this is attacked by Qur'anic spirits *(eljenan)* and goes insane. It was necessary for the person to go toward the great tombs and pray for what one needed and wished for. At that time, even the drinking water was at sites where two current villages are today [about five miles away]. One had to go there for it. One told us that in the past, there was a very deep well, but it no longer existed. A dog once came to drink at it, and ever since then, the well no longer existed; for because of that dog, the devil closed the well. That's what they told us when we were little.

After a time, there were taxes [imposed by the French colonial administration], and people came to stay here [to escape the taxes]. Before that time, there were Kel Nagarou [a descent group] only around here, around the end of the nineteenth century. After that, the Kel Igadmawen arrived, and the Kel Nagarou are the ones who left the Tamgak Mountains, then during Kaoussan's war [the Tuareg Senoussi Revolt against the French in 1917]. The Kel Igadmawen then stayed toward the Tenere, to drive the Tubus away during war, near Tabelot.[1] That was the time of Kaoussan. Other people left for Tanout [in present-day central Niger en route to Hausa regions farther south]. Imghaden settled fifteen kilometers east of Agadez, where they lived. That is the reason you see all the people in Aïr, their kinship is all around Agadez because they gathered around the Sultan for security from wars [of Kaoussan and also against the Tubu]. All people in this countryside still fear the Tubu. Always, they were on the brink of war. Kaoussan was chased by the French in this region, and afterwards, people ceased making war. This era of Kaoussan and war was about 86 years ago. Kaoussan caused a lot of devastation in the Aïr because the Ikazkazan, his combatants, followed in his wake. They fought, they killed people, anyone who did not help them, they killed. After Kaoussan, the French imposed taxes. Chiefs were elected and people remained calm, but the French installed authorities and controls.

I was born after [the era of] Kaoussan. One year, there was a famine, everyone caught crickets, they dried them and after that they took them, grilled them, and ate them. There was also a year called "the doum palm pit" year. People went to other regions in order to gather the pits of the doum palm to eat them. Another year [in our history], called *Kojaja,* was the time when people ate the wild fruits. These were fruits of the *acacia* tree that normally animals only eat; one placed them in water for one week to make them less bitter. Then people did not travel [as far as today]. In the morning, people went into the bush in search of food for their children. They gathered wild manioc, a root, like tomatoes [today], and then they ate it. The people in this region before Atkaki were at their pastures, then the herds diminished, then they made the lands into oasis gardens. Now, everyone is all mixed, in background. The Kel Zingifan left a village called after a dune shaped like a horse's back.

Each descent group has the name of the place where they once lived. The Tubu are related to the Tuareg. A long time ago, Tubu from Kewar arrived making war here. They abducted some Tuareg women and took them and their children to Bilma; others stayed here. They took them as captives first and then married them.[2]

In the past, people had fewer resources than we do. Youths today think they are better because of this [solely because of material things], but they are not. Clothing used to be all brought back [on caravans] from Hausaland. Before, all men were gone during the cold season, on caravans, and the women led their goats to pastures. Often, everyone in the family shared a single new shirt, waiting to wear it at a festival. Back in those days, there were fewer material goods, but since people shared, there was more *al baraka.*

In the past, therefore, Aghaly's and Hadia's village was designated as *al hima* or protected land, a term that also is an expression denoting the healing by *icherfan,* descendants of the Prophet. As Aghaly explained, it was believed that one would die if one cut a tree or dug a well there, because of the tomb of the prominent marabout-founder named Atkaki there. In order to do this without dying, one had to make a sacrifice and give alms (an animal). Aghaly and Hadia's village is one of the oldest villages around Mt. Bagzan, several centuries old. The oldest neighborhood, Moussabka, denotes "place of a step of camping (on caravan or nomadism)." Atkaki's marabout-founder and his clan are believed descended from the Baghdad caliphs.[3]

Hadia, as observed, also resided in this village. During her accounts of her life (as she termed this, "news of my life"), she added her own perspective of this region. Her perspective is not necessarily contradictory, and I do not include it as a corrective to Aghaly's history; rather, Hadia's view offers a different emphasis, one that includes her own and her family's subjective experience there. I include these two stories because they complement each other in ways similar to the way medicine women view their relationship to marabouts and Islam, the topic of the next chapter.

Hadia recounted her background:

> Before, I used to live in Tessouat near Ajirou. We left that place a long time ago. One followed the mountains of the Aïr, everyone. They were saved [from the war against the French] and went to Hausa country with their animals, their wives, and their children. All their animals, each man with his family. We were many people. We were with Kel Fares, we left up to Yaguiji [between Tanout and Zinder, towns in present-day central and southeastern Niger near Hausaland]. We made our homes there for several years. Homes were in woven straw *(paillottes)*. After we left there, we came up to Agadez, we lived there then. There weren't many homes there. There were only Agadezians there.[4] We spent one year there, after which we left for Tadulafaye [three kilometers from Agadez]. After Tadulafaye, we came to the Aïr *oeuds* (wadis, Tamajaq *egoras*, French *coris*) around here. We passed through Abardak, there were no people there then. The people of Talat were still in Hausa country.[5] The mother of the current chief of Kel Igurmadan in that region [whom I knew], everyone, stayed in Hausa country. And afterward the people were there, after their return, they became our neighbors. They even lived in Emdigra [45 kilometers from Agadez]. They also lived in Takibichere [located between two sedentary oases today]. At that time, there weren't many people here, there were not many whom one did not know [around here]. At that time, we had three goats. People returned, little by little, until they all came back to the region; each place was [re]inhabited.
>
> We lived in Atkaki, Nabarro. After that we returned to Atkaki, where we have remained peacefully. Also, when other people came back, they lived in Azday. After Azday, they came to Talat. Those of Abardak also returned [to this region] after we did. At that moment, we did not have many children. At that time, I was an adolescent. There was an old camp to the west of Talat; as far as I know, it was the only well of Abardak, and that of Assaqamor. At first, one passed by Atkaki without inhabiting it. Before, our village was in Nabarro [a nearby *oeud* or *cori*]. That which took me to Atkaki, was when Nabarro had a drought. At that moment, we had cows. My little brother was born in Atkaki. At that moment, I knew Anna [grandmother of Hadjiatou] only. Toua [Amoumoun's mother] was little. At that moment, she was not married [yet]. There was only the old one [Ouma, Amoumoun's maternal grandmother] there. Always we followed our herds, I was small, younger than Ouma. At that time, it was still war. I forgot other things.

Hadia did not relate her story in a linear manner; therefore, the events that occurred, in contrast to those described by Aghaly, were not necessarily in strict chronological order. She related events as they came to her, over several different meetings with me over a span of several years. She was first married at about fourteen years old. In contrast to most first marriages, Hadia and her husband were not close cousins, and her marriage was not arranged by her parents. Perhaps this was because of the political violence, migrations, and social upheavals occurring in the early twentieth century, when many Aïr populations fled from French military repression of the Tuareg Senoussi Revolt led by Kaoussan and escaped the battles and famines by going to the

South, where many families had social ties with merchants and clients in Hausa communities from caravan trade (Rodd 1926; Bernus 1981; Nicolaisen and Nicolaisen 1997). During the French massacres, some fled to the top of Mount Bagzan, and others fled to Hausaland (Rasmussen 2001a). Some Kel Igurmadan came down from Mt. Bagzan, but gradually, rather than suddenly or due to any single event. Most of Hadia's relatives were fortunate and escaped the violence. But her father was imprisoned by French soldiers shortly after the 1917 Senoussi Revolt. Sadly, no one heard from him again, and his fate remains unknown.

Like many, Hadia came to Atkaki for its pastures. Her husband died later, between 1974 and 1978, after another major drought which lasted from 1969 to 1974. Hadia's compound when I knew her consisted of one conical grass building, one small kitchen tent, and some goats; like other very elderly women, she had ceased to keep up her nuptial tent, brought by women to marriage as dowry.

In her over thirty years in Atkaki, Hadia had been happy. Two daughters had begun apprenticing with her but were less renowned than their mother. One married daughter resided, until her death in a malaria epidemic in 1992, in a nearby village. Another daughter left the region for the towns and married a non-Tuareg man; her story will be told in a subsequent chapter.

In the narratives and reminiscences of Hadia and Aghaly, they review their life career, in Myerhoff's sense, but also much more: in focusing upon their village and region and the historical events experienced there, they make connections between sacred place, cultural memory, and ritual protection. Beliefs concerning space or place here involve both literal geography and the more abstract, symbolic/semiotic space of cosmology, ritual, and myth, in particular consecrated *al hima* land protected by *al baraka*. The arrival of the founding marabout, Atkaki, brought *al baraka* to the region, whereas the invasions of the French and Tubu only led to sadness and deprivation: the jailing of Hadia's father, taxation, and the Tubu raids and taking away of Tuareg women.

Threat of pollution to this land came from an additional source: one of Hadia's daughters who gave birth out of wedlock was obliged to leave, perhaps because illegitimacy polluted the sacred land surrounding the marabout-founder's tomb. Yet notably, Hadia as the maternal grandmother was able to raise illegitimate grandchildren discreetly, as long as this was done out in the pastures, away from the mosque, tomb, and the marabout family. The *al baraka* of lands must be continually protected, never taken for granted.

Consecrated or sacred *al hima* lands are found in many Saharan regions. In a nearby village at the base of Mount Bagzan, the prominent *icherifan* in the maraboutique clan of Kel Igurmadan related to me how two brothers arrived there first, sank the first well, and built the first mosque. Although the men and marabouts emphasize these Islamic versions of their communities' founding, rather than the tales of female ancestresses, their mythico-history complements and exists alongside, rather than challenging or displacing, the mythico-history of herbal medicine women. The coexistence of these different histories of sacred terrains, which include "wild" as well as protected, consecrated spaces, establish the cultural groundwork for the ideally complementary healing roles of Islamic scholars and herbal medicine women, discussed in the next chapter.

Herbal medicine women, like more "official" heroes/leaders with accumulated *al baraka*, also acquire successive identities by traveling across familiar and distant terrains, and going back and forth between the sacred and the dangerous. Hadia, in her discreet raising of several illegitimate grandchildren in the pastures away from the settled marabout families, and herbal medicine women more generally in their gathering of medicines, also accomplish this feat, albeit in a different, more "low-key" manner from those more officially celebrated leaders in Tuareg battle legends such as Atkaki and Boulkhou. Medicine women in their gathering near tombs, sacred groves and forests, and ancestral ruins revert back and forth between the sacred and secular ground, the visible and the invisible, the known and the unknown, and the tangible and the intangible. While medicine women do not physically repel invaders, they nonetheless may be considered a kind of *taggagart* (masc. *aggag*), mediators between cosmological boundaries. Indeed, there is the idea of a "vibrating" dynamic in their cyclical alternation between tent and the wild.

As Parkin (1991) observes, territory can have no significance for humans unless it is in some way differentiated from other territories, whether or not through human settlement: people only identify areas in relation to other areas. Spatial categories and ritual powers do not, or do not inevitably, neatly correspond with social distinctions or encode themes, but are, as Parkin terms it, "worked at and constantly reinterpreted by people of a culture, sometimes being changed in the process" (Parkin 1991:6). Their constant reinterpretation is part of everyday practice. In times of crisis, many compete to impose their own definitions, interpretations, and agendas concerning what is "best" for everyone and what needs protection.

There is a proliferation of sacred but also contested spaces—in which leaders with special protective powers must mediate between these ideals and increasingly secular and material concerns. This does not always go smoothly. Lala, the most senior medicine woman, lamented: "Occasionally, outsiders deceive by pounding medicines and claiming they are mine, trying to sell them. But only if a real *tanesmegel* gives anything to someone, even a bit of earth, this contains and conveys *al baraka*. Also, in the past it sufficed to touch with our hands and we cured, like the *icherifan* (descendants of the Prophet), at that time they did not have many sins, but now they have many sins. Healers must not do any harm if they really have the true power of *al baraka*. But now, some do healing without inheritance."

Dangers to *Al Baraka* and the Sacred

Al baraka is destroyed by impurity. At night, when non-Qur'anic Kel Essuf spirits are active, marabouts' tombs with *al baraka* are believed to become dangerous with evil spirits and to attack passersby without protective metal, e.g., swords. Female herbalists cannot gather their medicines from tree spirits on Islamic holy days. Women who are menstruating are in some respects considered by marabouts (though not, to my observation, by many other Tuareg men) to be impure, and they are not supposed to come into contact with certain forms of *al baraka:* they should not drink the milk of animals who have very small offspring and not drink water from freshly tanned sacks (Nicolaisen 1961). For this reason, until recently only old (post-childbearing) women traditionally harvested crops in oasis gardens (Rasmussen 1991), and for this reason, also, only they should, if necessary, raise the illegitimate children of others or gather herbal tree medicines.

According to Nicolaisen (1961), the earth also is impure and undermines *al baraka* (though it also is highly charged with spirits), and this is why one must not pour milk on the soil. Even when one washes a milk bowl with water, this water must be poured on a stone or in a manner so as to avoid its direct contact with the earth (Nicolaisen 1961:122). One can add that similar taboos apply to the drums of chiefs that should not touch the ground and, among some groups, must not be touched by young (child-bearing) women. Here, however, there are hints that, rather than women "polluting" the *al baraka* of the drum, perhaps the powers of the drum might attract *djinn* spirits to the women, for *djinn* spirits are attracted to anything or person in life with high concentrations of *al baraka*.

Women's *al baraka* is less openly discussed, both among the Tuareg and in the anthropology of religion and gender. Most studies do not specify the deployment of *al baraka* by Tuareg herbal medicine women in context but rather emphasize its uses by Islamic scholars, in particular those in the esteemed *icherifan* clans who claim descent from the Prophet (Bernus 1969; Nicolaisen 1961; Norris 1975, 1990). Nicolaisen, for example, emphasizes male Islamic scholars' mystical power of *al baraka*. He hints at, but does not pursue, a possible relationship this has to older female curers: he reports that the moon, a prominent female symbol in Tuareg cosmology, is one source of *al baraka,* and that older, postmenopausal women are no longer considered "impure" in Islamic ritual (Nicolaisen 1961:113–62).

Tuareg herbal medicine women, as well as more officially prominent chiefs and marabouts, deploy *al baraka*-related medico-rituals and protection of the sacred, despite the medicine women's "low profile" in public, official domains. Although *icherifan* marabouts continue to enjoy more public prominence, nowadays additional persons who are not traditionally mediators in the local cosmology also seek to protect the land by appealing to *al baraka* (Rasmussen 2004). In performing the same roles, do medicine women do the same things? Oosten (1984) reports that Inuit male shamans engage in competitive rivalries and hold major public seances, but it is less clear that female shaman counterparts do the same thing. I ask, where no cultural distinction is articulated between Tuareg women's and men's healing and other protective uses of *al baraka* power in ideology, do some differences nonetheless emerge in practice?

Medicine women work in a religious and political setting in which *al baraka* converts into changing and disputed concepts of purity, the sacred, and danger in local mythico-history. This ritual force is deployed in different ways by Islamic scholar/marabouts and herbal medicine women, as well as other social and political leaders, to reiterate and reflect upon cosmologies and mytho-histories. *Al baraka* as a "barometer" of anxiety: there is greater emphasis upon increased human (particularly female) fertility, as the land, gardens, wells, and livestock herds lose their fertility. Yet there is also disagreement over the causes and consequences of these conditions and how to cope with them, and medicine women are significant in underwriting male leaders' *al baraka*.

The political and economic crises in northern Niger and Mali have created ambiguity and fear in which former rebels, stray militia, and unemployed youths stalk the regions, with uncertain sources of income. Legitimate itinerant merchants, NGO aid workers, sympathetic European expatriates, tour guides, police, or even former rebels (the latter now peacekeeping forces in the semi-autonomous zones) are not always clear-cut in their identity. The boundaries of ritual powers and their social agents are not predictable; some ex-rebels and militia alike become bandits. As Lala pointed out, some medicine women do not in her view have a legitimate claim to *al baraka*. In this predicament, the *al baraka* protection of self and others may sometimes be defined as effective, sometimes not, or it may have been diluted and dispersed, routinized in some contexts. During the robbery of a group of tourists in the Sahara, some youths reportedly tried to harass the women, while older men with them reprimanded their violation of a serious Tuareg taboo against raping women.

Herbal Medicine Women's Uses and Conversions of *Al Baraka* in Sacred (and Not So Sacred) Domains

Al baraka is ideally legitimately accumulated, indeed manifested through almsgiving and obedience. As Lala explained, "it is not enough to even have parents' authorization to begin professional practice; you must have a 'complete head'; sometimes, one can even be jealous of one's parents [who practice herbalism]. One also needs obedience *(adeleb)*."

Another herbalist, Mina, indicated that she practiced herbal medicine "in order to atone for her past sins" *(ibakaden)* and to seek pardon from God." She, too, compared practicing herbal medicine to giving alms. The ceremony when they are authorized to become herbal medicine women or *tinesmegelen* is very simple: "an older relative says you are ready, that you know medicine; (and then) you give dates and cheese as alms to children."

Before their medicine gathering expeditions, I saw medicine women give alms *(takote)* of millet and sugar to children in the family. As Mina explained, "If one has a problem or difficult task to do, one makes an offering to children: this may be a small amount of millet, milk, dates, candy, etc. In addition, millet offerings must be made to the tree before taking its products."

Milk, water, blood, and date symbolism connect *al baraka* to gendered cosmology and ritual spaces. Water is ideally never sold. Milk and blood are images used to describe degrees of kinship. For example, in order to say that a child resembles a relative, one says that he has a little of his blood *(azni)*. In order to designate someone as not in a kinship relationship, one says "there is no milk in her *(akh)*" (Ag Solimane 1999:22). In order to convince someone of the importance of doing something obligatory in a kin relationship, one uses the expression: "in the name of the breast that one shares"; this trope suggests extension of links of solidarity (Ag Solimane 1999: 22).

Milk is most firmly associated with *al baraka;* milk is produced from (based on) blood (Ag Solimane 1999:22). Sharing is also important; ideally, at least, one obtains *al baraka* from sharing, and from giving alms, particularly to children and on Friday, the Muslim holy day. It is necessary in order to survive in an austere environment. Milk is considered the most sacred of foods; one must not waste it, for one began nourishment at the mother's breast. Also, milk represents sustenance (i.e., is a staple). The first milk of an animal always goes to children; the child to whom the animal belongs distributes this milk to children of the camp or village, in order to protect his or her family from all misfortune (Ag Solimane 1999:23). Evil spirits enter the milk of an animal that has not been milked for more than forty-eight hours (Ag Solimane

1999:24). If one drinks this milk, this causes very violent illness. In order to render the milk drinkable, one curdles it or boils it. The milk from the first three months of the camel is not given, either to adult women or to strangers, for this would be a bad omen for the animal. If a woman having her menstrual period or a stranger drinks this milk, that can bring misfortune for the camel milked; this milk, which has a sweet taste, is called *akh zeggeghen* or red milk (Ag Solimane 1999:25). Priority in milk, however, is generally given to a breastfeeding mother. It is believed that if the milking of goats is not finished before the setting of the star of the shepherd, this latter will disappear with the *al baraka* benediction in the herds' milk (Ag Solimane 1999:124). One places the goats of the camp into their enclosure at sunset, and one also milks them at that moment. If one delays, their milking becomes more complicated, for one risks losing them in the night and their kids can thus profit from the situation and feed from them.

In alms and other presentations, objects should be given directly to another person from hand to hand, not thrown on the ground; this is the case particularly with sacred or sacralized objects, for example, the chief's drum, a saber sword, or the Qur'an. Also, a brush or comb should not be thrown, for these are in contact with the hair; hair also is considered sacred among Tuareg (Ag Solimane 1999:32). Before Islam, men did not cut their hair for this reason. In the Azawagh valley, there still remain today some families where men do not cut their hair. When a child has his/her hair cut, one must bury it beneath a tree, for as long as this tree is living, it also has a sensitive heart. If the child leaves his/her hair dispersed in nature, the child's intelligence will disappear like the hair.

In medicine women's gathering and treatment activities, the earth was revealed as important and not altogether a negative force for *al baraka;* rather, it emerges in this light as an ambiguous mix of positive and negative connotations because it is central to female ritual cures. Local ideas concerning the earth or ground *(amadal)* are somewhat contradictory: like trees, it is an abode of spirits but also a source of danger and pollution (for example, a chief's drum cannot touch it, yet babies are supposed to be born on the ground on clean sand inside the mother's tent). One must respect the earth because one is born on the ground and one returns to the ground. In one's daily life, one walks upright on it, it supports and nourishes. One is dependent on the earth or ground, from birth until death (Ag Solimane 1999:19). The ground is believed to absorb the illness from the patient and thereby to protect the medicine woman from contracting it in their empathetic healing process. Marabouts sacrifice animals crouched down on the ground. Yet, in order to protect *al baraka,* there often are taboos against certain substances touching the ground, such as milk, Islamic amulets, and blood (because this latter attracts spirits to the place where it is spilled). There are also taboos against throwing dates into a fire; yet *icherifan* marabouts, as well as smith/artisans, have a special relationship to fire: they can control it. For example, smiths are associated with hot fire spirits, and some *icherifan* marabouts are believed able to touch fire and not be burned (Rasmussen 2001a).

In this light, the logic of taboos surrounding pregnancy and birth is clear. When a woman is pregnant, one must not frighten, anger, or harm her. As implied earlier in Tata's treatment of Fatima and in Hadia's consultations with Takhia, medicine women counsel a husband to give a pregnant wife whatever she wishes. Otherwise it is believed she will have a miscarriage or a defective baby. The person who harmed her is held responsible in cases of a birth defect (Ag Solimane 1999:52). Since pride often prevents women from expressing their wishes, the man must guess what they wish and respond to these wishes. When an animal is slaughtered for a baby's name day, special parts of the meat (sometimes the liver, sometimes the lamb chops and meat along the backbone) are given to the new mother.

Nonetheless, despite the importance of motherhood, as already noted, Tuareg women's prestige does not depend solely upon marriage or childbirth. Until the recent ecological and economic disasters, most single women were independent and prestigious, if they had large herds. But many have lost herds and are now less independent. Until recently, single female status *(tamesroyt)* used to have positive connotations of independence. Now, however, this is becoming defined as problematic, almost pathologized, by NGOs. *Tamawat* denotes a female adolescent, but in some sedentarized communities this now has new connotations of being "too free." Qualities valued in a man are widely said to be generosity and having pretty daughters. There is now pressure upon women to bear more children. The term for infertile, *taquor* (feminine, "dry"), is used by men as slang for "dried up," to refer to childless women whose childlessness may, in fact, by due to men's sterility; but, as the case of Hadijiatou and Amoumoun revealed, women are increasingly blamed for this themselves.

There are various proposed solutions to these "problems" of anomalous females: single women (unmarried and/or widowed from deaths or exile of men during Tuareg Rebellion), unwed mothers, and married but childless women. Solutions include earlier marriage; marriage of noble women to Kunta and other Arab men and to marabouts; adult literacy; and artisan training programs. Yet literacy lesson themes, for example, illustrations in books, emphasize traditional gendered motifs and activities (e.g., milking livestock) from an era whose bases of security are now less certain. Some women, as well as men, are beginning to receive small compensation herds in repatriation programs by the UN *Haut Commisariat de Refugies.* UNHCR gave funds to PSRAK *(Programme de Securite Alimentaire)* for several women around Kidal, Mali, in 2002 who had lost their herds: one woman received from UNHCR ten sheep; another received five sheep and five goats; another received two goats; another, five sheep and 5 goats; another woman applied and was proposed but had not yet received compensation as of 2003; others received five goats and five sheep. PSRAK has a division for refugees. The United Nations organization also dug two wells: one for village refugees who had fled during the armed conflict and returned afterward, and one for more nomadic herders. The program hopes to compensate ten persons annually. Those who did not yet receive compensation will hopefully receive it in the future.

The point here is that residents are becoming dependent upon a much diluted, impersonal *al baraka* of a routinized leadership, of distant, outside agencies and their impersonal bureaucratized authority. For women, this is double-edged. In some ways, this is an advantage because it encourages new activities and wider associations, and in theory at least, brings new material benefits. In other ways, however, it brings greater surveillance. These contradictions, with manipulated imagery of *al baraka,* are shown in the broadcasting of Hawa Efanghela, head of an Agadez women's artisan cooperative and also a radio personality. In her program on gender and development issues, Hawa encourages controversial new policies such as tree conservation and girls' education. In her radio commentaries, Hawa emphasizes the need for all to work toward development.

She describes work metaphorically as an amulet, asserting that "work covers, protects in this world. Work will bring [back] *al baraka* to the Aïr region." In this, Hawa also emphasizes the values of advance preparation and foresight: "All Tuareg, you must run before thirst [attacks you]" (i.e., not wait until dangers arrive) (Rasmussen 2003).

Thus *al baraka*, life abundance and its ritual protection, has become a prominent part of wider economic and political discourses. Also, in its gendered imagery and uses, its sense is being drawn upon metaphorically in discourses promoting national reconciliation, repatriation, and "development" in Tuareg regions, by NGOs, the government, and the media and their leaders. The strategies for equity are contradictory. For example, on the one hand, there is encouragement of girls' education, but on the other, there is also encouragement of women to marry and be good wives. Posters make a connection between secular education and adherence to, rather than abandonment of, traditional values of family and religion; one poster, for example, reads: "I sent my daughter to school. Now she works, and she paid for my trip to Mecca!"

At the same time, however, women are also expected to carry the burden of child rearing and household work; for example, government pamphlets with health education themes address women, not men, as the persons most responsible for family hygiene and homemaking tasks. In the face of devastating losses, most women are encouraged to contribute work, cooperate, and share powers, rather than to compete with others or hoard power or wealth.

Many aged persons, including some medicine women, lament that Tuareg home spaces appear to be losing their benediction. Spittler relates how, during the serious drought of 1984–1985, many Tuareg asked why such a catastrophe hit them in particular: why did God send the drought to this country, rather than to Europe, the country of infidels? (Spittler 1993:301) Had sins increased so much that God sent the drought as punishment? Marabouts explained this as a withdrawal of *al baraka* in order to remind human beings that only God is capable of sending rain. They made a comparison to illness: "God sends illness to remind humans of his power to send health and illness at will" (Spittler 1993:302). Additional explanations were that God withdrew *al baraka* from the Aïr region because people there abandoned traditions. For example, many told Spittler that shepherds today prefer to stay in the oasis rather than in the wild outside it, and leave the latter with their goats and also prefer the company of others instead of going off alone in search of better pastures (Spittler 1993:303). Medicine women remarked to me, similarly, that "many young girls today prefer fine clothing and an easy life to apprenticing for herbal medicine practice." Many lamented to me, "Before, we were Muslim; now, we are less so. Youths go to bars in towns, etc. We have abandoned reserve (shame, respect)."

Sedentarization, war, and repatriation of refugees and exiles have brought greater regimentation, surveillance, monetarization, and overuse of land and other property, which leaders in the past tried to guard against. There are challenges to long-standing values of obedience, sharing, and redistribution associated with the conveying of *al baraka*. Medicine women and other leaders attempt to remind others of the precariousness of the old protections and the need to continually practice ritual and social precautions against harming *al baraka*. Yet many feel, despite problems, that life is generally better and perhaps there are benefits to some changes. Many say that now there is more food (although one needs money to buy it, and this is difficult); whereas in the past, one had to move around constantly to find food, and often there was not sufficient millet.

Medicine women and other respected persons attempt to strike a balance between long-standing (albeit changing) local religious and cultural values and emerging economic needs—in this, ritual protection and consecrated spaces remain important in consciousness, if not always in practice. Most medicine women view their mythico-history and contemporary roles as continuous with protecting sacred spaces and conveying blessings to patients, in the tradition of wider religious devotion. Medicine women promote these goals, in their view, through working in a partnership with marabouts. At this juncture, the following question arises: how do these ideals play out in practice?

The next few chapters pursue this issue of medicine women's interaction with wider powers: Chapter 8 examines their relationship with marabouts and the latters' and local cultural interpretations of Islam; Chapter 9 focuses upon their relations with the spirits of specialized divination; Chapter 10 details the experiences of some medicine women (thus far still a small minority) with clinic and hospital staffs, and analyzes the interaction between them.

The difference between herbalists and marabouts is like that between men and women who are married [explained Tana, the medicine woman whom we met earlier]. The illness that the *tanesmegel* treats is distinct, and that which the marabout treats is distinct. Each is complementary, like a wife and her husband. I referred the daughter of a smith who came to see me to a marabout, I touched her, I told her, "I cannot treat you, you have a spirit illness." Her mother got her amulets with Qur'anic verses inserted into them, and she was cured. One can choose any marabout . . . this [one] was her neighbor. Now she is cured. One does not know what sort of spirits *(eljenan)* she had, she was in bed. As soon as I touched her, it was spirits that I felt. She hid the sort of spirits [bothering her]. The amulets the marabout wrote on a tablet *(ardoise, assiloum)* she drank that, and she was cured. When she made an offering with the marabouts' medicine, that was good.

In this chapter, I explore Tuareg medicine women's ambiguous relation to Islamic science, ritual, and its symbolic repertoire of powers, as interpreted by local cultural values and Islamic scholars or marabouts. Despite explanations emphasizing a partnership, on closer scrutiny of this relationship there are some tensions in practice. Several medicine women listed certain taboos related to respecting Islam. Tima indicated medicine women cannot gather medicines on Muslim holy days. They cannot cook medicines on Thursday or Friday since these are Muslim holy days; if they violate this rule, their medicines will not cure. They cannot gather tree bark during the month of Biannu (a pre-Islamic and Islamic holiday) because during this time, harmful spirits haunt trees. Ideally at least, they must use a clay pot. They can accept cloth as a payment, but according to Amina, they cannot be paid with anything of a black color, since this color is associated with sorcery. Several medicine women stated that an ax is not good for gathering medicines, one must use stones instead. Also, recall how many medicine women indicated that their medicine "does not like metal, particularly iron"—here, the implication is that, the metal iron, as a potent weapon against spirits, ideally should not be used by medicine women because they wish to attract rather than repel spirits. This is a complex relationship; for nonetheless their relations with spirits are subject to constraint because of ambivalent feelings concerning the compatibility and potential conflict between the science of Islam and their own science. This uneasy truce parallels the compromises in wider Tuareg society between institutions antedating conversion to Islam and Qur'anic religious and Arabic culturally influenced institutions.[1] Perhaps, also, these ritual restrictions and other ambivalent attitudes and practices express a preoccupation with accommodation to Islamic leadership's powerful position in much healing, particularly in the countryside, where many marabouts are respected and act as doctors, psychiatrists, lawyers, and jurists.

Hadia added further insights into these roles and relationships: "Spirits of the mind are treated by marabouts. These include crazy people and their victims, for example, they undress, run about, and are antisocial and aggressive. *We tinesmegelen* treat only illnesses of the body. *Goumaten* (or Kel Essuf) spirits are less aggressive; their illnesses are outwardly bodily illnesses, but underneath is a problem of mind. I sometimes refer patients to the spirit possession rite. They have liver ailments. The liver is the seat of the spirits, the place spirits occupy. *Goumaten* (non-Qur'anic spirits, also called Kel Essuf) prefer the liver and they need noise for their cure. *Tende n goumaten* ritual exorcises by gestures, noise, and instruments."

Hadia's comments therefore appeared, on first scrutiny, to support the ideology of body/mind and organic/inorganic illness divisions, which are often identified with medicine women and marabouts, respectively. However, in Hadia's and others' practices, there is revealed a more complex relationship between these categories of illness treatment, thereby suggesting that these divisions are not so rigid as portrayed in the official discourse of healers and patients and in some previous analyses of Tuareg illness categories (Fiore and Wallet Faqqi 1993; Noel in Claudot-Hawad 2002). Hadia further elaborated that,

> During these last two weeks, I spent only one day without treating someone. I have also treated eight persons in two weeks, . . . all kinds of people. Some had *tuksi,* others wanted purging of the stomach, others had backaches, and others were vomiting *(tizoufnine).* For the large medicine pot, it costs 2000 CFA (US$4). The small pot costs 1000 CFA (US$2). There was a child who came, and I touched him and told him that "I have done all I can for you, you must go to the clinic." When he went there, he felt better, and later he was cured. I treated another man, Tahirou, at my home. His mind was affected (Tamajaq *alkhal,* French *l'esprit),* he was a bit crazy. He also had *tuksi* hot illness because he had taken too much maraboutage ink verses. He also had spirits. He was very afraid *(tikartou tessa).* There also may have been sorcery *(ark echaghel)* involved here, as well. I touched him to diagnose with my hand like a stick. Even by just seeing his head, one knew that he was not normal [it had diminished in size].[2] He could not sit still, and he walked endlessly. He sought healers. Every time Tahirou was sick, he believed that he was going to die.
>
> Tahirou visited me over three years. He took my medicine. I advised him to see marabouts for a cure. He spent a long time with two local marabouts. Each time he came to me, I prepared a pot of medicine for him. He drank that, and he returned. I touched his stomach and I saw nothing; in my opinion, he had been struck in the mind [i.e., shocked]. Others told him he was a victim of sorcery, that caused him fright. He [still] does maraboutage, but is not cured. He has spirits, but not in the stomach. He is nervous, only. If a person with *tuksi* hot illnesses takes the ink of a marabout, he will go crazy. It is spirits that one cures with [Qur'anic] writing. *Tuksi* hot illness, Qur'anic writing of a marabout does not cure. Also, one must do maraboutage in steps, in order. One must look for a marabout in whom one has confidence, he will make a medicine. Now Tahirou is better. He said he would return here. I do not write or read [different from marabout]. Each of us has a different role.[3]

Here, Hadia is careful to express respect for marabouts, but she nonetheless reveals that her own diagnosis and treatments involve some psychosocial counseling. Even for referrals, medicine women must have considerable knowledge of illnesses of the mind.

Lala, the senior medicine women on Mount Bagzan, commented further on the relationship between medicine women and marabouts: "The herbal medicine woman *(tanesmegel)* does everything (in medicine) that God taught her relatives (also denoting parents, *marawanet*). The medicine woman/diviner *(tamaswad)* also, she does her looking or seeing, because she has spirits who tell her something. The herbalist and the marabout each does what God taught them. Preferably, the medicines of the herbalists and the marabouts should unite together [i.e., be used in combination]. I have referred patients to marabouts."

Even those rituals peripheral to or outside "official" Islam are circumscribed and controlled by marabouts, or perhaps, self-controlled internally from within herbal medicine by religious devotion. Those medicine women who specialize in non-Qur'anic divining by dreaming must be authorized to do so by Islamic scholars. Medicine women are not, however, "marginal" in the commonly understood sense of low, deprived, or oppressed status. Marginality, therefore, can imply not negative, "minority" status, but rather, positive positioning, or mediating between different cosmological and social worlds, as culturally constructed in parallel local universes of knowledge and power. The spirits with whom mediumistic medicine women communicate will be shown to be socially important, and even these women ritual specialists are not antisocial sorcerers, but prescribe treatments that require patients to mend social relationships. In general, medicine women emphasized to me their need to respect and protect the natural and social sources of their remedies, as when they refrain from using metal to collect their tree barks, and as when, while gathering, they communicate with their matrilineal tree spirits, to which they offer libations before collecting or picking their medicines, and as when they give alms to children for their medicines to work.

Others elaborated further on these issues. Tanou explained: "The herbalist and the marabout, each has their work apart; they are not the same. The work of diviners, also, is not the same; each does the work they know. The marabout knows writing and *alestakhara* (a type of divination)."

Tata, who treated Fatima earlier, indicated, "I sometimes refer patients to the *tende n goumaten* spirit possession ritual practitioners. Their illness is that of spirits. The difference between marabouts' remedies and those of us *tinesmegelen* is that the former use writing, [whereas] the latter use herbs, such as tree bark. But some people first try both these two, and then they try *tende n goumaten*. But this treatment pattern is by choice; it is not a rule; some persons want to see all three practitioners (as shown in the case of Fatima). Even my own granddaughter once saw a spirit with a sword, during her "hot" illness *(tuksi)*. She saw me first, and then a marabout."

Anta added: "I touch patients and refer them to marabouts. For example, I touched a man named Ismaghil once, I told him that this illness I could not treat, he had to go see the marabout because it was evil mouth or eye. He is an older man. This *togerchet* symptom is located in the body between the bladder *(tezague)* and the belly button *(taboutout)*. Ismaghil saw a marabout once, he had little time, but he is now better, he is here in my village. He returned to me a second time, he told me he had a liver problem, and I would treat it. His liver was dislocated, and I told him to come back, I was going to give him some barks. At first, when he arrived, he said his entire body felt bad, particularly the stomach. He asked for more medicine, and I gave him some. I asked him, 'Did you do maraboutage medicine?' He told me, 'Up to the present, I have not had time.' He does oasis gardening. His wife died during the malaria epidemic (around 1992)."

In contrast to Hadia, Tata distinguished between, not illnesses of the mind and illnesses of the body, but rather between medicine women's use of herbs and marabouts' use of Qur'anic writing. But as I show soon, even this division can be bridged by a few medicine women. Anta also asserted she could not treat *togerchet,* but nonetheless, she could diagnose it. As shown earlier, *togerchet* itself involves very complex interconnections between mind and body, as do afflictions of the liver—seat of strong sentiments such as anger, love, and fear. All these observations reveal the "messiness" of idealized distinctions made in principle between herbal medicine women's and marabouts' patients, illnesses, and treatments.

In their statements, moreover, these medicine women emphasize their complementarity and cooperation with, rather than competitive relationship to, Islamic scholars/marabouts in healing. Many described these healers as being "like husband and wife," and indeed, they referred some patients to marabouts. In practice, however, there are sometimes hints of competition between them.

Islamic scholars or marabouts *(ineslemen)* are active in healing organic and nonorganic illnesses, many of which are defined as caused by spirits. They also do psychosocial counseling. Marabouts cure with the Qur'an, which has special verses that cure diverse illnesses. Marabouts make amulets from these verses, to be worn around the neck or against the skin. Many men and some women see marabouts, although some women feel intimidated by them; for women find them unsympathetic to certain complaints (usually marital problems) and often choose to undergo alternate cures. In the local idiom, there is face-saving in this; many spirit possession exorcism practitioners explained, for example, that women see additional healers "when their illnesses are caused by spirits who do not respond to Qur'anic verses' treatment" (Rasmussen 1995). In such cases, patients are referred to other healers, such as exorcism specialists who preside over that musical spirit possession ceremony called *tende n goumaten,* featuring drumming and singing believed to "please" and placate certain non-Qur'anic spirits alternately called *goumaten* or Kel Essuf, which afflict predominantly, though not exclusively, women. In an ethnographic study of Tuareg spirit possession (Rasmussen 1995), Rasmussen has analyzed how songs addressing the spirits also express critical social commentary.

What is one to make of all this? Multiple models can work within a single society, although some of these models are more subdued than others. When they diagnose and refer patients, herbal medicine women reinterpret Tuareg cultural forces in dialogues concerning women's bodies and identities. Medicine women intervene in confrontations between opposed interests surrounding women's bodies, which extend into more "cultural" interests; for example, the foregoing cases revealed how medicine women open up, and subtly suggest diverse interpretations of childlessness, illness causation, and social relatedness. In these processes, some oppositions may be mediated, although these often entail compromises in which women's property interests may sometimes be co-opted. Medicine women's powers are sometimes contained, if not marginalized. To what extent, then, are these compromises experienced and interpreted by the medicine women: Are they aware of some appropriation of their very diagnoses, let alone their muted role, by marabouts and other authorities?

I found there to be a close, mutually respectful, but ambivalent relationship between herbal healers, Islam, and marabouts. All herbal medicine women I knew described their relationship with Qur'anic scholarship and healing as complementary, and gave "lip service" at least to the prerogatives of marabouts in treating spirits and the mind. Yet I found, in practice (and in some discourse, albeit "between the lines"), actual overlapping and also hints of structural conflicts in this arena. Medicine women usually expressed the ideal of a partnership and strict division of labor, especially in reference to complementary powers, as when they indicated that they can transmit *al baraka* Islamic blessing like Islamic scholars. Indeed, there are numerous parallels between their rituals. Like marabouts, a medicine woman spits on the medicines in her hand when she administers them in order for her blessing power to be transmitted. Also like marabouts, in order to cure adequately, the healer must begin when she has no sin *(abakat)*. *Takote* or almsgiving to convey blessing is central in this. Mina, whom I accompanied on gathering expeditions, indicated that she cures "in order to obtain pardon from sins; curing is like almsgiving." She added: "All the medicine a woman learns is from God and relatives. . . . In the past, herbalists did no harm, but today some are impure and commit sins." Local residents say that a truly great marabout must similarly never do harm. Although many medicine women such as Tata distinguished their own role from that of Islamic scholars by saying, "Herbalists cure with tree medicines; whereas marabouts cure with writing," many others, such as Tana and Lala, emphasized herbalists and marabouts being "like husband and wife" and asserted that "Our medicine is (therefore) best in connection with that of marabouts," i.e., both are often needed in the same affliction; their medicines are best when taken together or in sequence.

I am aware of the need for caution here in addressing the widespread problem within the anthropology of religion and Islamic studies of distinguishing local cultural beliefs and practices from "official"—itself admittedly a problematic term—or Qur'anic Islamic dogma. This is no easy task at any time, but one even more complex today, with increasing pan- or global "Islamist" influences, as well, in many Muslim communities.[4] Thus I do not wish to oversimplify the portrayal of Tuareg Islam here; what I seek to do here is to analyze, as adequately as possible, Tuareg cultural interpretations of Islam, all the while keeping in mind that even these are not monolithic or unitary. Tuareg cultural interpretations of Islam include, but are not limited to, those of marabouts. Herbal medicine women and others also participate in actively shaping religious meanings.

Culture is therefore key here. Medicine women convert natural materials into cultural materials: for example, medicines they cook over the fire or steep in water for teas. It is in this sense that they combine pre-Islamic, Qur'anic, and "popular" Islamic ritual paraphernalia, acts, and spaces. Yet their overall relation to the total Islamic-Qur'anic symbolic repertoire of ritual powers is ambiguous, and despite their exegeses emphasizing complementarity, reveals at least some potential for conflict. For example, if herbal medicine women violate that taboo against cooking their medicines on Thursday or Friday, Muslim holy days, they believe that their medicines will not cure. The reason they cannot gather tree medicines during the month of Biannu, they explained, is that during this time, harmful spirits are believed to haunt trees, competing with Qur'anic spirits. Those herbalist/diviners who specialize in non-Qur'anic divining by dreams must, in principle, be authorized to do so by Islamic scholars who more often dream in Qur'anic divination.

Spaces where medicine women work include both the home space of villages and camps, including inside women's tents, and the wild of dried riverbeds, high mountains, and deserts where they gather. The latter are distant from home and are opposed to maternal tent, male-dominated mosque, and men's adobe mud houses, although near ancestral ruins and holy men shrines. Medicine women alternate between the culturally constructed wild and civilization, and these are not always so neatly separate or opposed. They cure in domestic spaces but gather medicines outside in the wild *(essuf)* near stone ruins *(ibedni)* of ancestral spirits. Before they leave to gather, they must circle millet and sugar three times over the heads of their maternal nieces and nephews. While as noted many medicinal trees are associated with matrilineal spirits, medicine women sometimes carry Islamic prayer beads along on their gathering, pronounce Bissmillah, an Islamic benediction, before some trees, touch the ground three times, and perform Islamic ablution motions and recite full Islamic prayers. In this activity, therefore, they combine many different cultural and ritual themes.

Some more devout women (some, though not all, medicine women are in maraboutique families) also write Qur'anic verses in the sand. In this context, therefore, although herbalists seek to attract, rather than repel, matrilineal spirits, they also display devotion to "official" (i.e. Qur'anic) Islam. The substances and spaces with which they work, and their social referents, are associated with unpredictable and potentially destructive powers, but also with their conversion and regeneration (McNaughton 1988; Rasmussen 1992, 1998b) into more positive forces. In controlling and mediating these forces, these specialists are able to successfully navigate dispersed and dangerous social and ritual territories. Their roles take on multiple nuances, as shown in the following narrative.

Mina diagnosed my neck, shoulder, and back aches as *tarzak*. As she treated this condition with massage, using each hand in a separate area of my back, which considerably relieved my pain, she elaborated on these themes:

> I am thirty years old. I was born in this village. I make medicine and I touch. In gathering from trees, I take alms with me gathering, and I place them on stones near all the trees for medicines one gathers. When one picks them, one must give an offering, for example, to the *kalgo, ashik najad,* and *tuwila* trees. I practice what I learned. Now for all of us to do medicine, usually our mothers must die. [But] my mother is old, now she does not touch, [so] I touch. If she gives you authorization, you can. In order to obtain authorization from your living mother, you go to your mother and tell her, "Mother, people come to me for medicine. You must give me authorization in order to treat." And then you have your work here. Anyone who wants to learn, is not prevented from learning medicine.
>
> I have been married for three years. I have three children. I also make medicine. I do medicine work because of God and in order to seek pardon [for sins; medicine is a form of alms] from God. It is not only for making a living. It is in order to save and guard people with what is needed. Also, the people at home

pushed me to practice medicine, they caught illnesses. It is for that reason that I began with [treating] people of the family at home. When they saw me treating people in the family, people who are far away, they began to come see me. I began to learn at about fifteen, and I practiced little by little. I learned from [women on] my father's side of the family. I completed about five years of apprenticeship with my mother. As I learned, whenever my mother sought medicines, we went together [to gather them]. Also, when we arrived home, I watched her. I learned the [medicines'] names when she placed them on the fire. I watched. Everything she did, I watched.

Mina belongs to a prominent family of marabouts; therefore she received some Qur'anic education, and frequently wrote Qur'anic verses, though she indicated she does not practice official Islamic scholarship or professional Qur'anic healing. In this regard, she stated: "In my opinion, a person who writes learns medicine easily, because each medicine you can mark its name and the illnesses it cures. So a person learns very easily who knows how to write and read. If you find a person who wants bark medicines, you can do writing of marabouts for them."

Mina knows some Arabic script and possibly, also, Tifinagh, the Tamajaq script; but since she is in a maraboutique family, she tends to emphasize Arabic Qur'anic scholarship more than other women, who are usually more proficient in Tifinagh.[5] This was shown when she wrote in the sand while gathering from, praying to, and making offerings to trees. Yet these trees represent matrilineal spirits. She does not, however, write Qur'anic amulets:

So someone like that [i.e., a very literate person], if I identify the illness, particularly spirits, I would refer the patient to a marabout. I know how to write Qur'anic verses, but I do not write them [for patients]. Even if the illness is serious, I do not attempt to practice a combination of herbalism and maraboutism. I do not treat the Kel Essuf spirits, either, because although I know Qur'anic writing, I do not have authorization [to do it in maraboutique healing]. That writing, also, has its authorization: he who does the work of writing goes to a marabout for its authorization. I could seek this [authorization to write Qur'anic verses]. But currently I do not agree to treat spirits, as that is dangerous, because they can contaminate me, since I am too young in age [i.e., older women are safer from spirits].

I do not do writing [i.e., Qur'anic verse amulets to heal spirits]. I tell you I do not myself like writing [this]. The only thing that is going to push me to write that is if there is not a marabout [around to do it]. Writing is the domain of marabouts.

To diagnose the illness, I touch the body of the person and I find the illness. I touch the stomach with my hand. With some illnesses, I feel something hard. Each illness has its symptoms. *Alafaz*, sorcery *(eghaghawe* or *echaghel)* it is those that are hard [in symptoms]. That is located in the stomach. *Tuksi* hot illness is soft. *Tessmut* cold illness is like seeds or grains to the touch. *Tuksi* refers to the ensemble of many illnesses, also. It can provoke heart problems *[tourna n ouwil]*, it causes indigestion or vomiting *(tezournine)*, or backaches. It provokes illness.

I only touch, do not divine by dreams or amulets. I do not chew perfumes [aromatic barks] or slaughter an animal as alms to diagnose illnesses. The only alms offering I make is what I make for God to facilitate everything I seek. If I want to do writing, I must make an offering; then [only], I slaughter an animal. Also, it is alms that makes medicines more effective.

I treat *tuksi, tessmut,* sorcery. I diagnose *ado* [literally denoting "wind"], that condition caused when the wind penetrates the woman, especially if she washes, and also when a woman has just given birth. This woman is vulnerable to several illnesses. The woman who gives birth does not resist illnesses well. If the woman has ceased her menstrual periods, she does not catch illnesses. She resists more than the other woman. I have touched people who had [afflictions from] sorcery and I told them to go to marabouts: Adam, Aghaly, for example. Those men came, I touched them, and it was sorcery that I felt. I told them to seek their medicine at marabouts'. They were treated, they are now cured. Aghaly took many medicines at the hospital and those of herbalists, but he was not healed. He came to my home and I told him "You have sorcery, you must go to marabouts." These people had many worries. They spent a lot of time in Tafadek [a natural hot springs]. I gave them all kinds of medicines that I know.

In Mina's next story, there are hints of women's reluctance to see marabouts for some problems:

There was one woman who called me over to her home whose name is Rahmou. I went to touch her, and she told me that she wanted me to treat her. I told her, "I touched you, but I cannot treat you. I have not your medicine [i.e., the Qur'an and its verses], you must go to marabouts." She told me, "You are going to treat it." She had confidence in me. She wanted me to treat her, but "I cannot treat you," I told her, "a marabout must." She left to see the marabout. But I do not know if she was near spirit places. She is a sweet woman, from nearby. She has headaches, body aches, she cannot stay at home [i.e., is restless]. She believed that her illness was serious and she could not cure it. Most of the illness was the head. Thus far, she has not been to a marabout, she is undergoing a *tende n goumaten* ritual. Of these four persons, only two have paid me, 1500 CFA (US$3) each. Anything one gives me, I accept it (like an offering). A person can pay little by little. Each person has confidence in some healer. God gave me these patients' trust. Sometimes people prefer someone who inherited medicine from her parents. In my case, it was my grandmother who did medicine. After her, my aunt and mother did this.

Here, Mina's comments also reveal some contradictory attitudes concerning writing, treating illnesses of the mind, and afflictions of the spirits. There are indications that many afflictions have overlapping causes and symptoms and etiologies, as shown earlier, in several cases. There are also hints that many women prefer to see medicine women for a variety of problems, but Mina referred them to marabouts. Their reluctance to see marabouts suggests that medicine women are the preferred, first caregivers women seek.

The survival of herbal medicine women's profession stands in striking contrast to the fate of some herbalists and midwives in the West. Tuareg Islamic scholars have not overtly opposed medicine women in the way that the Christian Church in early modern Europe persecuted herbalists and midwives, or in the manner that some more recent established biomedical systems have restricted them (Szasz 1970; Chesler 1972; McClain 1989; Sargent and Brettell 1996; Orion 1999). However, although Tuareg herbalists are respected, competing medical practitioners could restrict them if they found it in their interest to do so. Thus the question arises: why have they not restricted or persecuted herbalists more stringently? This is, I argue, precisely because Tuareg medicine women are perceived as not threatening—in effect, because although competent and in demand, they are powerless outside their specialized niche. On one level, this seems to be true when herbal medicine women emphasize refraining from intrusion into marabouts' "turf" and deferring authority to them, and observing those ritual restrictions expressing respect for Islam. On another level, however, cases in this book suggest that medicine women, in fact, do also treat some "illnesses of the mind." In their actual practice, medicine women emerge more as collaborative, that is, as one step in the healing process, for many patients with a variety of problems spanning organic and nonorganic. Also, as I show in the next chapter, when medicine women venture too far into special mediumship, they risk censure.

While marabouts never speak out against herbal medicine women, evidence suggests that they do indirectly contain their practice, albeit in benign ways: as seen, they circumscribe it to times and places that do not compete with marabouts' own practice. Marabouts also guard Arabic Qur'anic writing; many tend to disdain Tifinagh, and some Tuareg indicated to me away from their presence that they believed the reason for this was that marabouts feared economic competition, since their incomes derived from writing Arabic Qur'anic verses. Marabouts thus guard against appropriation of their own monopoly over some forms of divination and amulet-manufacture, since these latter, many local residents acknowledge, bring much economic remuneration.

Among herbal medicine women, there appears to be less emphasis upon competition than among male chiefs and marabouts. Most medicine women in their ideology state they refer patients to marabouts for many mind- and spirit-related illnesses: one must find a marabout who treats this, and go through curing steps gradually, in order, with that marabout. Among the herbal medicine women, there are fewer if any sorcery or "witchcraft" accusations or victims. Whereas by contrast, among marabouts and those aspiring apprentices to maraboutage, who are predominantly men, there is often sharp competition, and occasionally new practitioners are accused of trying to "take on" too many or too "advanced" Qur'anic verses (Rasmussen 2001a). As a result, such persons are sometimes accused of practicing sorcery themselves or are believed to become victims of sorcery themselves, from jealous marabouts guarding their *al baraka* force and other professional "trade" secrets. The brother of a prominent local chief was once such a victim in these struggles over maraboutage. The result, in the local view, was that two of his children were born mute. Another man, who allegedly attempted to take on too many Qur'anic verses too quickly in studying maraboutism, suffered from problems attributed to malevolent spirits and sorcery, and "blue" or "black" spirits.[6]

Among the Tuareg, Islamic scholars (called marabouts or *ineslemen)* are predominantly men. In principle, they treat both men and women patients, but more usually men. They use Qur'anic verses and amulets, treat many types of illness (including those believed to be caused by those spirits mentioned in the Qur'an, usually called *el-jenan* or *djinn*), and also practice Qur'anic forms of divination. Each Qur'anic text contains a remedy for illness; texts are numbered and named. Each verse *(Surat)* is numbered, and each is a potential cure: when ritually activated, it heals a specific illness, or relieves a social grievance, complaint or misfortune. In addition, the marabout often works within the social networks of the community to mediate the problem, and thus, like medicine women, conducts psychosocial counseling as well. The marabout writes numbers in red or some other ink—often vegetal—next to the verses that correspond to the patients' age and other characteristics. In marabout treatment, a patient may drink the vegetal ink used to write verses on a prayer board, or they may wear amulets containing verses copied by the marabout from the Qur'an and inserted into metal or leather packets by smiths. Some inherit special talents of laying on of hands, healing by conducting their *al baraka* power alone; they are usually in the *icherifan* clans.

What exactly do some marabouts themselves say about these issues? According to Kadi, who specializes in *alekhustara*, a type of divination done in dreams while sleeping,

> When marabouts treat, they must measure the patient, in order to know the illness. If it is caused by spirits, if it is evil mouth or eye or sorcery, you will know [by measuring]. If you use *alekhustara* in order to sleep, you do it and in the morning you will know what is wrong with the patient. I use this method when a person wants to know his/her illness. One reads or writes Qur'anic verses as amulets, places them under one's pillow, and pronounces some prayers and sleeps after that. During sleep, you will discover the illness of the person who came to see you. There are those also who do not need Qur'anic amulets. You only read verses to them. That is *alekhustara* that I use. The person does two *raquarattes* [Islamic prayer motion]. You read after these motions. And the person advises the route or course of action. My patients tend to mostly have one of three types of ailments: *togerchet* or *imi n dunet* evil eye or mouth, *eljenan* spirits, or *echaghawe* sorcery. These illnesses are the most common [that I treat]. In the Qur'an, each illness has a remedy.
>
> I use measuring in my work. I take three *coudes* (a local measure; the term derives from French denoting "elbow"; three *coudes* equal approximately fifty centimeters or the length of one forearm) and I spit on the cloth, and say an illness name each time I measure to divine illness. Each time the three coudes of cloth increases, that is the illness [i.e., when cloth enlarges as a marabout pronounces the name of an illness, that is the illness]. If you measure the three coudes and there is not enlargement, this illness remains unknown, and this illness does not have medicine.
>
> Medicine women who divine *(tchimaswaden)* use non-Qur'anic (Kel Essuf) spirits in their work, that is what distinguishes them from marabouts. Each healer uses their own systems or logic: divination (seeing or looking, *asawad*), stars *(itran)*, dreams *(alekhustara)*, and touch *(edes)*. Medicine women touch the stomach of the patient to find the ailment. They can diagnose spirits, evil eye or mouth, and sorcery, but not cure them; for a cure, they must refer patients with such illnesses to marabouts. But they can touch to know the [required] medicines. Some

stomach ailments are caused by evil mouth or eye, sorcery, and spirits, and these patients come to me. Payment is negotiable; it depends on which illness. One slaughters an animal (a goat or rooster) and gives the meat away. Or a camel or bull of about five years old. Now many also pay in cash.

I studied with my father. I began at about twenty-five years old. You must obtain authorization to practice fully. You must know how to read and translate the *Surats* of the Qur'an. During dreams, you compare good and evil; you choose the truth and the good road. It is done not only for ill persons but to advise on actions, for example, for contracting lucky marriages. During the dream, I see if there is luck (in the match) or no luck. The man who is marrying asked me, because in principle men choose their wife. In our region it is not the woman who chooses; she does not ask man's hand in marriage. If the marriage is not lucky, it results in divorce.[7] I also use some wood, for example, *alghod, jawid, almissik, manzakar,* they smell good, perfumed. The Qur'an also contains medicine. The spirits are treated with scented wood sometimes, since they respond to good odors. If one burns the wood, this relieves, but not necessarily cures, spirits.

Another Islamic scholar/marabout, whom I'll call Ahmed, showed me his book (a compilation of selected Qur'anic verses called *el kebir*). On the cover of this book was an illustration of a lion and sword. Ahmed explained its significance as representing the occasion when the Prophet rode a lion while carrying a sword. Ahmed uses this book to cure in *itran* (star) divination and also guides the patient's finger to the appropriate verse after ritually spitting on the latter's finger (to convey *al baraka*). *Itran* denotes the stars; this, somewhat like our horoscope, is the result of calculating number of the Surat for cure from letters in the patient's name. There is the local belief that each person has a star, which constitutes the path to a cure.

Ahmed spoke about his life and work:

I was born here in this small village, my descent group *(tawsit)* is Igurmadan. I have eight children. I treat several kinds of illnesses related to my profession as a marabout. Sometimes I do writing, and I mix this writing with certain trees. I do *albourouj* (like *itran*) with the name of the person. *Albourouj* is *itran* with a board (wooden tablet). Everyone who sees me, I must do *albourouj* in order to know his/her star. That is what helps me to find their illness. Sometimes with the aid of numbers that contain the name of the person I treat. If I find the result, I know what verse he/she needs and in order to know the illness. For example, there is your name, I write it and I find the result and I look for the Qur'anic verse that treats the illness. For example, your name is 72, and the *Surat* that will treat will be written 72 times. Each person has his/her illness and his/her *Surat* for healing. Sometimes, I also have my little cloth that I measure. It is to identify the illness. I measure and call out the name of illnesses until I find it. With the spirit illness, if I measure three forearms *(coudes)* length, it changes length. I read nine verses, and I spit on the cloth. As with the cloth used to diagnose the *goumaten* or Kel Essuf spirits, if it enlarges, that means the spirits are disorienting the head of the person.

In addition to this, I also treat evil eye or mouth *(togerchet)*, it is with this forearm-measure cloth *(coude)* that I identify it. If it is diminished, by the difference of a finger, that is evil mouth. There are verses for this which I write [to cure it]: for example, *Tabarakatine* of 9. For example, there was one person named Almoustafa, son of Haya: during the malaria epidemic, one day he got up in the morning and could not move. His hands did not bend. They took him to the Agadez Hospital for three months. They brought him to the Tafedek hot springs. At that time, I was away on travel, they came to look for me. I rushed back here, and told them: "I must do fifteen days of seclusion with him and afterward, I can give him medicine. Before, I was their marabout. With the three months in Tafedek, in all he spent six months hospitalized [in those treatments]. I went and placed him in a place where people did not see him [i.e., in seclusion]. I treated him, but people did not see him. Always I did Qur'anic writing for him. One day, he began to walk, he was cured. He had spent forty days without people seeing him [in seclusion with me].

I do this work because it is my life. I was eighteen years old when I started it. There was a book that marabouts learned: the book that contains all the calculations of the stars. This was invented by the wise Prophet. It took me twenty-five years to learn. Anyone who has studied and knows the translation, who has sought out someone to teach him, he learns. Some learn and abandon it.

[But] only men, no women, do *itran* divination. The reason for this is that there are days when women do not pray, and a person can be ill because a woman does not pray [during her menstrual period]. At that time, she cannot touch the Qur'an.

I learned about the power of this injunction, yet also some flexibility in its enforcement, on one occasion while I was staying with a maraboutique Tuareg family in Agadez. One day, during their absence from the compound, a violent sandstorm suddenly broke out, followed by a downpour. I noticed they had left their beautifully illuminated, leather-bound copy of the Qur'an and some prayer beads out on the open windowsill of their house. I was in somewhat of a quandary, as I was aware that a woman should not touch them. After some hesitation, I decided that the "lesser evil" in my own reckoning was to rescue the Qur'an and the beads. Gingerly, I moved them inside to protect them from the wind and rain. Upon the family's return, two of the men were grateful, but a bit ambivalent because I had touched these items. Upon learning that I had moved them, they thanked me and were not at all angry, but flushed slightly, laughed, and seemed at a loss at what to say and do. They were obviously flustered and anxious—laughingly, they said, "Thank you, everything is fine," but glanced at each other. Undoubtedly the men were caught in a dilemma: of discomfort over a woman—a non-Muslim and of apparently childbearing age—having touched these items, but also feeling relief that they had been saved from ruin. In fact, later when we discussed how women in principle should not touch men's Qur'an and prayer beads and amulets, they admitted there "might be an exception to this rule in an emergency case." Herbal medicine women's practice is, similarly, constrained in principle, but in certain situations, as shown, their actions may in fact overlap with those of marabouts—there is tacit agreement on this, though neither party overtly acknowledges it.

Ahmed continued:

> When I do *itran*, when I begin the treatment, I make an offering. I slaughter a
> goat or a sheep given by the patient, part of the payment. For example, with the
> illness of spirits, the person cannot even begin the work without making an of-
> fering. If he does not make the offering, the marabout catches the illness. He pays
> me one camel, between one and two years old. I treat evil mouth, spirits, *albarass*,
> which causes tearing of the skin and paralysis. In the past two weeks, there was one
> person who came, he had an eye problem. He told me that he needed an operation.
> I did writing for him, and I told him that "If you see that it is not cured, come
> back." The illness was spirits who had entered his eyes during travel. He spent three
> months ill. It was something that had entered the eyes, like an insect. I treat every-
> one. But I must first do the *itran* (horoscope or stars) method.
>
> A *tamaswad* (medicine woman specializing in dream divination) has relations
> with spirits. Someone who has relations with the spirits, when one calls them,
> they reply. One gives spirits an offering, but spirits are not always in their head.
> Medicine women also learn medicine at their elders. The reason many medicine
> women tend to be older is that certain trees have a scent that if a young woman
> smells, she will not have children. Also, an older person really knows medicine.
> But they also need inheritance and apprenticeship.

Thus Ahmed confirms that not solely gender, but also age factors, are significant
considerations in medicine women's specializations. There is concern with distancing
childbearing women from certain practices and substances, that is, ideally one must
keep separate certain domains: those of fertility and infertility; active motherhood and
successful motherhood; and youth, elders, and ancestors. Again, the senses of touch
and smell as well are significant here: certain persons only must touch certain objects,
such as the Qur'an, prayer beads, and amulets. Certain persons and not others are able
to smell certain substances, such as the herbal tree medicines mentioned that allegedly
make childbearing-age women infertile. Certain types of knowledge, power, and vulnerability, somewhat like "trade secrets," must in principle be kept apart in order to be
controlled and protected and to work properly. Yet these ideals are always negotiable,
and as medicine women's and my own experiences revealed, sometimes there is tacit
acceptance of variations on these principles. There is, in effect, a hierarchy of needs á la
Maslow in which overlaps of power and knowledge are strategically necessary, such as
when some women (as Hadia and Mina observed) prefer to see herbal medicine
women even for illnesses in principle treated by marabouts.

While the medicine women dutifully referred such women to marabouts, there are
hints that these patients rejected or resisted such referrals. Other cases (for example,
that of Fatima earlier, and that of Amoumoun and Hadjiatou) revealed a treatment sequence and cooperation (albeit not without disagreement on illness causes and treatments) between medicine women and marabouts. In other words, input or intervention from medicine women, when the grounds are justifiable, is not ignored or
minimized in effect. While Mina minimized her expertise in Qur'anic writing and
amulet manufacture, she nonetheless knew this well; perhaps her deferring to
marabouts in that skill was only a matter of modesty.

Another marabout, whom I shall call Malam Moussa, also does curing, but not *alekhustara* or *itran*. Rather, his specialty is called "calculation," or *lisafe*, a kind of divination done in the sand. This method involves mathematics with the name of the person concerned. Its purpose is to find the day of birth. Each letter from the name corresponds to one number. The marabout adds them up with letters of the name of the person's mother. Then, he divides the total by 12. In one year, there are 12 months. The resulting number and what is left over represents the destiny of the person from the day of his/her birth until his/her death. Information for this is found in a book called *Abbou Maghchare Al Falaki,* and also, Malam Moussa consults *Al Kabir*. Malam Moussa explained *itran* as follows: "You need this when you are sick, so the marabout knows how to cure. Each star *(etri)* requires a different cure. This, however, is not always used in curing illness; it is also used when someone is merely curious to know his/her future, called *alghoumour.*" He compared this to our astronomy and astrology in the West and asked if our astronauts needed to know this.

Malam Moussa described additional divination/diagnoses and treatments of marabouts. These include *Igazen,* a method of divination in the sand done by marabouts; such a specialist is called *amegazo*. *Imegazen* (pl.) are sand-diviner specialists, apart from other marabouts; this subspecialty is inherited and passed down in apprenticeships in certain clans. One specialist performed this for me and told me, "your mind is happy, but your body is tired." This is therefore also used for psychological advice. Locally, there were several, all men as far as I was able to ascertain. *Alekhustara* is done for good luck. It consists of prayers for invoking God, and is also done to identify an illness. The name of a person is divided by seven, and the rest indicates the illness. *Ghuneb* refers to the horoscope-based process of divination. It is used to predict marriage compatibility and for strength against sorcery. Each person has a star that represents the sun, wood, animal, water, fire, etc., that contains a person's future and character, according to which day of the week he/she was born on. Illnesses Malam Moussa recognized included evil eye or mouth, indigestion, and *izafnen,* denoting microbes. Malam Moussa, like many medicine women, also emphasized the importance of modesty. He commented, "a marabout should be a reflection of God, calculate with God *(lisafe ser Allah).* We marabouts should not seek glory."

Despite their renown and skill at amulet protection and divination, however, marabouts do not enjoy a complete monopoly on these skills. Some people occasionally "sidestep" them and seek other practitioners for these needs. One Tuareg man in a noble maraboutique clan from the countryside, who worked as a merchant and resided part of the time in Agadez, needed advice concerning business, travel, and romantic liaisons. But he did not consult a fellow marabout, instead selecting an Agadez man who was renowned for his "sorcery-like" powers to do *alekhustara* for several days before he traveled to the countryside. This specialist, though Tamajaq-speaking and considered Tuareg, was called a *boka* (Hausa for "sorcerer"/healer) in this multiethnic town. He was of servile descent and came from outside the region, around Tahoua. This man also sometimes swept the Tuareg man's compound and washed and pressed his clothing. He was also active in some Hausa possession *bori* rituals in Agadez. He performed some divination with cowrie shells for me, as well. He stated, somewhat teasingly, that before my visit to Agadez, he had predicted that the noble man "would be visited by a European woman who would bring him good luck."

The Tuareg noble man in the marabout family had to maintain a delicate economic and emotional balancing act between his two co-wives in the countryside, who, fiercely jealous of each other, resided in neighboring villages, and his Tuareg sweetheart who resided in Agadez. He had to please all three women equally, particularly the wives. Perhaps he avoided other marabouts in this process and instead turned to the *boka* as an outsider he believed would be "safer" as a confidante than local marabouts in his own social network. By 2002, however, the Tuareg man had experienced conflict with that *boka:* he suspected the *boka* was involved in theft of a suitcase of a relative staying with him. Henceforth, he no longer consulted him in divination or employed him in housework.

By contrast, the same noble man, in his consultations with herbal medicine women, never experienced any such conflict. In the countryside, he and his wives turned to them upon their children's illnesses; Tata, for example, healed his son's diarrhea. Another medicine woman relieved the suffering of his married daughter following a difficult childbirth, though her baby died. To my knowledge, no herbal medicine woman was accused of wrongdoing or antisocial actions by local residents, whereas certain *bokaye* and marabouts are sometimes accused of subverting their powers, even practicing sorcery (Nicolaisen 1961; Rasmussen 2001a).

The point here is that *bokaye,* in contrast to *tinesmegelen,* seem to become more easily embroiled in social conflicts. Their sorcerous powers are more morally suspect and allegedly, at least, more prone to negative uses because they do not employ as strict ritual restrictions as herbal medicine women in regard to maraboutique injunctions. *Bokaye* in their relations with the Kel Essuf stand completely outside the popular Islamic ritual complex system; whereas herbal medicine women, even those who specialize in divination, seem to have "tamed" their spirits to accommodate Islam. As shown in the next chapter, medicine women more effectively build followings within that system.

Key issues here concern the wider implications of marabouts' competitors, in particular, herbal medicine women's roles. Are Islamic scholars requiring them to conform to their logic, or does this work the other way around? There appears to be little acrimony, but rather more cooperation and mutual respect in their relationship, on both sides. To what extent and how are compromises experienced and interpreted by the medicine women, and how far are they aware of these processes?

Medicine women, as observed, combine pre-Islamic and Islamic substances, actions, and spaces. Yet in these practices, their relation to the Islamic symbolic repertoire is ambiguous and, despite explanations emphasizing complementarity, reveals tensions and an "uneasy truce." This was illustrated by ritual restrictions and requirements of herbalists against cooking their medicines on Thursday or Friday, and against gathering their tree barks during the Muslim month of Bianu, because during this time there are believed to be harmful spirits haunting trees. Those few herbalists who specialize in divining by dreams, as shown in the chapter on divination, must in principle also be authorized by Islam: one such famous diviner or *tamaswad,* who cured many patients following her ten-year illness, was said to have practiced with both cowrie shells (a pre-Islamic symbol of fertility) and Qur'anic verses, which she miraculously learned suddenly, never before having been literate.

Although medicine women and marabouts often refer patients to one another, I noticed that in practice, herbalists often do diagnostic work early on in patients' healthcare histories, and then send patients to marabouts in later phases for more intensive treatment, more frequently than vice versa. This is often the pattern, for example, in spirit possession (Rasmussen 1995) and was also illustrated in the case of the couple's childlessness. When medicine women diagnose women's stomach trouble as due to spirits dancing in the stomach, which will soon travel up into the head, they send most but not all of these cases to marabouts, who attempt (with varying success) to treat them first with Qur'anic verses, before reluctantly acknowledging an altogether different ailment with the need for possession exorcism rituals—and sometimes, even sending them back to the medicine women.

Yet despite contradictions, overwhelmingly, herbalists verbally emphasized the complementarity between their roles and those of marabouts. Perhaps this was merely politeness, perhaps it masked the way they really felt, or perhaps they were actually unaware of competition between these healing roles; I do not know. Many Tuareg express ideas indirectly: nobles emphasize *tangal,* denoting speech by allusion or metaphor, and elders tend to be reticent with most youth (Rasmussen 1997; Casajus 2000). Yet the beliefs and statements of local residents are important and cannot be ignored. It is also important, however, to contextualize local statements and beliefs in the dynamic system of constraints and possibilities, not merely the ideal system (Rasmussen 1998b). In approaching these issues, therefore, I take into account local statements of beliefs, including their idealized system of opposed categories, but also analyze them as they exist within the system of power relations and as they are negotiated in diverse contexts.

In the countryside, where marabouts are respected and influential, it is through their "low profile" that Tuareg herbal medicine women guard their professional role. They must be resilient to protect their special powers in the face of both long-standing contradictions and recent change. Yet they cannot overstep certain limits. Thus the role of herbalists in treating diseases, particularly those afflicting women's bodies, is resilient but precarious, and their future uncertain, in a community where men and women experience changing social relationships and property balances, and where all suffer from ecological, economic, and political crisis. Like some other mediating figures, such as African griots, hunters, and smith/artisans (Arens and Karp 1989; McNaughton 1988; Sáenz 1991), medicine women broker male/female concerns, in a sense similar, though not identical, to some ambiguous gender roles such as the *waneng aiyem ser* (female ritual leader) among the Bimin Kuskusmin of New Guinea (Fitz Poole 1981) and other older women healers, as among the Hausa of Nigeria (Coles 1990). They are, as shown, often marital counselors. Medicine women use natural and cultural materials both literally and metaphorically to refer to, but also negotiate among, sometimes opposed spheres in the local ideal system of categories. But they do much more, as well. In their managing of female biological fertility, cultural/legal descent issues and interests of men and women, and cooperation with Islamic scholar/marabouts, medicine women subtly comment on and reinterpret important issues in Tuareg society: matrilineal and patrilineal property institutions, and pre-Islamic and "official" Islamic worldview. Local residents themselves make distinctions, and sometimes oppositions, among these domains; but they are not always rigidly opposed. Rather, they become intertwined and sometimes reversed in herbalists' work. Nonetheless, they stand in continual tension. In herbal medicine women's translation and negotiation of men's and women's interests in fertility, descent, and property, there have been shown to occur compromises and appropriations. But most Tuareg, including most herbal medicine women themselves, perceive these healers' role as bridging and reconciling others' interests rather than betraying them.

Perhaps marabouts are aware that medicine women may venture dangerously close to their "turf" of power and expertise. Certain stones and metals are believed to have protective and healing properties, but these same substances are believed dangerous to all except ritual specialists who "really" know them. Iron and other metals are more closely associated with hot fire spirits with whom smiths work: iron is considered close to, but also to repel, spirits. After all, as noted, medicine women are supposed to avoid iron precisely because they do not wish to repel their own tree spirits. Yet on the other hand, this taboo could be interpreted as restraining their spirit from challenging or competing with other ritual specialties. When Amina explained, "the ax is not good for gathering medicines; one must use stones or rocks, because the medicine does not like metals," here, she used the term *amagal*, not *eljenan* or Kel Essuf spirits; but this euphemism includes spirits. Thus here, medicine and spirits are collapsed into a single meaning in this euphemism. Smiths, close to the world of "hot" fire spirits believed to live underground, are a special, protected group, handling iron and other metals in their work with fire at the forge (Nicolaisen 1961). Mythical "fire spirits" are portrayed as living in subterranean grottos in the wild, working on miniature forges, and are feared for occasionally playing tricks on humans, as are human smiths in the countryside. Possessed women during spirit exorcism rituals hold an iron sword, believed to "cut and separate spirits." Both spirits of the wild and smiths are opposed in local symbolism to official Islam, and marabouts express greater ambivalence toward them openly than they do medicine women, toward whom marabouts express, almost always, benign attitudes and respect. Marabouts clearly reveal the wish to demarcate differences between all these specialists, however: they attempt to distance smiths and possession specialists from the mosque and to control times and places where exorcism and smithing are practiced, and also, they discourage medicine women from gathering their medicines in certain places (near marabouts' tombs and shrines) and times (Muslim holidays) and attempt to restrict (though not forbid) their writing of Qur'anic verses.

Implications

Most medicine women apparently, therefore, accept a specialized niche, in order not to challenge male Islamic authorities. Yet many, in their practice, mediate symbolically, socially, and materially between a series of dynamic powers in Tuareg society. In their touching, particularly, medicine women connect body and mind. On the one hand, herbal medicine women contribute to maintaining the status quo, through their practice as negotiators in the somatization of gender and wider conflicts around the central issues of fertility and displacement of matrilineal continuity by patrilineal affiliation. Local residents emphasize compromise and cooperation in herbal medicine women's role, and medicine women construe their role as that of mediating agents. This adjustment appears acceptable to most medicine women, one they can endorse without themselves perceiving (or at least, without voicing) contradictions, in spite of the possible erosion of their role as healers (of both bodies and social relations) in Tuareg society.

On the other hand, there are hints of conflict and even contestation, as shown, for example, in those rare cases of nonconformist medicine women who seek to pursue more powerful careers in their subspecialty of divination but who experience some obstacles to doing this, in mildly negative sanctions and penalties. If such women became too numerous and powerful, they would undoubtedly create rival power centers and compete, rather than cooperate, with Islamic scholars. For the vast majority of medicine women, their compromise with marabouts is an asymmetric one, which entails control and possibly subtle discouragement of the herbalist diviners. Many practices of medicine women in their relationships with spirits, patients, and marabouts may therefore be seen as strategies in the face of a dominant power that they have come to terms with in their work. Tuareg women have therefore strategically preserved their position as herbalists by collaborating with male Islamic healers, even in situations that may compromise the interests of women as a group. Although this allows them to remain viable and important within Tuareg society, it also contributes—along with central state tensions, ecological disaster, and economic scarcity—to their possible future marginalization.

Yet it must be recognized that, thus far at least, herbalism, its mythico-history, and its healing practices remain resilient in the face of change and crisis, through herbalists' avoidance of direct competition or open resistance. They achieve this by subtly evoking and commemorating aspects of Tuareg culture that tend to be submerged in everyday contexts. In herbal medicine, I argue, there is still a feminist reinterpretation of Islamic and maraboutique healing and science, though not a direct challenge to them. Herbalism yields insights into the formation of religious, philosophical, and scientific thought in terms of gender critiques. Herbal medicine emerges as a story of some women's intellectual efforts to reinterpret the canons of local authoritative knowledge systems. This was shown in rites of passage that remind participants of the importance of protecting women's interests. They also fulfill a real material need, relieving much pain with remedies that are inexpensive and easily available to local residents. But as also shown, herbalists' diagnoses and referrals in cases not responsive to such remedies may be reinterpreted and subverted. It is evident that herbal medicine women, wittingly or unwittingly, contribute to a kind of "panoptic gaze" and surveillance of the body, in that they act as brokers in a distinctive way: by also translating, facilitating, and converting the memories of pre-Islamic matriliny, encoded in medicine for women's bodies, into forms more acceptable or palatable to Islamic legal and medical influence. Further light is shed on these processes in the next chapter, in a closer examination of their more specialized mediumistic powers.

9—Medicine Women and Other "Shamans"

Herbalism, the Spirits of the Wild, Divination, and Power

"I do not work with dreams, because some dreams are false."—Zara

"Diviners work with the spirits. Herbalists and bone-setters touch."—Tana

"I am both an herbalist *(tanesmegel)* and diviner/medium *(tamaswad)*. I use dreams. The use of the dream *(targat)* is to tell the difference between good and evil, since if I dream of that which is good, I am happy. I dream for patients and I dream for myself. I must sleep to dream. It is sufficient that I sleep, I do not eat anything special or give anything in particular. It is my relatives who do that. There are nights when I do not dream, Thursday and Friday [Muslim prayer times], and sometimes Monday. There are also days I do not cure, for example, the 21st of the lunar month and the 28th of the month. Good times for curing are in the morning, because the two types of blood—good and bad—are apart [separated] at that time. Also, the patient I treat should not take milk or *eghale* for three days. There exists a medicine for vomiting *(tezufnin),* which purges the stomach. There are some persons for whom I do not dream because my spirits do not like the person. For example, that happened when there was someone who was bad.

"I dreamed for my daughter that she was going to bear a child and the child would not be normal. And she had that child, and the child was not normal [i.e., had a birth defect]. And I also dreamed *(orgata)* that the son of a man I knew would be killed by thieves, and they killed him, in Hausa country. The thieves killed him with a gun. They stole two hide sacks of dates. The child who was not normal was not killed. That child was not normal because of *tourgoum,* a pregnant woman's anger when someone, especially her husband, displeases her. When the woman is angry and she is pregnant, that happens."—Tina, an herbal medicine woman with additional, more powerful specialized divining skills

Tina, who lives in a small village near Timia at the summit of the Bagzan massif, was originally from the small village at its base where I resided long-term in my research. Tina is both an herbalist and a medium or diviner who uses dreams. As already observed, most medicine women use some basic divining methods in diagnosing for certain afflictions: namely, touch and spinning the pot for *karambaza,* that stomach ailment believed caused by smiths' anger. But most deny they divine by any more powerful means, such as dreaming. On one occasion, as Tina was treating two women patients suffering from hot illnesses or *tuksi,* she expressed the belief that a pregnant woman's anger *(tourgoum)* can sometimes cause the birth defect of having incomplete sexual organs. On the same day, Tina also examined a man briefly for cold illnesses or *tessmut* and treated me for a sore throat with bark from trees in Hausa country, called collectively *ilaten n tuksi:* these are from trees called *kedenya* and *tekaka.* *"Tessmut,"* Tina explained, "is associated also with the bitter taste, as well as the category of cold."

Tina continued: "Amulets (grigris, *ciraw,* or *elkhejjab*) will work only for those who believe in them. Bones contain powerful concentrations of *al baraka.* Medicine women who divine practice marabout divination, advice, and medicine only for people they know well; they must be kin or like kin."

Tina had treated eight persons within the two weeks before our interview. They had illnesses such as the hot conditions of *tuksi,* and she touched them to treat them. She continued to discuss her dreaming *asawad* method: "I dream without being asked. If someone requests dream divination, first I dream and divine that person's character before all else. If the person is honest, and whether he/she will pay. I do not do *alekhus-tara* because that does not resemble my dreaming; that is in the Qur'an. I do not have tools, I only see the patient. I am not the same as those who descend from the Prophet, the *icherifan.* But I am related to some of them distantly."

Tina also spoke of giving hope to patients, pointing out one woman in particular, who had recently suffered from marital problems with her husband, the deaths of several children, and also, economic reversals:

I dreamed that this work of curing Fatimata will go well here. Fatimata became ill in adulthood, about five years ago. She never went to the hospital. First, she was crazy and had the *goumaten* spirits. She has six children. She is of noble origins and has goats. In my opinion, since she came here to me, she is better. Before, I am told, she even struck her relatives. Now, she likes people, drinks water, and eats. Before, she neither drank nor ate.

I do not use cowrie shells, I only use my hand for this work. I touch and do medicines, my profession from my relatives. My relatives (parents) themselves gave me medicine. But medicines cannot cure Kel Essuf spirit affliction. There exist some illnesses that need doctors and their medicine—urinary problems, blood lacking or anemia, for example—here we need a clinic and antibiotics. Some medicines which are less strong, I give to women and children; the stronger ones [are] for men.

Usually, I touch the part of the body with my hand to diagnose the illness. *Anoughou* (a change in the usual routine) has caused your sore throat. Fatimata learned that I am here, and her daughter and older sisters accompanied her here. Fatimata is spending about a week here in treatment with me. They [her family, specifically, her cousins accompanying her] are paying me about 2500 CFA (US$5). If I touch the body of the patient, I must touch the earth in order not to catch the illness. [She demonstrated this by feeling the stomach of a man who had come to see her while I watched; she then diagnosed.] That is cold, *tessmut* that you have, inherited. You should place this medicine in the teapot and place it on the fire.

I am about 56 years old, Kel Ajirou and Kel Igurmadan. I have three children, two girls and one boy. My husband has been dead for a long time. He was a camel caravanner. I touch and make medicines to drink, and I also dream *(etaga targat)* when I sleep. If I touch the person and sometimes, I tell the patient, "You must be patient [phrase used if cannot cure, to give hope]." It is my inheritance from my parents, touching, the medicines, the dreams, everything. It is the medicine of a great need, if I work, I receive my compensation. Also, I do it to ask God's pardon for me. I did nine years of apprenticeship. When I received authorization, I offered alms in a small ceremony. A marabout read verses for me.

Tina and a male *boka* from Tchiluzduk were currently camping in a small seminomadic community for several months in order to treat local residents there. Often, well-known and highly regarded medicine women attract many patients, who come to them; but many also are itinerant and travel to patients' homes or throughout regions in different seasons. At that time, Tina was treating three women, all related to Mariama, the wife of a local chief who was cured by Hadia earlier. Tina's female patients suffered from *tuksi* and *tessmut*, and all were seeking a male diviner *boka's* purging medicines, as well as Tina's treatments. Tina added, "Fatimata suffers from these [illnesses], and also from Kel Essuf spirits and *togerchet* (evil mouth/eye)."

Fatimata, about 35 years old, was widely considered to be insane. Local residents warned me that she sometimes struck people. She had also undergone the spirit possession *tende n goumaten* rite, as had her cousin Mariama and her now-deceased mother, who had been frequently possessed. Fatimata and her accompanying female relatives camped apart from residents of the village. Tina, who was staying in a small conical grass building during the rainy season in that village, visited the women with her medicines. Fatimata's husband had a second co-wife in a village about half a mile down an unpaved road from the village of Fatimata. He spent most of his time with the second wife, however, and acquaintances indicated the couple was not divorced, but informally separated. She and her husband had a total of six children, some of whom died under very stressful circumstances: the husband had purchased magic from a spirit in Nigeria to make him become rich but had neglected to sacrifice the necessary chicken weekly, and so the spirit, it was believed, had caused several children to die. Fatimata had seen a marabout to "undo" the spirit curse, and this was accomplished, but at a price: the couple had become poor.[1]

Since medicine women believe that each person has two blood types, good and bad, separate in the morning, the morning is considered the best time for herbal pursing treatments that cause the bad blood to leave the body. Tina cooked her medicine overnight in a pot over the fire, and carried it over to the shady *ebizgen* trees where Fatimata was camped with her two relatives. Shortly before dawn, Fatimata drank this herbal concoction and allegedly felt better.

Some medicine women's more specialized non-Qur'anic divination, called *timaswaden* or *timanai* (from the verbal noun *asawad*, denoting "to look or see"), uses predominantly non-Qur'anic techniques such as herbs, perfumes, cowrie shells, mirrors, and other paraphernalia. Non-Qur'anic diviners, like Islamic scholars/marabouts, may call on spirits in private dreams. But whereas Islamic scholars dream by placing Qur'anic verses beneath their pillow, the tutelary spirits of sleeping non-Qur'anic diviners respond to them only after they offer them alms of perfume or animals. The most basic, standard divination/diagnosis most herbal medicine women use, called *takabar*—rotating a pot to diagnose for one type of stomach ailment believed caused by malevolent powers activated by an angry smith who has been refused a request for gifts or compensation for work—is much more widely practiced and also is the least controversial form of divination by medicine women. *Asawad* in dreaming is practiced by far fewer medicine women and is more controversial. Mina, the medicine woman who discussed Qur'anic writing earlier, added perspectives on this: "A diviner has relations with spirits (the Kel Essuf term was used here). Spirits are like a husband; with a contract, the woman does things for them, for example, she slaughters an animal. Otherwise, she loses her menstrual periods, or her child dies. That is why many prefer an old woman to have these relations with spirits for divination. For this interrupts marital life. For example, the husband of Tina died, and that of a famous deceased diviner, Toua, divorced her. For news the diviner asks the spirits for their reply." After this warning to me, she fearfully concluded: "I cannot give more news of diviners. I make bark medicines. I do the work of the medicine pot. The marabout works with his writing. That is why the marabout does *alekhustara* divination."

Another woman I knew, who resided in Hadia and Aghaly's village near the founding marabouts' tomb and sacred grove, allegedly began relations with spirits in order to divine. But she reneged on her promise to sacrifice a goat intermittently. This obligation nowadays is particularly difficult, in the wake of droughts and diminished livestock herds. As a consequence, the spirits allegedly "closed her door" (this expression local residents used meant that they caused her female genitals to vanish and made her asexual), and this, allegedly, prevented her from having children and ruined her marriage.

Another woman, now deceased but still famous throughout the region, had greater success in a mediumistic career. Toua of Ajirou knew Qur'anic writing cure, as well as divination. Hadia the medicine woman who resided in Atkaki, told me more about Toua:

> I knew Toua's relatives, though not Toua herself. Her village is called Aghatchere, it is next to Tilia, to the north of Affassas, near the Tenere desert plain. She began her divination after she had a serious illness for a long time, lying down without speaking, eating, or drinking. Throughout all this, people thought she would die, [but] she did not die. She remained there, she stayed alive, until she became very thin, thin as a rail. One day, people saw her install her covers, she told them, "You must bring me a sheep and slaughter it for alms." They slaughtered the sheep, and she said, "Now I am cured," and she began the work of divination *(asawad)*. Each thing she told them, they saw it was true. A child who was my nephew left to tell Toua, "My little camels are lost, you must divine for me." She divined and she said, "You must not go looking for them, you must stay at home, you will have news [of them]." He stayed at home, one day there were men who arrived, so he asked them, "Have you had news of my camels?" They replied, "Yes, they are over there, next door, for a long time."
>
> Toua was married, she had three daughters. Her husband left for Hausa country, he remained there for a long time. He returned, but he refused to stay with her. They separated. At that time, she was not quite right in the head (French *toc-toc;* Tamajaq *achelague*). Toua was part smith and part servile in origin. After that, always, wherever she lived, there were clients there. There were many people who sought her divination. All who were disoriented, they went to see Toua, to obtain the result or guidance. She even did [Qur'anic] writing, but no one taught her. Sometimes she referred people to marabouts. There was a

man from Berger who left to see her, and she referred him to me for medicine because he had been to the hospital several times, and then even to marabouts. She told him, "You are not cured, but your medicine is available from a woman named Hadia. She lives in an area where there are doum palms." When he came to me, he said, "I will tell you the truth, it was Toua who referred me to you." And I treated him. And I did not see him again. I asked news of him and was told he was cured. Another man also came to see me, and I told him, "I cannot treat you, I cannot." He went to the Agadez Hospital, where he died.

Here, Hadia expresses both admiration and some subtle envy of Toua. She seems proud that Toua referred patients to her and boasts that she ultimately cured a man who had seen Toua beforehand. Generally, all the foregoing comments and vignettes suggest that divining by dreams is unusual among medicine women. Yet as already noted, many medicine women perform another type of divination very routinely: that conducted by rotating the pot, called *takabar*. Wasu described this practice: "I do *takabar* divination with the pot. I place a hide on the ground and I place the wooden bowl on it, to identify [the source of] smiths' anger *(tezma)*. *Takabar* is uniquely for *tezma* illnesses. If there is someone who needs touch, I refer them to Lala. The old one does not refer patients to me. Sometimes I refer someone to her to touch, and the person returns to me for [other] medicine. I cannot treat the person except if she has been referred [to me] by the old one. She identifies [diagnoses] the illness and I treat it. Within the last two weeks, I have treated one person who came, but I did not have medicine for their illness. I did not have time to gather it. I said, 'You must go to the old one [Lala] or to someone you trust.' People pay me about 100 CFA (US 20 cents). One day I shall raise the price."

Even in practicing the method of *takabar*, therefore, are hints of the need for authorization and certain criteria for different healer apprenticeships and patient referrals. Wasu further explained:

The healer chooses the apprentice, and people choose the medicine if the practice is good. Other people sometimes crush barks and take them to other localities and they say, "It is the medicine of old Lala." They sell them, and it is not true. (They lie.) There is also a difference between those who divine and those who make bark medicines. Also, the herbalist works with the aid of her hands. A diviner is a confidante, she will divine all the spirits contained and all that clients seek. The medicine woman treats the person and feels changes in the organism. Medicine needs security. The marabout also identifies hidden illnesses, such as spirits, evil mouth/eye, and afterward the patient seeks medicine. . . .

I once referred the patient for whom I did *takabar* diagnosis/divination by the pot to a marabout. I also use the *takabar* divining by spinning the pot for my own children. I sent them to a marabout for Qur'anic verses. One time I did that for a neighbor, I told him to see his elder for Qur'anic verses afterward. When he first arrived, I did *takabar* for him and then he left. One time, I did *takabar* for old Tamalete. Her little camels were ill. I used the *takabar* pot divination, and I cited the names of the foods, and I called out all the names in order to identify which one she had been attacked for, and I told her "it was the millet." On her return, she did not save her little camel, he died. He had severe diarrhea. However, this *tezma* came, not [as usual] from a smith/artisan [denied the millet], but from a noble man unrelated to her.

Here, Tamalete lost camels to the anger of someone—not a smith in this case as usual—whom she had alienated. Most often, *tezma* is generated in local belief, automatically from a smith's angry heart when a noble patron fails to provide food, tea, or cash on demand or for services such as singing at rites of passage, arranging noble marriages, or manufacturing tools or jewelry. Residents explained to me that occasionally, however, nobles can generate very strong *tezma*. The point here is that *takabar* divination with the pot is used to diagnose problems related to economic competition, guilt, or jealousy, or from neglect of obligations.

In some more specialized medicine women's divining by *asawad* dreaming, perhaps there is potential competition with marabouts and other diviners such as the male *bokaye*. I do not wish to overstate a "conflict model" here, because local residents did not emphasize this to me, and cooperation, as shown, is also characteristic of their relationship. However, over a long-term process and in many contexts, while marabouts do not openly condemn or restrict herbal medicine women who become diviners, they do act in subtle ways to protect their own profession.

Thus it is not surprising that Hadia, Mina, Wasu, and others regarded the most specialized medicine woman diviners such as Tina and the late Toua with awe, but also some fear. They related problems befalling those few herbalists who became *timaswaden*: mainly marital instability and divorces. In this light, the woman whose "door was closed" (i.e., her genital organs were believed to disappear), upon her acquisition of these skills may have perhaps gained substantial influence; I do not know. But clearly, in effect, this woman's fate involved a curtailment of powers that had perhaps became too threatening to the healing "establishment." What is clear is that a few herbalists, while in conversation and other overt acts deferring to official authoritative knowledge claims, may indirectly express dissent or dissatisfaction, or at least feel ambition (locally articulated as a "calling" by spirits, sometimes inherited), and become more specialized, pursuing divination by dreams. But when they do this, there is a price.

The Tutelary Spirits and Essuf or the "Wild"

There are many empty, abandoned places in more nomadic Tuareg regions. Upon my residence among more nomadic Tuareg in northern Mali, I was able to better understand why Tuareg believe Kel Essuf enter places once full of people and now empty. I came to feel myself the power of this concept of *essuf* from my own wanderings in these vast spaces. Nomads often move, and as a result, tents are there one day and gone the next, or still there on the same spot but left empty for weeks at a time. I was left with the impression of a mirage. This was very disconcerting. Even if tents remain, but are unoccupied or half-disassembled (their parts are portable), the effect is one of desertion and abandonment: not just physical but also psychological. While undoubtedly as an outsider I was more affected by this, still, there is more at play here than mere "culture shock." For local residents, also, express similar sentiments. In some regions, even houses are spaced far apart and stand empty for much of the year, as nomads follow animals out to pastures with the arrival of the rains around late July. The more well-to-do sedentarized people often have large compounds in their village with large interior courtyards, with their houses located deep inside and far from outer doors.

In the high winds (which occur almost daily), one cannot easily hear hosts or visitors. Striking here are the vast spaces, dotted with wells without concrete linings or rims into which children (and also many non-Tuareg visitors unfamiliar with the environment) sometimes fall.

One morning, upon my first arrival in a more nomadic community in northern Mali, I announced over tea to my host family that I was looking forward to taking a walk around the area. Suddenly alarmed, they quickly arranged for an adolescent to accompany me. I now realize the reason for this: the first action to protect a guest is to have someone accompany him or her on their first walk, in order to avoid these wells! Of course as an outsider, I was more vulnerable to these hazards. To the new visitor, this terrain appears undifferentiated at first scrutiny, but to local residents, at least adults, there are clearly demarcated features and bounded zones, some safe and others dangerous.

There is spirituality here, but also loneliness. Spaces once peopled and vital are apt to suddenly become empty and solitary: this is *essuf*. The human social group should ideally be marshaled to fill this dangerous void. To grasp the full meaning of *essuf*, one in effect needs to wander. Hawad, the modern Tuareg expatriate poet (1989), frequently compares his poetry composition to wandering. *Essuf* is therefore both a literal place and a psychosocial state. *Essuf* is extended metaphorically into wider social and political symbolic spaces. Herbal medicine women are associated with the wild and affliction, the spirits, and yet also with conversion into healing and cultural knowledge, and the maternal tent. They in effect make the wild less threatening, in taming it, *"bricoleur"*-like, with their materials at hand, but they also act as philosophers and psychiatrists.

Usually Kel Essuf non-Qur'anic spirits are considered evil, but some say not all such spirits are evil. Certain persons are believed to have a pact or contract with some Kel Essuf, who aid them. Such persons, sometimes called "friends of the Kel Essuf" (Rasmussen 2001a), almost always have several spirits with them, speak to these spirits in their special language, and execute mystical actions with their aid. They can help other humans by giving them advice against illness, or they can find things or predict future events by sending their Kel Essuf spirits who travel far very rapidly (Nicolaisen 1961). As shown, Toua the medicine woman with special divination skills helped someone find lost and stolen camels.

The concept of *essuf*, which denotes "the wild," and by extension, sometimes, also "solitude" or "nostalgia," is used, not solely in public spirit possession ritual contexts, but also in mediumistic divination and healing outside possession rituals, and is therefore most central to more general divination (Hawad 1979; Nicolaisen and Nicolaisen 1997). Relevant here are conceptualizations of trance and altered states of consciousness (ASC), which are so central to classic shamanistic/mediumistic healing in many cultures (Monnig-Atkinson 1992; Winkelman 1999, 2001). Yet the outcomes of trance vary: some persons who are possessed by the Kel Essuf become healers, whereas others do not (Rasmussen 2001a).[2]

There exist special methods of contacting the Kel Essuf through the following rules: one must be very clean, because Kel Essuf detest dirt; one must sacrifice a sheep or goat every seven days, because the Kel Essuf like blood; one must speak directly to the Kel Essuf by not pronouncing the Islamic *Bissmillah* benediction conveying *al baraka* during sacrifice; and one must not marry without authorization of one's spirits (Nicolaisen 1961:129).

The Islamic and pre-Islamic spirit pantheons are both powerful in mediumship and healing. The Qur'an mentions *djinn* spirits, appealed to by Islamic scholars in their written verse healing and divination methods, but there are also non-Qur'anic spirits, including those matrilineal, ancestral, and other spirits appealed to by all herbalist "medicine women." Others, the Kel Essuf, are appealed to by those gifted with special mediumistic powers. In much previous Tuareg ethnography, however, there is a neglect of the tree spirits and medicine women's relationship to them. As seen earlier in the chapter on arboreal imagery, during their gathering all medicine women—even those not specialized in dreaming—directly address personified tree spirits hinted to have anthropomorphic ancestral and matrilineal kinship roles.

Thus divining is a matter of degree and specific context. There are subtle nuances to these powers. Medicine women's more specialized "shamanic-like" mediumistic powers in many contexts derive from an interweaving of, rather than rigid opposition between, hierarchical "official" and nonhierarchical unofficial religious cosmologies. Medicine women specializing in the most powerful form of mediumship—*asawad* dream divination—are not exactly disapproved of, but there are strong hints they are feared, regarded ambivalently, and need to be regulated. Although many marabouts conduct divination by dreaming with Qur'anic verses beneath a pillow, nonetheless, dreams as authoritative knowledge are somewhat controversial; local residents tend to disagree about their reliability or truth value.[3]

Toua, the deceased famous female herbalist/diviner who had been gravely ill, divined where lost or stolen property was located, and like Tina, the living diviner medicine woman we just met, predicted birth defects. This ability to predict birth defects believed caused by a husband's angering of his pregnant wife is a crucial power of medicine women in their mediating marital conflict and protecting women from domestic abuse. Significantly, Hadia and others emphasized that Toua later also began to combine non-Qur'anic and Qur'anic divination. Yet equally significant is their marveling at how Toua continued the more common non-Qur'anic practice of divining with cowrie shells, however, and they considered this complementary rather than opposed to her Qur'anic healing/divination. In drawing upon both "shamanic"-like powers and the Qur'an, therefore, this diviner/medicine woman integrated the cosmological systems of the Islamic God, Qur'anic spirits, and non-Qur'anic, matrilineal ancestral spirits.

Women who become diviners face dilemmas, however. For since the Kel Essuf spirits are like a husband, the diviner has a contract and obligations to them, and this may compete with and damage her sexual relationship with the human spouse, or may drain off property resources from the domestic household. Ideally, however, as Tina explained, dreaming is done "in order to distinguish between good and evil, foretell the future, and diagnose illnesses." When she indicated that the diviner must also know the patient very well, and must like them by dreaming first to divine the patient's character before proceeding with additional diagnoses, Tina implied the strong pressure to imbue these skills with moral legitimacy. Indeed, Tuareg debates over the uses of dreaming to divine and diagnose resemble some debates in the West over the uses of scientific research, such as cloning and stem cell research. These powers, in other words, are viewed as awesome but fearful, and they must be channeled. Divining medicine women address (often implicitly and obliquely, rather than directly) relationships between men and women: for example, love, marriage, and property concerns.

Women's empowerment is promoted (if not always successfully, at least in intent) by the matrilineal symbolism of herbal and diviner healing, with an overlay of social criticism, as shown in Hadia's and Tina's warnings about *tourgoum* and birth defects resulting from husbands' mistreatment of pregnant women.

Kel Essuf possession is one kind of illness of the soul, in its initial manifestation. In the local medical system, an illness of the soul is a state, or more precisely, a place of alterity, where one takes refuge, torn between two choices or universes that are different and irreconcilable (Hawad 1979:82). It is that desolate space and its condition called *essuf*: solitude or, as Hawad terms it in his more modern poetic works (Hawad 1989), nostalgia. At first, when the person is attacked by the Kel Essuf, initially he/she is torn between the moral community of humans with its rules and the worlds of the evil spirits. Hawad (1979:82, 1989) calls this a "cultural and social desert" that makes the patient sensitive to the calls of the Kel Essuf. Elements of divination and possession rituals encourage the possessed to make a choice between these worlds. For example, the songs in the *tende n goumaten* assist the patient to choose to return to cultural sources of support. Often their first phrases sing of loneliness and desolation, and their last phrase sing of the joys of social life, ideally bringing the ill person back into the community. Or, alternatively, one becomes adept at controlling the Kel Essuf spirits of the wild and solitude, and, cured, begins to practice divination/mediumship in a contract or pact with these spirits.

Here, as in many studies of shamanism and related processes such as possession and mediumship, one faces the issue of control, or power. Where women dominate in the shamanic ranks, shamanic prominence has often been subsumed by political and religious centralization. However, early interpretations of this pattern as women's peripheralization and deprivation (Kennedy 1977; Lewis 1971) have now been challenged as mechanistic and inapplicable in many cases (Lewis 1986; Boddy 1987; Rasmussen 1995). For example, there is also widespread cross-dressing among male shamans, interpreted by some theorists as a means whereby men attempt to tap these special female qualities. Among the Tuareg, male *bokaye* most often wear henna; but female *tchimaswaden* diviners do not wear this, nor do they dress as men.

In understanding the relationships of gender and "shaman-like" divining power, therefore, both need to be understood as parts of wider sets of discourses and practices specific to particular regions and histories instead of predictable outcroppings of a general physiological and psychological substratum (Monnig-Atkinson 1992:319). Shamans both create and sustain, and also disrupt and decenter natural and social order as well (Taussig 1987). Exploring the dialectics of shamanic power in relation to gender must take into account the ambiguities and multivalences of shamanic power and anticipate related complexities in gendered ideas and practice (Monnig-Atkinson 1992:319).

Problematic as the term *shaman* may be, some (though not all) Tuareg medicine women divine, and their forms of ASC, while not absolutely identical to classic shamanistic healing, closely resemble it. Although the Tuareg are a seminomadic pastoral (livestock herding) and oasis gardening (and, increasingly, also, labor migration) society, nonetheless, gathering was once an important source of food, and today it remains a significant source of medicinal herbs for many in rural communities. Tuareg mediumistic healers do gather medicines and ritual paraphernalia in their healing methods. Medicine women's narratives, comments, and actions in context suggest that one important preoccupation and goal of theirs is to continue to gather—and this is sometimes a challenge. Importantly, there is more is at stake in this than the material medicines: cultural memory and knowledge are also bound up in their gathering. In effect, gathering—while no longer the general activity of all Tuareg—serves as a mnemonic to remind other Tuareg of the importance of physical and spiritual connections to the medicine complex, which constitutes part of their more general pastoral nomadic cultural heritage. Herbal medicine women act to promote this heritage and all it evokes.

Regardless of gender, anyone's altered state of consciousness involving spirits is initially defined as an affliction. It becomes empowering and leads to special mediumship/divination skills in some, but not all persons (Rasmussen 2001a). Less fortunate persons remain ill or even become "crazy" according to local cultural formulations and remain so, without developing mediumistic powers, that is, their illness does not lead to diviner status (recalling the case of the Korean woman who did not become a shaman, analyzed by Marjorie Wolf). How do these processes occur, and what accounts for their different outcomes? In particular, how do Tuareg medicine women attain close relations with the Kel Essuf spirits, but also maintain control over the spirits and empowerment in the human social sphere? This is an important criterion for medicine women diviners such as Toua and Tina, since the call of the Kel Essuf usually leads to efforts to pull humans back into the social community, or they are lost (Hawad 1979).

In Tuareg medicine women's routine and more specialized divination, diagnostic, healing, and referral work, therefore, are hints of contradiction and conflict. *Asawad* divination by dreams is regarded with mixed fear and admiration, considered a special gift difficult to attain, of uncertain moral value, and risky. For it often follows a serious illness, such as Toua's, and also requires a contract with spirits whose demands cause a drain on the diviner's time and resources, distracting her from her domestic responsibilities. *Shamanism,* if indeed the Siberian term may be used in the Saharan context, herbalism, and spirit mediumship are therefore inseparable among the Tuareg; these are a matter of degree of specialty and also of degree of influence in the social network—by implication, acceptance by the powerful maraboutique clans, as was evident in Mina's comments. Some persons inherit or cultivate or purchase a "pact" with the spirits, bringing them under their control through offerings and observance of certain ritual restrictions, and acquiring mediumistic/divining and healing powers. Some medicine women, although not exactly equivalent to the prototypical gloss "shaman," approximately correspond to some widely distributed characteristics of shamans, in their recruitment and activities. Some medicine women, such as Tina, may, like marabouts, call on spirits in private dreams, but whereas Islamic scholars dream by placing Qur'anic verses beneath their pillow, the tutelary spirits of sleeping non-Qur'anic diviners respond to them only after they offer them alms of perfume or animals. The tutelary spirit is believed to mount the diviner. Both specialists, however, must establish trust and credibility if their authoritative knowledge systems are to be held in equal, parallel esteem.

Shamanic power generally manifests itself in trance. As a concept, however, trance constitutes a naturalist gloss or cover term that somewhat inadequately describes a range of altered states of consciousness and should be distinguished from other similar states, involving finer nuances of meaning, in different cultural interpretation. Possession, for example, has frequently been contrasted with shamanism in anthropological literature (Eliade 1964:6; de Heusch in Lewis 1986:81–83). In this view, shamanism is seen as voluntary mystical flight, possession as involuntary experience of descending spirits. Yet as I. M. Lewis has argued, this opposition is misleading. It is, for example, through the intervention of spirits that an individual first recognizes his or her vocation as a shaman or medium (Lewis 1986:84–91). Thus the issue is how those Tuareg medicine women who dream attain a state related to trance and how this process is related to their "friendship" with the Kel Essuf.

Among the Tuareg, non-Qur'anic diviners differ from marabout Qur'anic diviners in the nature of their relationship with the spirits and how this is expressed. Although both do divination and healing, the types of divining and trance differ. Instructive here is a focus on the performance aspect of shamanic trance. There is a compelling poetry of shamanic chanting (Siikala and Hoppal 1992): spirit-evoking songs help shamans enter trance, with key mythic metaphors. Rasmussen (1995:130) emphasizes how important the aesthetics of the sung poetic verses are to the therapy of exorcism: local participants in the spirit possession rituals stated that the songs soothe illnesses of the heart and soul and distract the possessed person from troubles. As Malam Moussa explained, marabouts describe themselves, ideally, as a channel, mouthpiece, and magnet for God. They divine through several means of interpreting astrological numbers and letters and verses from the Qur'an. Non-Qur'anic diviners call on the spirits in private dreams after they offer their tutelary spirits alms. While most medicine women usually diagnose through touching for illnesses locally defined as organic (i.e., physical or "naturalistic"), the boundaries between "natural" and "psychosocial" afflictions, as I have demonstrated, are hazy, and some herbalists have been shown to possess special mediumistic powers and divine for not solely organic but also psychosocial or nonorganic, afflictions. This was vividly illustrated earlier, in the cases of the medicine women's divination for evil mouth/eye and for smiths' *tezma*-caused stomach *karambaza*, both of which are connected to wider beliefs concerning the causation of misfortune, which sometimes serve as "leveling mechanisms." *Tezma*-related beliefs, for example, tend to limit the accumulation of too-concentrated wealth in the hands of too few persons, thereby tending to encourage economic reciprocity and redistribution. In those contexts, medicine women's diagnoses served to transmit cultural values of sharing and mutual obligations, crucially important in rural communities in the Sahara and its Sahelian fringes, where resources are often very scarce and uncertain, and people are understandably tempted to hoard items for security.

Implications

Thus by performing various types of divination successfully (that is, without challenges from others), medicine women wrestle with but also manipulate the spirits and, in effect, "turn around" misfortune and suffering, bringing into the open latent psychosocial and interpersonal conflicts and diagnosing their causes and prescribing their remedies. Some challenging was implied in the case of the couple's childlessness: Hadia and the marabout, in effect, were seen in alternation and their opinions were contesting ones. But in general, successful diviners underline and remind others of important values in public consciousness.

The question arises here of exactly how effective in consequence are these reminders? In their warnings against domestic violence in rural communities, medicine women appear still effective. In the Tuareg countryside, there remains a strong taboo against wife-beating, and as far as I was able to ascertain, most men obey this. On the other hand, violence is more frequent in the towns. Moreover, as the foregoing cases and vignettes show, some rural men, while not physically violent, inflict much psychosocial violence upon women, particularly in men's threatened and actual polygyny.

Throughout the more specialized divining of some medicine women like Tina, who warned of *tourgoum* and birth defects, there were shown to be hints of spirits and humans competing for the diviner's attention, and of difficult demands made upon these shamanic healers in their pact with the Kel Essuf. What is the meaning of these beliefs? Since the diviner must make certain sacrifices and give them as alms to the Kel Essuf and also to other humans (for example, maternal relatives and children) to reinforce their medicines and preserve the contract with the spirit(s), by extension, she must establish trust in the social sphere. There must be concern for human welfare beyond the immediate household and one's own gain. Above all, however, people must come to trust all healers who claim special relations with the spirits. This is what distinguishes their ritual/therapeutic practice from ordinary illness, mental deficiency, or other personal problems. All diviners—not just medicine women, but also others in the pluralistic healing system described by Rasmussen (2001a), in fact, must ideally display dignity, reserve, and generosity. They must follow special rules and observe taboos: for example, male diviners are not supposed to see prostitutes or take lovers. One male *boka* sorcerer stated: "You must love one woman, [the one] you are married to; you must wear henna, for spirits like henna [on fingernails, toenails, hands, and feet], you must make other offerings to the spirits and to people" (Rasmussen 2001a).

The point here is that the attainment of a legitimate pact with the Kel Essuf, as with much shamanism and other healing specialties, despite some nonconforming and anomalous characteristics, does not really result from "marginality," but rather, this requires a secure network of social support transcending the immediate possession ritual context and professional credibility based on personal character credentials. Medicine women, in other words, may stand on the boundary and periphery, but they cannot venture too far out into the wild. They cannot fall over the abyss. Tuareg women's activities imply that mediating, more broadly, does not create simply "alternate" scripts or "dissonant discourses" (Boddy 1987; Abu-Lughod 1993) but rather may often require exemplary conduct to produce a parallel authoritative knowledge system.

As Fabrega and Silver (1973) point out in their study of shamanic healers in the Mayan community of Zinacantan in Mexico, the professional success of folk healers depends upon the healer's interpersonal skills, which are in part reflected by his/her ability to emotionally arouse others and especially by his/her ability to influence and manipulate their behavior in line with particular decisions related to treatment he/she administers. These skills stem from persuasive or "charismatic" personality attributes. A practitioner's success also depends on what could be termed his/her "clinical judgment" (Fabrega and Silver 1973:8). In other words, patients of successful practitioners should more often improve than not. These authors surmise that perhaps healers select and treat only those persons whose underlying medical problem is likely to remit or improve. Recall that Tina the diviner medicine woman only divined for some patients, and only after dreaming to ascertain their character. Clearly, Tina was more sensitive to physical attributes and manifestations of illness that relate to prognosis. Tina and other more "clairvoyant" medicine women are believed to have special powers and responsibilities, furthermore, because their territory includes principal sacred landmarks or zones, as also reported among the Mayans studied by Fabrega and Silver (1973:38). Tuareg medicine women continually invoke similar credentials.

Most medicine women have therefore "carved a niche" for themselves within official Islam. How exactly do they fare with other more powerful systems, namely, the wider infrastructure, dominant in the towns but also encroaching in the countryside, of Euro-American established allopathic medicine or biomedicine?

10—Changes in the Wind

Medicine Women's Relations with Established Biomedicine

We herbalists [Tana asserted] can cure some illnesses that hospitals cannot: for example, cold or *tessmut;* we also can feel spirits. One person, for example, searched time and again for medicine against *tessmut* at the hospital. He could not find it. There are also illnesses that the hospitals can cure that herbalists cannot: these include *taghrawe* (smallpox), *kourji* (or *lumat,* measles), *zigagh* (chickenpox), and *akissiwe n azni* (approximately denoting a deficiency of blood, often translated as "anemia"). For good health, one needs antibiotics from the clinic, in order to facilitate our curing, if the hospital is nearby, and if there is also a marabout [i.e., one needs to supplement traditional healing with Western biomedicine for certain illnesses]. I have never been to a training session on the large oasis near here. I would like to go, if given the opportunity. I would like to increase my experience, to learn about childbirth and the care of newborns. . . .

Once I was in a nearby village. I saw Adima, the mother of Halalo, as she crushed her *eghale* to go to Agadez, because Halalo often has childbirth problems each time she has a child. I touched her, I told her, "That does no good, even if you crush *eghale* [to travel to Agadez], you must not go to Agadez. The child in the stomach, he is better, leave him alone, she is going to give birth here. The other herbalists recommended that she go to Agadez, not me." They told her that the child was not normal. The following evening, she gave birth. The child was normal, however, except for a twisted foot. [Here, it is unclear whether Tana meant that the woman's usual reproductive problems included difficulties in giving birth, as well as having children with birth defects, or birth defects in her children only.]

According to Zara, the medicine woman specializing in massage whom we encountered earlier,

during a session of [first-aid] training for medicine women, the state nurse *(l'infirmier d'etat)* at the clinic told us when there is a birth, one heats water and keeps different foods nearby. Whenever she [a woman] gives birth, she eats them. If the pregnant woman is swollen, you must place two pillows on either side, at the head and the feet. You give her soap with which to wash, each time she urinates, she washes. If there is an older child, one heats water and places a little sugar in it, and gives that to the child to drink before he breastfeeds. One gives the woman hot water and soap to wash.

We went four times [in a training program for *tinesmegelen*] to the large oasis town about twenty kilometers from here. On our first trip, we spent fifteen days there, and each day we received 1000 CFA (approximately US$2). We lodged in the village, sometimes at the primary school there. There were seven women who did the training project, and it interested us. We left [to return to our villages and camps] by a small truck. Me, I still wish the other organizations would come [return again] to help us, as before.

According to Amina on Mt. Bagzan, "there are some illnesses that medicine women can cure, but hospitals cannot: cold illnesses or *tessmut,* because the medicine woman touches [to diagnose this] and the marabout cures this. Also, an herbalist must cure hot illnesses or *tuksi* [i.e., illnesses requiring touch are the domain of medicine women]. The hospital can cure skin irritations with shots *(atinfousse),* and headaches, sores, and fever. For better health here, we must have a doctor in the village. I have never gone to school or to training sessions, and do not want to, because I have no time. Now, however, the bark medicines are difficult [demanding to obtain] because they are on the mountain, one must find them on the mountain. Also, if it does not rain [in drought], they do not grow. Also, people are old, they cannot climb."

Wasu explained, "in order to have a medicine woman's medicine work, one must guard against *ezziz* (the illness from sitting on hot sand or mats), the wind, and cold water. One must use tepid water. Illnesses that medicine women, not hospitals, heal are the heat *tuksi*-related illnesses. Some sores on the interior of the body herbalists cannot cure, only hospitals. For good health, however, one needs a clinic. [After this study, later, a clinic was built near her village.] . . . Once, they [clinic personnel] held a training session in the large oasis to the southwest of Mt. Bagzan for herbalists, but I did not attend because I was not invited."

Mina, the medicine woman I accompanied on gathering expeditions, explained, "Illnesses that herbalists can cure and clinics cannot cure include *anoughou, tezoufnine, tuksi, eziz*—their medicines are tree barks. Clinics can cure other illnesses that herbalists cannot; for example, skin problems, some more serious such as *kourji* sores, fevers. There are three types of fever: *alafaz* (from falling); *awissa* (from running) and *edichi* (malaria, literally denoting "mosquito"). In my opinion, for better health here we need doctors of the hospital—all the products at the hospital. I have never participated in the training sessions in the large oasis. I would like to. I hope to increase my experience, knowledge, and intelligence. And then, I believe that I also want to know certain illnesses that I do not know. The biomedical doctor *(lokotoro)* knows certain illnesses that we do not know here. I can learn all of them."

Tanou commented, "I have never referred anyone to the hospital. The hospital cures knee problems better than herbalists, but herbalists cure *tuksi* better than hospitals. *Tuksi* medicinal products are easy to find. Shots, antibiotics *(tchibloulagh* or *tchiwadaqen,* also pills) and a clinic are needed for better health here. I have never been to a training session in Tabelot or Agadez. No, I do not wish to do this; I cannot learn there."

Many medicine women emphasized to me that some women are ashamed to answer personal questions in the presence of their husband. This is contrary to what some urban biomedically trained staffs in hospitals and clinics told me: the latter believed that women are less ashamed to answer these questions when the husband is present to translate. The problem here is one of control: how much choice do women have in this situation? To local Tamajaq speakers in northern Niger and Mali, in particular rural residents, medicine women are important social and ceremonial, as well as medical, specialists. As in some other cultures, such as among the Navajo of the Southwestern United States (Trudelle-Schwartz 2003), medicine women formulate their own type of legitimacy and authoritative knowledge within their own small-scale communities of face-to-face contacts, intimate social networks, and shared cultural knowledge. Within predominantly Tamajaq-speaking rural communities, medicine women renegotiate authority and legitimacy in practical situations. As shown, this system constitutes a parallel authority system, neither superior nor inferior to that of Islamic scholars/marabouts. Beyond this context, exactly how dominant is their own system of authoritative knowledge? How do they fare in more multiethnic settings such as larger sedentarized communities and the towns, in closer encounters with Western state and NGO powers of Western allopathic medicine?

Only within the last fifteen years have hospital and clinic staffs in Tuareg regions of Mali and Niger consulted Tuareg medicine women as intermediaries and go-betweens in their medical consultations with local Tamajaq-speaking women. Until recently, many hospital and clinic staffs in the northern regions were predominantly male and of outside ethnic and regional origins. In previous analyses of the pluralistic medical system, Rasmussen (1994, 2001a) has described details of the political processes and local attitudes concerning medicine and healing in historical perspective. In the past, many Tamajaq speakers tended to fear hospitals and clinics. Attitudes are changing: many now increasingly go to hospitals and clinics for treatment of illnesses. However, many women in rural northern Niger and Mali still prefer to give birth at home and take children to medicine women as a first choice.

Since the peace accords ending the Tuareg nationalist/separatist rebellions during the early 1990s in Niger and Mali, some state and international NGO-sponsored aid programs have been emphasizing greater collaboration with local healers in the semiautonomous northern regions of Aïr and the town of Agadez in Niger and Adragh-n-Ifoghas and the town of Kidal in northern Mali. While these policies have initiated fruitful dialogues in training programs for some medicine women and other health workers, problems remain. Sometimes there are collisions between their different knowledge and power systems.

Davis-Floyd and Sargent (1997) have, correctly in my view, pointed out that there is never one single system of authoritative knowledge, but several. In any particular frame of observation, the dominant system either better explains the experienced world to its actors, or it is associated with a stronger power base. All logical systems coexist with varying degrees of cooperation and conflict. People seeking help often move from one to another, and practitioners borrow techniques from each other. Jambai and MacCormack (in Davis-Floyd and Sargent 1997:443) describe how, in Sierra Leone, Mende women's Sande secret society high officials are also traditional midwives and healers. Thus the issue explored in this chapter becomes, how do Tuareg medicine women feel about sharing power with government-trained clinic and hospital personnel? How are respectful working relationships negotiated? Tuareg medicine women work in an environment of increasing pluralism but also conflict, contradiction, and change. Indeed, even in rural communities, as shown, they face changing and contested local interpretations of their authoritative knowledge. Some philosophical and technical resources of Tuareg medicine women remain effective, yet others are increasingly being marginalized by dominant state and NGO-sponsored health care.

Reactions to the relationship between medicine women and biomedical personnel and training programs are mixed, and the effects of these trends are double-edged. Future trends are difficult to predict. Thus far, Tuareg medicine women's strategies have protected them from being overtly persecuted by official religion or established medicine, in contrast to some other herbalists and midwives. But their emphasis upon accommodation in their local community may not protect their roles from being eroded, by national and transnational forces, whether secular, biomedically trained medical personnel representing central governments, or those representing broader-based Islam. Most Tuareg herbal medicine women remain peripheral in their relationship to established medicine in countries where they live. Other health practitioners enjoy a much higher profile outside rural areas, drawing upon a symbolic repertoire more widely understood throughout the nation-state. Medicine women's low profile, as well as ecological and political crises, the marginal position of Tamajaq speakers throughout Niger and Mali, and the low budgets of their central state governments have all caused these women to be only minimally included in health programs.

A few first-aid and midwifery programs based at the Agadez Hospital in Niger have occasionally offered training, supplies, and certificates to rural herbalists. In Kidal and several other nearby sedentary towns in Mali, there are similar programs, for example, an ambulance schedule. But these programs have been sporadic and irregular in follow-up support because of economic austerity throughout these countries (for example, severe shortages of medicine and devaluation of the local currency) and also from isolation of their northern regions, not solely during the recent Tuareg political conflict with the central government, but also more long-term, due to difficult geographic access; where roads exist, for example, they become impassable for even large trucks and four-wheel-drive landrovers during the rainy season, and in many more mountainous zones, there are only walking paths studded with volcanic rocks. Medicine women tend to move about in seminomadism, gathering in more remote mountain areas, and use predominantly local plant medicines sometimes threatened by drought. Also, as shown, medicine women tend to be modest, to be reticent toward youths, and to defer publicly to respected persons. These conditions suggest that, while rural communities have never been hermetically sealed or "timeless" places, nonetheless, some theories tend to exaggerate the extent of globalization and to assume its effects are homogenized, when they are not.

Even when medicine women occasionally purchase medicines on the outside markets, they tend to do this through intermediaries, usually male relatives on caravans and labor migration. Indeed, many medicine women are reserved toward all outsiders, particularly youthful outside (non-kin) males—who are frequent representatives of established biomedicine and aid programs. Narratives in this chapter and throughout this book reveal that medicine women in many situations can be quite assertive: for example, in conversations and interviews with me and in sessions with patients, they did not hesitate to request antibiotics, and they generally wished to increase their knowledge. Nonetheless, evidence also shows that medicine women prefer to treat in private and often express their opinions indirectly—among women, close kin, or to men who stand in joking relationships with them, such as cousins. Medicine women express sympathy with wives in private consultations but refrain from openly criticizing husbands in public, and they also tend to defer to marabouts' opinions in public.

A variety of medical practitioners provides local residents with a modicum of choice, as long as there is not coercion toward some channels at the cost of others. Limited access to established medicine shields local women from some more oppressive effects of medicine, such as pressures to undergo unnecessary reproductive surgery (Rasmussen 1994). Perhaps too much intervention, however well intended, may further restrict or co-opt local medicine women's roles. Yet in conversations, interviews, and narratives, medicine women never objected to male state nurses, nor did they express any wish to become state nurses themselves (though Tana expressed a desire to train as a midwife); rather, most favored cooperation and sharing some useful knowledge but retaining their own niche. Yet one must remember that local cultural values, especially among persons of noble origin, discourage direct expression of one's wishes or opinions.

Only a few Tamajaq-speaking medicine women have become licensed midwives in the towns. One such medicine woman, whom I'll call Mama, resided in a large sedentarized village in the Kidal region of Mali. Mama, a midwife whose mother had been an active herbal medicine woman, related some of her experiences and impressions: "I am twenty-seven years old and have practiced this profession [midwifery] for about five years. I learned it in a training session in Kidal for three months in 1996. I do this work because they built a maternity [here], and women are afraid without a female midwife. There was a Bambara midwife *(sage-femme)* who was brought here by the Malian army, for two years, but women were intimidated by her."

In Mama's village, there had been a tense situation during the Tuareg nationalist/separatist rebellion, although there were efforts to repatriate and compensate local residents upon their return from Mauritania and Algeria, where they had fled in the early 1990s as refugees. There was much political conflict surrounding the closing of the modern well near the military camp. There was renewed military and civilian competition over wells during the more recent occupation by the army in the 1990s, the volatile era of the more recent Tuareg nationalist/separatist rebellion in northern Mali and Niger. There was pressure to give priority to the military in water use. Women, in particular, still deplore the inexploitabilty of the truck-gardening wells from lack of technical assistance. They often have to walk long distances to wells, and they express resentment over the military's use of much local water. This use also interferes with the water availability at a local clinic, Mama indicated. Although the army post was due to leave that village, it had not yet moved. Mama and her husband resided near the local clinic. They had several children. Her husband was originally from southern Niger, and in contrast to most residents of their village in Mali, who were predominantly herders and merchants, he tended a small garden plot in his compound and also baked bread for local sale.

Mama indicated to me somewhat wistfully that her mother used to practice herbal medicine, but "the plants are scarce in our region, so she was not too specialized." Other women in that region told me that herbal medicine women occasionally come through as itinerant rather than locally based healers. This suggests their healing involves less knowledge of intimate social networks than that of the Aïr region medicine women. Perhaps because of her extensive travel and mixed social origins, as well as her training in midwifery, Mama expressed a synthesis (though not a complete hybrid) of knowledge concerning women's health:

In the eighth and ninth months of pregnancy, the woman needs light food. I give her porridge, meat broth, and *gombo* (okra) and butter. That makes the birth easier. The baby is thin. [There is a belief, widespread in Sahelian communities as well, that pregnant women should lose weight to avoid a heavy baby and thereby reduce childbirth difficulties.] She should avoid salt, hot pepper, and heavy burdens. From the seventh month onwards, sometimes I use the medicine *azargar* mixed with meat, which gives the mother strength. Widespread problems for women in pregnancy and childbirth include anemia, heart problems, and miscarriages because of fear. I am sometimes called in to assist at home. Only seven or eight women in my village per year go to the clinic to give birth. Most women still prefer to have close female relatives present at birth and to give birth at home. In Kidal, the hospital organized and appointed women in charge of twenty-one women in *sage-femme* (midwifery) training sessions. For better health here, we now need vehicles, mattresses, and buckets. We have only one ambulance here, which goes between Kidal and Gao. We also need biomedicines [i.e., pharmaceutical antibiotics].

Medicine women gladly accepted first-aid supplies, however limited, from the government- and NGO-supported clinics and hospitals, acknowledging that herbal medicine can cure some problems, but not others. Recently, however, with financial problems from the restructuring, privatization, and debts, these programs have suffered. As in Europe and America, for those who have difficult access to both herbal and antibiotic treatments, there are new alternative medicines. Noel (in Claudot-Hawad 2002) reports that among some Tuareg, certain industrial products now have a place in local treatments: brake liquid on open cuts; some industrial car repair solutions for stopping bleeding; battery fluid; and Nescafe or bouillon cubes, which give a hot sensation (Noel 2002:156). This author also mentions that Magi cubes replace meat juice in some maternity rituals during the postpartum period, with the goal of regaining strength and heat in an anemic woman, but especially to purify by eliminating from her stomach "dirty" blood. Nonetheless, in this instance, despite the change of therapeutic object, the basic logic is the same. I noticed that sometimes, fly-tox insecticide is used for scorpion stings. Mohammed Schotz, a Malian Tuareg orphan adopted by an American family, reportedly treated his leg wound with gasoline while on the streets of Gao, Mali, where both traditional herbal and Western biomedical remedies were beyond his reach (*60 Minutes* television segment, 1980s).

The foregoing trends do not imply, however, that urban Tuareg have ceased to use the services of medicine women or other "traditional" healers. On the contrary, many patients, both rural and urban, combine different healing strategies, seeing a variety of practitioners. It has been acknowledged that African traditional medicine not only represents an affordable health-care delivery system but constitutes a dynamic and evolving system, one that is turning into a lucrative business enterprise and becoming a major part of the informal sector in urban Africa (Good 1987; Green 1999). It was often belittled during colonialism by Europeans and local elites. But today, it is becoming more respected and once again widely sought out. There is sometimes an emergence of a new stratum of healers who use the very "tools" with which the orthodox standard biomedical practitioners gained their dominance, while rejecting those characteristics that stigmatized them. In so doing, they have also distanced themselves from other healers and replicated the same dominance against which they resist, by placing themselves in a position of dominance with respect to other healers and the latter's patients. They usually practice in herbal clinics devoid of rituals of the more traditional herbal medicine. Bureaucratic "props" used include signposts to and at clinics, record-keeping on patients, and labeled prepackaged or bottled herbal preparations.

Tuareg herbal medicine women sometimes receive government-distributed first-aid kits, but these usually go unreplenished. A few training programs have also given medicine women printed pamphlets with illustrated health lessons, but few herbalists read these publications' Roman-scripted Tamajaq or French. Tuareg medicine women express mixed sentiments regarding Western biomedical institutions; their comments and actions display elements of resistance, cooperation, and integration or incorporation.

For many patients, as shown, medicine women remain the first "opinion"; they do not, however, always have the "final say" in treatment. They continue to fill a gap where their herbal and psychosocial treatments are needed and effective.

The question here is how the greater collaboration between Tuareg medicine women and other health practitioners (both local Tuareg and outside specialists in the countryside and towns, who are trained in allopathic medicine) will proceed, and whether this will result in advantages or disadvantages for herbal medicine women and their predominantly female clientele. The popular media and some studies (Green 1999) tend to portray a "rosy" picture of such collaboration. Others (Sargent 1989) recognize that, while traditional practitioners (for example, midwives in Benin) still play a very vital role in African health systems, many face challenges. Many traditional practitioners work either in rural areas or in urban areas in poorer neighborhoods.

The Tuareg case suggests contradictions and uncertainty. Additional, more ambivalent attitudes concerning relations with more powerful outsiders came to light, not in interviews, but in more informal unstructured conversations I heard during medicine women's consultations. In one of her morning consultations/examinations, Hadia in her village was treating a young, recently married woman from the large oasis where the recent training program for medicine women had been held. She diagnosed her with the hot illness, *tuksi*, the muscle pain around the back and shoulders called *tarzak*, and other aches in the body. The patient, approximately twenty-two years old and the daughter of Hadia's younger brother, was not eating well. She had sought Hadia's care once before. The woman said that these aches are due to aging, despite her childbearing age. Upon my questioning, the patient indicated that although she came from that large oasis with the clinic, she had not been to its clinic because she preferred herbalists and was afraid of shots, and she remains a patient of Hadia's. In her responses, therefore, this patient emphasized her fear of biomedical personnel and some of their techniques, such as injections, and also hinted at a certain loyalty to Hadia. Hadia, however, commented that, "Clinics can treat sores that increase on the skin. For good health here, we need shots and clinic biomedicines [antibiotics]."

Striking here is how this patient avoided the clinic, even though it was not geographically distant from her home—indeed, it was in her own village. This patient's session with Hadia also reveals the kind of "haven" offered some patients by medicine women, in the comforting network of kinship relations (though of course, these may at times, as also shown, become acrimonious). This combination of herbal and psycho- medico-ritual techniques administered by the medicine woman, as well as the confidentiality surrounding this treatment, and the patient's shyness, could not have been easily accommodated in a clinic setting. Doctors and nurses are not accustomed to retreating but in fact remain dominant and omnipresent throughout the treatment. On the other hand, one wonders why women have not sought to escape the intimacy, but also the prying eye of kinship networks, and move toward more impersonal health-care networks which can offer another benefit: of anonymity away from familiar, but also prying local social networks. I did not find any cases of women doing the latter; perhaps this will change. One possible reason is that, despite a series of training programs for local medicine women, most hospitals and clinics tend to remain dominated by male nurses and doctors, toward whom most rural Tuareg women say they feel shy.

Additional reasons for this are economic. Most countries where Tuareg reside today are poor. For example, Niger has one of the lowest per capita incomes in the world, estimated at U.S. $260 in 1987 (World Bank, *World Development Report,* 1989:14). This income has declined in the past decade from World Bank–imposed economic austerity measures. Mali's GDP in 1998 was $2.5 billion, and Mali's per capita income for 1998 was $270 (*Background Notes: Mali*, U.S. Department of State, June 2000:2). Life expectancy in many countries where Tuareg reside is low; in Niger, for example, this was estimated at 45 years in 1987, and the infant mortality rate was estimated to be 135 deaths per 1000 live births (World Bank, *World Development Report*, 1989:226). More recently, infant mortality was estimated at 123 per 1000 births (U.S. Department of State, *Background Notes: Niger,* July 1994). The central government budget in Niger in 1994 was estimated at U.S. $291.4 million (adjusted for devaluation in 1993 of the French West Africa C.F.A.). The 1994 investment budget (capital and development expenditures) was $190 million (U.S. Department of State, *Background Notes: Niger,* July 1994). In Mali, the average annual salary of skilled workers in 1998 was $1,200 (Background Notes, Mali, June 2000:2).

The governments of both Mali and Niger embarked on a series of structural adjustment programs in the early 1980s, intending to reduce budgetary deficits, public enterprise operating losses, and public sector problems. Under an economic reform program signed with the World Bank and the IMF in 1988, there has been privatization of various business enterprises. These measures have had negative effects on health care, in particular, for the poor (Martin and O'Meara 1995; Rasmussen 2001a). Private medical insurance and other benefits are not available to the vast majority of patients in many countries where Tuareg reside. Governments do not reimburse hospitals directly for the care of their employees, so the programs for government employees are in effect exemptions from payment. Throughout Niger, for example, public facilities administered by the Ministry of Public Health provide most of the biomedical health care. There are two tiers of prices: private sector patients pay higher fees than public sector patients for private hospital rooms, diagnostic exams, and surgical procedures (Weaver et al., 1994:566). Only a tiny percentage of the population is employed by large companies and receives insurance benefits from them (Rasmussen, 2001a:13).

In principle, women and men have equal access to medical care, both traditional and established biomedically trained clinics and hospitals, throughout life. The problem of unequal care principally affects, not gender or age, but ethnicity and region:

many northern Tuareg, regardless of gender, tend to suffer from less health-care access, until recently marginalized within the nation-state and residing in geographically inaccessible rural communities. The primary factor now is the general poverty of those nation-states where most Tamajaq speakers reside. In a study of medical pluralism and sociopolitical processes surrounding Tuareg medicine (Rasmussen 2001a), Rasmussen describes reasons for local fear of hospitals: like schools, hospitals appeared implicated in colonial and postcolonial schemes to dominate and control; for example, many medicine distributions were accompanied by census counts, taxation records, and political speeches, with soldiers standing by with guns at the ready. Some, especially women, viewed hospital and clinic staffs as unsympathetic and hostile to the local culture.

Many people are nowadays less fearful of hospitals and clinics, partly because their staffing, since the peace negotiations in Niger and Mali, includes more local and Tamajaq-speaking personnel. Most rural people still go to traditional local medical practitioners before going to clinics and hospitals because of difficult access to hospitals, located only in the major towns—and travel there is often difficult. However, as shown in the case of Hadia's patient, geographic distance is only one factor. Other kinds of distance are nonliteral: for example, kinship relations will bring a patient across great geographic distances to see a medicine women and cause the patient to avoid more convenient treatment locally, even close by, by unrelated clinic staff if the latter are perceived as intimidating, or if their medicine is too expensive. Prescription medicines are irregularly stocked and expensive. Some pills of uncertain identity and origin are now sold at cheaper prices on vending tables in urban streets of these countries; these are often dangerous, uncontrolled, and unlabeled. Private medical practitioners have sprung up in capital cities, but most Africans cannot afford their fees. Previous studies of the pluralist medical system (Bernus 1969; Noel in Claudot-Hawad 2002; Rasmussen 1994, 2001a) reveal that specialisms overlap, many practitioners refer patients to each other, and most patients consult more than one practitioner for a given illness. However, when one examines herbal medicine women's practice more closely, one finds that there is a hierarchy of preferences and priorities, and not all specialists are trusted equally.

Despite their recognition of needs for some Western biomedicines and surgery in their narratives and comments, medicine women's experiences with biomedicine reveal some appropriation and challenge to their system of authoritative knowledge. Medicine women's *al baraka* can now be withheld and even stolen, thereby becoming a finite and "limited good" force, whereas once it could be freely given and absorbed without being taken away or completely co-opted for private use. How, exactly, does this occur? The experiences and comments of several herbal medicine women from rural origins who now live and practice in the town of Agadez, Niger, are instructive in this regard.

Dabo is an herbalist from Tchighozeghine (a large sedentarized village and seat of the regional sous-prefecture) now living in Agadez. I met her and first interviewed her in 1995, and interviewed and visited her several more times in 1998 and 2002. She belongs to the Kel Ferwan confederation and is of noble social origins. Like her rural counterparts, she touches and knows many of the *ten* medicine pot recipes/combinations. Dabo obtained a certificate from the Agadez Hospital in 1987, and she acts as a liaison between the hospital staff and local Tamajaq-speaking female patients in the multiethnic town of Agadez. She indicated there were still some herbal medicine women practicing in Agadez and also many informal healers.

Dabo has eight children. She learned herbal healing from her grandmother. She also weaves and sells mats, and she keeps a few goats and chickens inside her compound. Her elderly mother still resides in Tchighozeghine. During the afternoons, Dabo treated predominantly women and children patients who came to her. For example, she treated two babies during one of my afternoon visits. One was the child of a Tuareg smith woman from Azel, a village near Agadez, and the other was the child of a Hausa woman who lived in Agadez. She used suppositories on each child to treat their stomach conditions, after she diagnosed their illnesses by touching the stomach of one child and the back of the other.

In the evenings, Dabo's tent and compound were usually filled with visitors, young people of diverse ethnic backgrounds, who chatted and drank tea as she also continued to treat children brought to her. But these sessions, also, revealed subtle healing, informally without tangible medicines, during sociability.

Dabo was often also visited by a troubled young man, an illegitimate child of a now-deceased French colonial administrator who had founded one of the nomadic boarding schools in the Aïr region. This young man, although intermittently employed as a mechanic, appeared slightly disoriented. He often related how he had been to France and seen his relatives there, and he claimed that his French relatives were "nomads." Away from his presence, mutual acquaintances claimed that he had never traveled there, and that he had been, sadly, never recognized or supported by his father, who had never married his Tuareg mother. Acquaintances referred to him as "a child of the road." Dabo treated him kindly, however, and listened with interest to this man's stories, thereby providing some soothing comfort as a nonjudgmental audience. Several other persons who visited Dabo also appeared in some respects to be socially marginal; one woman, for example, had traveled to Gao and Europe and worked in bars there, an occupation many tend to scorn and associate (not always accurately) with prostitution. Dabo therefore provided some psychosocial therapy in listening to others' problems, in this respect continuing the roles of many rural medicine women. Dabo also continued to share many other medicine women's traditional beliefs, as when she explained, "a childless woman cannot be a *tanesmegel;* the requirement of having children is, even here in the town, crucial."

Dabo described to me some current problems many Tuareg face:

Often, women here have syphilis. They do not protect themselves. They also have many stomach problems and the back problems, and they go out in the wind and sit in hot places. Many men, also, come to me with back problems; one cannot drink anything bitter or sour. Before, our [health] problems included dirt [i.e., less sanitation—Tamajaq term used is *wa jarga*], but nonetheless, we had fewer illnesses then because we drank more milk. [Now milk is scarce from deaths of livestock during a series of droughts.] . . . Also, nowadays, food does not satisfy; it is now too light (refined). The most important changes within the last twenty years among the Tuareg are no more herders, many want to come to town and establish shops. Everyone is free. Even the youths, they depend less on their parents. Before, we had livestock and gardens. Now we need money.

I noticed some interesting features of her practice that distinguished it from that prevalent in the countryside. After a brief joking debate with her daughter, Dabo omitted the usual ritual incantations of benediction and actions of touching the earth done to convey *al baraka,* refer to spirits, and protect from communicating the illness, which herbal medicine women unfailingly do in the countryside. As Dabo gave me a massage to relieve my neck and head aches, her daughter commented mockingly, "Mother, you should say *'Bissmillah!'*" Dabo did not reveal the reason why she omitted these actions. At first I surmised that perhaps it was because I was an outsider and a non-Muslim, but I noticed that she also omitted all these ritual incantations and actions with her local patients. Perhaps she simply did not consider them important in her current treatments. Since she no longer practiced in her rural village, and my study is not, in its ultimate goal, a rural/urban comparison, but rather a study of predominantly rural *tinesmegelen,* systematic comparison of Dabo's actions in each setting was not feasible. Perhaps, alternatively, Dabo felt ashamed of these actions as too conservative, an impression from her training sessions with the hospital and clinic personnel. My educated guess is that this latter was the case, for some of her other comments soon revealed these biomedical staffs' condescending attitudes toward her practice.

Consider, for example, the following impressions, which reveal mixed attitudes of Western-trained staffs toward her skills. Dabo described to me her encounters with biomedicine: "Once, my father had urinary problems and he was hospitalized, and after twenty days, I gave him a combination of [my traditional medicine pot] treatments, and he was cured. I have connections with state nurses at the hospital, and they call me over there sometimes to assist with difficult births. During the training session I attended, I did three years exchanging knowledge at the Tchighozeghine clinic."

Although Dabo termed this program a positive "exchange of knowledge," its effects were not entirely symmetrical or equal. She complained to me, for example, that town functionaries did not take her seriously because they did not want to consult in her "dirty" tent; she said she needed a "larger and cleaner house" for consultations. Indeed, despite her competence, Dabo tended to attract few functionaries as patients, and more of the poor and also women from rural areas who came into Agadez on other business.[1] Although of course her value in providing these services should not be underestimated, nonetheless, it reveals her collision with the Western allopathic emphasis upon different notions of "cleanliness" (i.e., "hygiene"—not pollution). Dabo's more psychotherapeutic treatments of those of her patients with nonorganic illnesses reveal, however, her continuing effectiveness in that domain. Notwithstanding her psychosocial therapy in cases of nonorganic illness, she appears to have dropped the additionally protective rituals accompanying many treatments.

Dabo also discussed her conflict with nurses who held different beliefs regarding advice to pregnant women. She expressed more long-standing Tuareg beliefs that a pregnant women should avoid "heavy" and "hot" foods like dates, wheat, and milk, "because they make the stomach "dirty" (*ta jerga)*—and cause the baby to grow too heavy, thereby causing a difficult birth." In this context, her sense of "dirty" does not correspond to the Western notion of literally "unsanitary." Rather, it translates here as approximately harmful or dangerous—and is therefore closer to the local sense of pollution or endangerment to women and children. Dabo recognized that some

Western-trained health education programs disputed this belief. Indeed, many health workers told me that one problem they encountered among many African pregnant women was their intentional curbing of weight gain in order to limit the baby's birth weight. While the local women's reasoning was quite logical, in that this measure minimized a difficult labor, in the biomedical staff's perspective, it threatened both mother's and child's nutrition and health and produced a baby with a very low birth weight. Other pregnant women complained that despite local Tamajaq-speaking liaison agents and midwives such as Dabo and Mama, they disliked giving birth at clinics and hospitals, not solely for these reasons, but also because of the dominant male personnel and also because these staffs compelled them to lie down to give birth; whereas as noted, among the Tuareg women customarily give birth seated with elderly female relatives and/or medicine women holding their shoulders. This method is, indeed, considered more comfortable in many other cultures.

Some of Dabo's experiences therefore suggest ways in which the traditionally comforting *al baraka* of herbal medicine women, as well as their protective social practice of buffering against potential domestic violence toward women, is being appropriated into a more "hygienic" discourse by outside NGOs' cooperative aid projects, in otherwise constructive collaboration programs between traditional local herbal medicine women and clinics and hospitals emphasizing Western biomedicine. In other words, the problems of patients in the version of the Western allopathic medical viewpoint Dabo encountered, at least, cannot be remedied by *al baraka* or battled as pollution with additional rituals besides herbal medicines or antibiotics, but needs additional revisions in authoritative knowledge: specifically, advice to women patients. Paramount in this latter are concepts of physical hygiene and deferral to established doctors and nurses. Other local medicine women's experiences with the biomedicines—as shown, for example, in a depleted first-aid kit and the stolen kits during the militia raid—indicate that material theft, as well as theft of ideas, are very real concerns, as well.

Therefore while Dabo enjoyed her work as coordinator for the linkages program between *tinesmegelen* and the Agadez Hospital and the Ministry of Health, and indeed continued to treat patients, her actions and more informal comments to me revealed underlying tensions, as when she indicated that "traditional healers need better places to examine patients, such as a new house with waiting room" and when she surmised that functionaries do not see her because "they refuse to enter my crumbling compound and 'dirty' tent." In other words, the standards of what is dirty and what is clean, what is safe and what is unsafe, and what is dignified and what is shameful, have all been challenged.

Also instructive in this regard is the experience of another herbal medicine woman currently residing in Agadez whom I shall call Chimo, the daughter of Hadia in the countryside. I knew Chimo since she had apprenticed with her mother during her youth. But nowadays, Chimo tends to practice more informally and less regularly, for several reasons. In contrast to Dabo, Chimo does not work in any collaborative programs. When I first met Hadia and Chimo in the early 1980s, in what was then a very small nomadic camp of about four households near the shrine of the founding marabout, Chimo was still residing with her mother, learning these skills, and spending much time also herding goats. Between sessions with her mother, she would lead the goats to pasture. I recall how Chimo refused to treat patients who came to her if her mother was absent, carefully observing the norm of respect toward the older healer.

Then, sometime around the mid-1980s, her life took a different turn and threatened to fall apart: Chimo allegedly had a love affair with an American aid worker, and gave birth out of wedlock. Local women, in their gossip, considered evidence for this to be the child's allegedly blue eyes. At that time, Chimo and her mother owned many livestock. Some local men, in their own gossip, felt that Chimo "did not need to marry" for that reason and appeared to grudgingly respect her independence. Nonetheless, the important marabout clans of the villages were sure to shun them socially unless the child was kept hidden from view. So Chimo left the child with her mother to raise at distant pastures in the "wild," a frequent pattern in cases of this shameful action, and decided to leave the countryside. Unlike Asalo, Rahma's daughter, the less fortunate woman in a similar situation who was poorer, less able to change her situation, and later went insane, Chimo had sufficient resources at that time to migrate.

Like many Tuareg women in such situations who flee to the large towns, Chimo eventually married an outsider, a Zarma merchant from Niamey who at first sold watches from a table around the Millet Market and later expanded his business and became more successful. She and her husband later moved to Niamey, the capital of Niger, where they resided until around 1994, and then returned to Agadez. They had three children. Their oldest son, upon adulthood, eventually became a marabout in that town.

Although Chimo still remembered the herbal medicines and treatments she had learned from her mother Hadia years earlier, she explained to me that she no longer practiced this profession regularly because "I am not yet an old women." She did not mention the past events in her life history, but I am certain that the out-of-wedlock birth also influenced this path—although that event did not negatively affect her mother Hadia's career, since the child was kept out of view, beyond their home mosque and tents. Chimo later built up a small clientele in Agadez, however. She showed me her bark medicines from Mount Bagzan, supplied by her mother through traveling kin, and identified some of the *ilaten* plants' Tamajaq names for me. Chimo indicated that she prefers Agadez to her rural village "because there are more products here and less arduous work. Life is hard there—women have to haul water and wood, pound millet, etc." Yet she also subtly critiqued the biomedical staff there, in saying that, in her opinion, "the hospital knows children's medicine but not women's medicine." Although Chimo was less specific about this issue than Dabo, here, again, are hints of collisions between ideas of the hospital personnel and those of medicine women concerning women's needs, and of conflicts between the hospital staff and female patients.

Chimo's reasons for curtailing (though not completely abandoning) herbal medicine practice are complex. During her youthful apprenticeship, she became socially marginalized in her community, early on, as a single mother. Though not rejected by her own mother, she was nonetheless obliged to leave rural practice. Single women among the Tuareg may receive suitors in courtship, but in principal are not supposed to have premarital sex, particularly among the *ineslemen* maraboutique clans influential in that region, who tend to restrict women a bit more than some other Tuareg groups. Virginity is usually not important, though among these clans some men express the desire for their wives to be virgins on marriage. Perhaps, also, Chimo's infraction was believed to pollute the sacred site of the marabouts' tomb in her village. She was obliged to flee rather soon and consequently did not complete her apprenticeship with her mother, although she appeared to retain much of their cultural and medical knowledge. Her cryptic remark that "the hospital knows children's medicine but not women's medicine" is a semantically loaded phrase. It implies that the problem for many women is indeed still intimidation by many nurses and doctors trained in Western biomedicine.[2] In Chimo's life history and comments, therefore, are hints of resistance (or at least resentment) toward both the powers of official religion and established allopathic medicine. Ultimately, Chimo found contentment. In so doing, however, there was a price: she acquiesced to the role of housewife in the town, wife of a successful merchant and mother of a marabout, primarily dependent upon her husband and son economically, and she curtailed the role of practicing *tanesmegel.*

In sum, these experiences, impressions, and sentiments of several medicine women in more urban and multiethnic settings, while not representative of all of them, nonetheless reveal much about some medicine women's encounters with powerful state and NGO institutions such as clinics, hospital personnel, and training programs. In these encounters, what occurs is not so much a hybrid of old and new, traditional and modern, or "clear-cut" replacement of one system by another; but rather, there occurs a selective remembering of cultural knowledge by different persons, depending upon individual life histories, directions, and subjectivity, as well as "objective" constraints of the wider infrastructure. In these processes, struggles and dilemmas inevitably occur.

Conclusions

Herbal Healing, Modes of Thought, and Gender

In this book, I have analyzed the symbolism and the diverse and changing social and medico-ritual practical contexts of medicine women's knowledge. Medicine women illuminate other domains of Tuareg culture and memory, and vice versa: other domains of Tuareg culture and memory shed light on medicine women. More broadly, their practice contributes to wider issues in the anthropology of religion and gender and medical anthropology: in particular, the cultural construction of knowledge and epistemologies—gendered and cultural—and the relationships between knowledge and practice. Rather than showing how "others, too, are rational," now largely a truism and itself condescending, and rather than seeking to translate exactly, or the alternative—equally problematic, of showing how all humans can "irrationally" accept cosmologies despite their uncertainties (Herzfeld 2001), I have sought to show how humans elaborate on the themes of rationality and uncertainty in endless ways, which defy exact translation but nonetheless merit efforts of interpretation. Indeed, showing how all humans accept cosmologies despite their uncertainties need not imply universal irrationality, either. Moreover, the forgoing chapters have also shown that not all humans accept all aspects of a single cosmology but may dispute it, and in fact there is a range of interpretation within each cosmology.

Herbal medicine women use both natural and cultural/symbolic materials, both literally and metaphorically, to treat organic and nonorganic illnesses. They symbolically delineate, but also socially negotiate among, sometimes opposed spheres in epistemological knowledge categories. In their managing of female fertility, physical suffering, and social conflicts (in particular, in their protecting against potential domestic violence) between women and men, in their cooperation with Islamic scholarship, their cautious forays into divination/mediumship, and their alertness to change, medicine women treat the body, but also do more: they comment on and reinterpret important issues in Tuareg society. In these processes, powerful forces sometimes viewed as opposed and discrete become interlocking and sometimes aligned in herbalists' work. These specialists translate and negotiate women's and men's concerns, bridging and reconciling conflicts. But their translations, reminders, and negotiations in turn remind anthropologists of the need to accept the approximate meaning in all translations of modes of thought and the variable subjective experiences of their practitioners.

During their treatments, medicine women use touch and massage, contacting not solely the female patients' stomach but also the earth in order to take the disease out of both patient and healer; these actions constitutes an effort to unburden both parties. Medicine women display much fortitude in adversity and inspire others to do so, as well. Yet they are also vulnerable through their intense empathy with others' suffering. Medicine women see many patients who come to them for personal attention and resolution of marital difficulties, and some medicine women have marital and other difficulties themselves.

Their mythico-history relating the female founding ancestress/cultural heroine, in the etiological account of the origins of their profession, serves to remind others of the importance of their own authoritative knowledge system, one that is parallel rather than muted, subordinate, or "alternate" vis-à-vis other powerful systems.

The most senior medicine women enjoy a status that, in effect, brings a state of being "full of prayer," albeit not in the androgynous sense of completely relinquishing their prior feminine gender constructs or in the sense of exactly imitating men or "official" Islam in all respects. Qualities defined as "feminine" and "maternal" are not so much relinquished as they are redefined and adapted to the cultural alignment of physiological processes, cosmological memories, and social roles evoked by herbal medicinal practice. There is a transfiguration of symbolic referents of wellness and illness. For many Tuareg women, in particular, subjective experiences of wellness and illness are shaped by an interplay, rather than rigid opposition, of Qur'anic, pre-Islamic, and popular Tuareg cultural interpretations of Islam, science, and medicine. Physiological, ritual, and social states are integrated in treatments that resist neat classification into either "medical" or "ritual" process.

In their legitimate though constrained curing practices, herbal medicine women do not seek to repel spirits, but to attract them. Despite (or perhaps because of) their concerns with cultural memory, knowledge, and legitimate property, paradoxically, they can approach the nonlegitimate (for example, illegitimate, disenfranchised, and "marginal" persons) more closely than some others. As marabouts are medicine women's metaphorical "lawful-wedded" husbands, spirits are their metaphorical lovers. These relationships explain many restrictions, privileges, and other ritual practices of medicine women, for example, why they ideally avoid iron and why they gather barks in the presence only of females or immature males, not grown men, the latter perceived as closer to the God of Islam. Yet, one must beware of simplistic equations and oppositions here, as well. For as shown, medicine women also display great devotion to Islam, and, like many other African Muslims, most of them do not view this as problematic or contradictory. Like Tuareg artisans, herbal medicine women also stand on a boundary. In appealing to locally recognized symbols, they make sometimes conflicting sources of power and credentials appear more compatible. Yet these achievements sometimes come at a price; for these forces are not merely static but have indeterminacy and potentially transformative qualities, and a capacity for redirection. While it is true, as shown, that medicine women evoke, commemorate, and mediate, they also comment upon and redirect these forces, socially, facilitating their reinterpretation by others according to need and context. Medicine women sometimes translate women's interests into more domesticated forms in men's accepted definitions, but throughout, there is a subtext of resistance in possibility of alternative understandings. Herbal medicine women in this regard resemble, but also differ from, smiths, who traditionally buffered noble families from threatening outside forces (unworthy suitors in marriage, feared government agents, and potentially predatory travelers). Herbal medicine women, as shown, do not always succeed in buffering their clientele from invading forces, sometimes they even facilitate the surveillance of women's bodies. Their own position is in subtle ways circumscribed, and vulnerable to marginalization as well. But they serve to check potentially abusive powers in their powerful knowledge of both medicine and history.

There are complementary and conflictual aspects to medicine women's roles in relation to wider powers, of professional Islamic scholarship and Western biomedical or allopathic medicine. Their survival paradoxically requires some containment of their knowledge and powers.

There are finer degrees of medicine women specialties among the Tuareg than English translation conveys. Also, as shown, typical of much *tinesmegelen* treatment is a simultaneous use of "natural-empirical" and "ritual" remedies. These complex processes reveal the inherent inadequacy of these labels and categories transposed across cultural contexts or used universally. In Tamajaq-speaking communities, as in any historical or cultural setting, science can coexist with laboratory manipulations of imagined, even metaphorical and "fanciful" cosmologies and other explorations (Mudimbe 1991; Tambiah 1990:29; Karp and Masolo 2000). The danger, in my view, is to reify or compartmentalize such phenomena as astrology, alchemy, magic, and so on, as well-defined, neatly bounded systems, or to view their contours, motivations, and propensities as delineated ahistorically and or in a context-free fashion.

How should anthropologists identify elaborations of these logical processes without establishing rigid reified categories and dividing lines, whether in defense of one or another classification scheme? Tuareg herbal medicine women offer suggestions. They stand at the nexus of several different modes of thought or "authoritative knowledge systems" and act to mediate them. Their practices act as a reminder to anthropologists that, as Malinowski long ago argued, magic, religion, and science are indeed all present and practiced simultaneously in all places, at all times, by diverse agents—albeit, the present book adds, in different ways and not in a homogenized form, or a form whose meaning is solely based on function, or meaning in the anthropologist's mind. When rigidly classified, these modes of thought remain conceptualized by some anthropologists as distinct. Of course, we have moved beyond Malinwoski's view of these systems in purely functional terms, as technologies—they are this, but much more as well; in their symbolic and ritual as well as medical content, they act in tandem. Yet even this important insight is insufficient. If all systems may be interpreted and represented endlessly in hermeneutic "circles," then, what are the limits of interpretation and representation? Social contexts of practice are needed (Ortner 1996; Ahearn 1998) in order to provide some guidelines for otherwise endless possibilities of interpretation.

In "translating" herbal healing, therefore, I intentionally did not consider these specialists as simply "herbalists" or "ethnobotanists" here because I wished to avoid slippage in such domains as the "natural" vs. the "supernatural." Tuareg herbalism suggests a critique and refinement of these categories, as well. For the idea of spiritual power of herbalists is important, also, in certain older herbal medicine women's capacity for conferring the Islamic benediction or blessing power of *al baraka*, just as the Islamic scholars/marabouts do, although the former tend to activate this somewhat differently than the latter.

In contrast to some other healers such as *curanderos* in the southwest United States and Native American healers, Tuareg herbalists do not face outright cultural disapproval from outsiders when they discuss sacred aspects of local healing. Yet the data have shown that there exist some challenges to their profession, particularly in more sedentarized, urban, and multiethnic communities where encounters with Western biomedically trained staffs offer a mix of opportunity (in training programs) but also some revisions of medicine women's knowledge. Herbal medicine women are aging, and few replacements are coming along. Many medicine women are aware of these problems, as when they stated that "young girls nowadays do not want to live as we live; they want nice clothes and an easier life." Droughts and wars have diminished not solely livestock herds but also valuable herbal trees and plants in the Saharan mountain massifs where they were formerly abundant. There is some ambivalence, but also accommodation and resourcefulness, toward outside interventions.

Rather than attempting to show the presence or absence of various logical categories such as "rationality" or "science," and rather than arguing for or against glosses such as "shamanism" among the Tuareg in herbal medicine, I have tried to explore the forms these modes of thought take and how they are embodied in the practices of medicine women. What, then, should be the goal of studying "indigenous" systems, if it is no longer constructive to demonstrate either others' similarity or others' difference from our own systems of thought? This book has attempted to offer alternatives. Traditional and contemporary ways of healing need not be in conflict with each other nor replace each other; rather, they can be complementary and parallel even within a single specialism (rather than in the plural system). Each definition of wellness, illness, and curing is not necessarily unitary. There is internal contradiction within medicine women's system itself. Hence my preference to refrain from forcing these processes and their significance into Western categories of rationality or empirical logic, advocating instead accepting them on their own terms in the local system of causation (Olkes and Stoller 1987; Stoller 1989; Horton 1993). In some settings and interactions of herbal healing, knowledge is hierarchically distributed; in others, it is horizontally distributed. Situations are defined so that one or another (or plural) knowledge system(s) ascend(s), as needed. Different authoritative knowledge forms become privileged according to context, not solely within pluralist medical systems but also within the herbal medical specialty itself. Yet in encounters with some more powerful officials—Islamic scholars and biomedical staffs—others give shape to and to some extent redefine medicine women's knowledge. But medicine women remain important gatekeepers to most female patients' treatment.

Medicine women's healing tradition therefore constitutes one of several authoritative knowledge systems for both men and women, albeit in different ways. Male patients, also, respect and consult them. Among the Tuareg, there is a continuum and range, rather than a rigid contrast, between a healing discipline emphasizing accessible authoritative knowledge and one that "vests all knowledge in "experts" (Beisele in Davis-Floyd and Sargent 1997:474–90) the concern is with spiritual, transformative aspects of authoritative healing, and among the Tuareg this is still viewed by many as a paradigm of healing. Thus medicine women's work stands at the nexus of sometimes adversarial, sometimes parallel and complementary systems. Tuareg medicine women are important in their own parallel system of authoritative knowledge.

Hence the duality but also the overlap between social, natural, and spirit worlds—of past and present, myth and history. These meetings of different "minds" mulling over the crossroads of different causal forces enable redefinition of nonorganic as well as organic illnesses and moral issues. In effect, medicine women must continually appeal to the moral sensibility of their community and walk a tightrope of power. They must approach the wild in order to tame it, but this brings perils of falling into an abyss. In this, Tuareg medicine women grapple with existential dilemmas common to all humankind.

Notes

Preface

1. *Akh huderan* (denoting "living milk") is property compensating female heirs for male heirs' inheritance of two-thirds of property in Qur'anic law, the latter called *takachit*. It is variously described as inheritance, endowment, and "gifts"—this has usually consisted of livestock herds, date palms, and occasionally, a house—though most houses, as well as oasis gardens, are built and inherited by men as men's property. Living milk property is not supposed to be sold but should be transmitted only to sisters, daughters, and nieces. Until recently, this property, along with jewelry given by mothers and husbands, and the tent (the latter built and owned by married women, brought to the household by the bride as dowry) provided economic security for women. In some regions, nation-state and Qur'anic legal institutions have challenged this form of property (Oxby 1990; Keenan 2003).

Deconstructing and Recasting Female Healing

1. These problems recall wider philosophical legacies in anthropology, such as the Cartesian dualistic "mind-body" opposition.

2. Since a series of droughts and the rebellion, the UN and some international NGO agencies have attempted to compensate returning refugees for their stolen or lost animals, to reinstate the *akh huderan* pattern of transmission, and to encourage alternative sources of income for women, such as artisan work and tailoring.

3. Over a period of nearly thirty years, I have resided and worked in Niger for approximately seven years, initially in Peace Corps and local teaching contract projects (1974–1979), and later in social/cultural anthropological field research (1983, 1991, 1995, 1998, 2001). More recently, I conducted research in Mali and briefly, in France (1998, 2002). The present book differs from some previous pioneering works on healing in Tuareg communities. Rasmussen (2001a) examined the plural (multiple) healing system, traditional healing generally, and sociopolitical processes surrounding Tuareg attitudes toward medicine. A previous ethnography analyzed Tuareg spirit possession (Rasmussen 1995). The present book focuses primarily upon these *tinesmegelen* medicine woman specialist practitioners. Additional works on Tuareg healing include articles and chapters within edited volumes (Bernus 1969; Fiore and Wallet Faqqi 1993; Figueiredo-Biton in Claudot-Hawad 2002; Noel in Claudot-Hawad 2002). I acknowledge my debt to these previous works. Here I hope to build upon and refine their data and to render them more theoretically informed by an understanding of current anthropological issues.

Chapter 1

1. For example, Davis (1983) analyzed the role of local "folk" theories of the menopause in relation to local gendered practices and to theories of established biomedical models; Martin (1994) analyzed changing notions and tropes of the body and resistance to illness in the United States. Sontag (1978) offered valuable insights into American imagery of tuberculosis and AIDS in historical perspective. Douglas (1996) applied classical "pollution" theories to comparative and historical analyses of attitudes toward leprosy and environmental pollution.

2. Tuareg men, not women, wear the face-veil/turban, called *tagelmust* or *asinker*. This headdress protects from pollution from spirits, and it conveys respect and reserve. See Murphy (1964), Claudot-Hawad (1993), and Nicolaisen (1997).

3. There are long-standing pollution beliefs regarding smiths' allegedly malevolent, "witchcraft-like" powers, believed to be activated automatically by a smith when a noble bypasses the client smith's services, or when he/she refuses a smith compensation. These practices by nobles operate as "leveling devices" discouraging excessive accumulation of wealth by anyone. See Nicolaisen 1997; Rasmussen 1989, 1992; and Sáenz 1991.

4. Precolonial political organization was based on regional confederations, each led by a sultan or *amenukal* elected by the noble descent groups within his confederation. The sultan maintained peace for the caravan trade and mediated among the warring noble descent groups and clans.

5. Lewis has in later work refined somewhat his earlier arguments that women (and also some "marginal" men) in such cults are consciously compensating for "female deprivation" in a kind of "sex warfare" expressed in their activities as adepts in possession. Others who have also revised deprivation theory have nonetheless recognized that possession expresses dissonant discourses or alternative scripts (Boddy 1987; Rasmussen 1995; Stoller 1997).

6. There is disagreement regarding the etymology of the term *Tuareg*. Many scholars believe this was of Arabic origin and denoted "the abandoned by God," a reference to some Arab travelers' disapproval of the Tuareg, whom they considered too lax in their adherence to Islam. See Rodd 1926; Nicolaisen 1961.

7. As early as the seventh century CE, there were extensive migrations of pastoral Berber peoples related to many contemporary Tuareg, such as the Lemta and the Zarawa. Invasions of the Beni Hilal and Beni Sulaym Arabs into Tripolitania and Fezzan pushed the Tuareg southward.

8. Slavery was officially abolished at midcentury. Tributaries gradually accumulated weapons and large livestock (Keenan 1976). Nobles and smiths in some rural regions practice a patron/client relationship: smiths manufacture weapons, tools, jewelry, and household items, perform praise songs at weddings and name days for their noble patron families, and serve as go-betweens and oral historian/genealogy specialists in noble marriage negotiations. But there has been considerable change in these social relationships (Bernus 1981; Claudot-Hawad 1993; Nicolaisen 1997; Bouman 2003).

9. Since the imposition of French colonial and independent state rule, the *amenukal* has tended to become backed by state forces and is now in charge of tax collection and school registration (Claudot-Hawad 1993, 1996, 2002).

10. Most women are not secluded or veiled, and most inherit, own, and manage their property independently. Women own the tent, may initiate divorce, represent themselves in legal matters, travel, and may visit and receive male visitors even after marriage. Musical festivals feature mixed-sex flirting and courtship. Premarital and extramarital affairs are tacitly permitted, but these must be discreet and not result in out-of-wedlock births. See Murphy 1964, 1967; Worley 1991; Rasmussen 1995, 1997, 2000.

11. In some regions, "aid" programs and land-related legal policies destroyed long-standing irrigation and well systems, replacing them with artesian springs that attracted mosquitoes, and installed gasoline-powered pumps that disrupted the balanced distances between herds, pasture, and water. Colonial policies also taxed subject populations, Tuareg as well as others, and coerced some Tuareg into sedentarization, forcing them and other peoples to grow cash crops, which were hard on the soil and led to the displacement of many populations farther north into pastoral zones of Mali and Niger. See Fugelstad 1983; Rasmussen 2001a.

12. Since these peace accords in the mid-1990s, the northern regions of Niger and Mali have been to varying degrees administered as semiautonomous zones.

13. Many young men who returned from labor migration, schooling, and rumored military training no longer wished to marry according to parents' preferences, or worse, could not marry at all for lack of bridewealth. See Dayak 1992; Claudot-Hawad 1996, 2002.

14. In contrast to Tuareg men, Tuareg women do not cover the entire face, but married women must cover the nape of the neck and the hair.

15. These policies have had varying receptions among the different confederations in the different regions. In the Aïr region in northern Niger, oasis gardens and date palms have been very important for several centuries.

16. There are numerous practices to ward off these problems: the use of amulets made by both smiths and marabouts, and the observance of many ritual restrictions.

Chapter 2

1. Among the Tuareg, mature adult social status is achieved upon marriage and parenthood. Older adult status is achieved when one's children reach marriageable age or marry. See Rasmussen 1997 and Bouman 2003.

2. *Amagal* denotes medicine in general, whereas *ilaten* refers specifically to plant remedies and, sometimes, vitamins.

3. For an extended case study of this boy's illness and his family's more long-term responses to it in sociopolitical context, see Rasmussen 2001a.

4. Botanical lexicons or glossaries for medicinal plants in Niger and Mali are rare. Those available, with few exceptions, do not include many Tamajaq terms translated into French and Latin. One pioneering work (Ikhiri, Mahamane, and Mounkaila 1984) contains names of plants from the southern regions of Niger in the Hausa and Zarma languages. Tuareg consultants and assistants with whom I conferred were unfamiliar with those plants. Many trees and remedies predominate in specific localities and are not yet all cross-listed in the few valuable lexicons and glossaries with Tamajaq terms (Bernus 1969; Schulz and Aboubacar Adamou 1992). My primary concern in this book is with the context of these remedies' use and their local exegesis. I am not concerned with their "etic" biochemical properties, nor with their medicinal action physiologically, in ethnobotanical or pharmacological terms. Likewise, with Tamajaq illnesses, I do not seek an exact or equivalent translation, only an approximate description of symptomatology from the local viewpoint.

Chapter 3

1. Touch and perfume are also used by predominantly male non-Qur'anic diviners called *bokaye*. See Hawad 1979 and Rasmussen 2001a. The brief references to medicine women in the ethnographic literature tend to emphasize their use of plants but neglect their use of touch.

2. As in many rural communities, there is a lack of written birth records. Age is calculated by reference to special events and eras.

3. Music, song, and poetry are greatly appreciated. Islamic scholars, however, tend to disapprove of nonliturgical music, associating it with illicit love.

4. The socioeconomic status of former slaves and persons of servile descent is today highly variable. Those who attended schools sometimes have obtained more remunerative jobs such as functionary positions in the towns; others, who remain in the countryside, sometimes continue menial work for past noble owners, for low pay.

5. For analysis of rites of passage in the wider context of aging and the life course issues, see Rasmussen 1997 and Bouman 2003.

6. For analysis of mortuary rituals and afterlife beliefs, see Rasmussen 1997; for analysis of tombs, see Nicolaisen 1961.

Chapter 4

1. For accounts of additional matrilineal origins and female ancestress/culture heroines/founders in some other Tuareg groups, see Norris 1975 and Worley 1991.

2. During the nineteenth century, there were Tubu raids for property and slaves into the Aïr region around the Bagzan massif. Some local residents there have some Tubu ancestry.

3. This tale also relates the origin of date and salt caravans in the Tenere in the eastern Sahara.

4. Upon burial, the head of the deceased is turned to face toward Mecca.

5. These beings are identified as the former inhabitants of the Sahara, and ruins of their residences and tombs dot the landscape.

6. Many local residents are somewhat shy and fearful of outsiders because of the intermittent armed conflicts and massacres in the region.

7. Kaoussan, leader of the 1917 Tuareg Senoussi Revolt against the French, fled to Libya and was killed. Following French suppression of the revolt, there were widespread military massacres, famines, and refugeeing (Rodd 1926).

Chapter 5

1. See Rasmussen 1995 and 2001c [2004] for additional descriptions of spirit possession songs, their origin, their transmission, their aesthetics, and their more general role and relation to possession during exorcism rituals.

2. I am in sympathy with these efforts. Buckley and Gottlieb, for example (1988), correctly in my view, prefer to use the term *menstrual cosmology* rather than *menstrual taboos,* thereby conveying the complex and multiple meanings—not simply either purity or pollution—underlying these beliefs and practices. Rasmussen in an earlier interpretation of Tuareg menstrual beliefs and practices (1991) similarly conveys the need to recognize finer nuances by using the term *ritual restrictions.* In some contexts, such practices often protect women, rather than protecting others from women.

3. First marriages in the countryside are still often arranged by parents between, ideally, close cousins, or "family marriages." These sometimes result in divorce, with subsequent marriages between distant kin or unrelated persons; the latter marriage, based on choice, is often called "a man's marriage."

4. This longitudinal case study/history is a much extended, expanded, and updated version of a briefer and earlier history of this couple (see Rasmussen 1998b:147–71), somewhat similar to Crapanzano's technique in several of his works concerning a married couple over short and long-term association (Crapanzano 1992).

5. Early in the twentieth century, many noble Tuareg resisted the boarding schools established by French administrators as part of their policy to control local populations. Nowadays, attitudes toward schooling are more positive (Keenan 1976; Dayak 1992; Rasmussen 1997).

6. In the past, noble women tended to shun direct commercial activity and markets, but they have always participated indirectly in commerce by sending trade items with male relatives.

Chapter 6

1. Only a few medicine women expressed this fear, of someone else stealing and selling their medicines. No medicine woman requested that I not mention any of her medicines, only that I not sell them as my own. All medicine women were aware that I intended to write about them and gave me consent to do so.

2. In many Tuareg groups, particularly in Aïr, initial postmarital residence is uxorilocal for approximately the first two to three years, until the groom completes bridewealth and groom

service, and "pleases" his parents-in-law, particularly the mother-in-law. At this point, the couple may decide to move near the parents of the husband, and many men see this as an advantage and pressure wives to reside virilocally. Until recently, many women resisted this.

Chapter 7

1. A large oasis town and center of Qur'anic learning in Aïr.

2. The Tubu in the nineteenth century raided the Aïr region around Mt. Bagzan.

3. These claims—of descent from the Prophet in clans called *icherifan,* of origins in the East, and of Arabic and/or Turkish descent—are widespread in the Sahara and Sahel. The first Sultan (*amenukal*) of the Aïr in Agadez is believed to have come from Constantinople. See Rodd 1926; Norris 1975, 1990.

4. Agadez, today a multiethnic town in northern Niger, was originally Songhai. See Rodd 1926.

5. "Hausa country" (in Tamajaq, *Agala*) as used here refers to Damargou or present-day southern Niger; Damagaram refers to present-day northern Nigeria.

Chapter 8

1. These interrelationships are complex and not subject to facile "pigeonholing" or sequential chronology. Many Tuareg and other Berber peoples initially resisted Islam from mountain strongholds (Norris 1975, 1990).

2. During diagnosis for spirits, possessing spirits are believed to change the size of the head (Rasmussen 1995).

3. Marabouts write Qur'anic verses and amulets in Arabic, although they speak Tamajaq, and most are Tuareg, with some Arabic ancestry. In a few regions, such as the Kidal region of northern Mali, many marabouts are Kunta Arabs.

4. Thus far, as of this writing, these influences are minimal in Tamajaq-speaking communities, though a few outside religious orders have established mosques in northern Mali and Niger.

5. Many women in the *ineslemen* (maraboutique) clans, in fact, denied they even knew Tifinagh. Other Tuareg women, by contrast, enthusiastically taught this researcher Tifinagh characters.

6. The spirits of Tuareg possession are less personalized than those of the Hausa, Songhai, and Yoruba (Rasmussen 1995).

7. Marabouts usually work for the family of the man in marriage negotiations, and smiths work for the family of the woman.

Chapter 9

1. For a more extended case study of this woman's husband in a different analytical framework, see Rasmussen 2001a.

2. My findings, like those of Wolf, suggest that social networks and trust are crucial to successful diviner status; but my findings also differ, in that they suggest a Tuareg cultural ambivalence toward divination exists generally.

3. For detailed discussion of local attitudes toward dreams, see Rasmussen 2001a.

Chapter 10

1. Many Tuareg alternate in residence between the town and the countryside. Rural women are free to travel alone, but urban Tuareg women must ask their husband's permission to travel.

2. Recently, there have been efforts to place Tamajaq-speaking health personnel in northern regions, but the majority of them are male rather than female.

Works Cited

Abu-Lughod, Lila
    1986   *Veiled Sentiments.* Berkeley: University of California Press.
Ag Erless, Mohammed
    1990   "Les populations nomades du Nord du Mali et le dromadaire: Approche socio-culturelle." *Études maliennes* 42:3–18.
    1993   *Writing Women's Worlds: Bedouin Stories.* Berkeley: University of California Press.
Achterberg, Jeanne
    1985   *Imagery in Healing: Shamanism and Modern Medicine.* New York: Random House and Boston: New Science Library.
Ag Hamady el Mehdi
    1988   *Nosographie tamacheque des gastro-entérites dans la region de Toumbouctou.* Bamako, Mali: Thesis, École Nationale de Médecine et de Pharmacie.
Ag Solimane, Alhassane
    1999   *Bons et Mauvais Présages: Croyances, Coutumes et Superstitions dans la Société Touaregue.* Paris: l'Harmattan.
Ahearn, Laura
    1998   "A Twisted Rope Binds My Waist: Locating Constraints on Meaning in a Tij Songfest." *Journal of Linguistic Anthropology* 8(1):60–86.
Arens, Willliam, and Ivan Karp, eds.
    1989   *The Creativity of Power.* Washington, D.C.: Smithsonian Institution Press.
Bamberger, Judith
    1974   "The Myth of Matriarchy: Why Men Rule in Primitive Society." In *Women, Culture, and Society,* ed. by Michelle Zimbalist Rosaldo and Louise Lamphere, pp. 263–81. Stanford: Stanford University Press.
Bernus, Edmond
    1969   "Maladies humaines et animals chez les Touaregs Saheliens." *Journal de la Société des Africainistes* 39(1):111–37.
    1981   *Touaregs Nigeriens: Diversité dans l'Unité Culturelle.* Paris: l'Orstrom.
Bledsoe, Caroline
    2002   *Women and Marriage in Kpelle Society.* Stanford: Stanford University Press.
Boddy, Janice
    1987   *Wombs and Alien Spirits.* Madison: University of Wisconsin Press.
Bouilley, Pierre
    1999   *Les Touaregs Kel Adagh.* Paris: Karthala.
Bouman, Annmarie
    2003   *Benefits of Belonging.* Amsterdam and Utrecht, Netherlands: University of Utrecht.
Bourgeot, André
    1990   "Identité Touaregue: De l'aristocratie à la révolution." *Études Rurales* 120:129–62.
    1994   "Révoltes et rébellions en pays Touareg." *Afrique Contemporaine, Études* 170(2):3–19.
Brenner, Suzanne April
    1998   *The Domestication of Desire: Women, Wealth, and Modernity in Java.* Princeton: Princeton University Press.

Brown, Judith, and Virginia Kerns, eds.
1992   *In Her Prime: New Views of Middle-Aged Women.* Urbana and Chicago: University of Illinois Press.
Buckley, Thomas, and Alma Gottlieb, eds.
1988   *Blood Magic: The Anthropology of Menstruation.* Berkeley: University of California Press.
Cardona, G. R.
1993   *La Foresta di piume.* Bari.
Carrier, James
1992   "Occidentalism: The World Turned Upside-Down." *American Ethnologist* 19(2):195–213.
Casajus, Dominique
1987   *La Tente dans l'Essuf.* London and Paris: Cambridge University Press.
2000   *Les Gens de la Parole.* Paris: Éditions de découverte, textes a l'appui/série anthropologie.
Chesler, Phyllis
1971   *Women and Madness.* Garden City, N.Y.: Doubleday.
Childs, Larry and Celina Chelala
1993   "Drought, Rebellion, and Social Change in Northern Mali: The Challenges Facing Tamacheq Herders." *Cultural Survival Quarterly* Winter:16–20.
Chodorow, Nancy
1974   "Family Structure and Feminine Personality." In *Women, Culture, and Society,* ed. Michelle Zimbalist Rosaldo and Louise Lamphere, pp. 43–67. Stanford: Stanford University Press.
Classen, Constance
1997a   "Foundations for an Anthropology of the Senses." *ISSJ* 153:400–10.
1997b   "Engendering Perception: Gender Ideologies and Sensory Hierarchies in Western History." In *Body and Society.* London: Sage Publications.
Classen, Constance, Davis Howes, and Anthony Synnott, eds.
1994   *Aroma.* London: Routledge.
Claudot-Hawad, Hélène
1993   *Touareg: Portrait en Fragments.* Aix-en-Provence: Edisud.
1996   *Touaregs et Autres Sahariens entre plusieurs mondes.* Aix-en-Provence: Edisud.
2002   *Voyager d'un point de vue nomade.* Paris: IRMAM, Éditions Paris-Méditerranée.
Coles, Catherine
1990   "The Older Woman in Hausa Society: Power and Authority in Urban Nigeria." In *The Cultural Context of Aging,* ed. by Jay Sokolovsky. Westport, CT: Bergin & Garvey Press.
Corbin, Alain
1986   *The Foul and the Fragrant.* Cambridge, Mass.: Harvard University Press.
Crapanzano, Vincent
1980   *Tuhami.* Chicago: University of Chicago Press.
1992   *Hermes' Message and Hamlet's Desire.* Cambridge, MA: Harvard University Press.
Crapanzano, Vincent, and Vivian Garrison, eds.
1977   *Case Studies in Spirit Possession.* New York: John Wiley.
Crick, Malcolm
1976   *Explorations in Language and Meaning.* New York: John Wiley.
Davis, Donna
1983   *Blood and Nerves: An Ethnographic Focus on Menopause.* St. John's: Memorial University of Newfoundland Institute of Social and Economic Research.
Davis-Floyd, Robbie, and Carolyn F. Sargent

1997 *Childbirth and Authoritative Knowledge*. Berkeley: University of California Press.

Dayak, Mano
1992 *Touaregs: La Tragédie*. Paris: Éditions Jean-Claude Lattes.

Decalo, Samuel
1996 *Historical Dictionary of Niger*. 3rd Ed. Lanham, Md., and London: Scarecrow Press.

Delaney, Carol
1988 "Mortal Flow: Menstruation in Turkish Village Society." In *Blood Magic: The Anthropology of Menstruation*, ed. Thomas Buckley and Ama Gottlieb, pp. 75–94. Berkeley: University of California Press.

Di Leonardo, Michaela, ed.
1990 *Gender at the Crossroads of Knowledge*. Berkeley: University of California Press.

Douglas, Mary
1966 *Purity and Danger*. London: Routledge and Kegan Paul.
1975 *Implicit Meanings*. London: Routledge.
1996 *Culture and Risk*. London: Routledge.

Durkheim, Emile
1976 [1915] *The Elementary Forms of the Religious Life*. London: Allen and Unwin.

Durkheim, Emile, and Marcel Mauss
1963 [1903] *Primitive Classification*. Trans. and ed. Rodney Needham. Chicago: University of Chicago Press and London: Cohen and West.

Eliade, M.
1964 *Shamanism: Archaic Techniques of Ecstasy*. New York: Pantheon Press.

Evans-Pritchard, E. E.
1950 *Nuer Religion*. Oxford: Oxford University Press.

Fabrega, Horacio, Jr., and Daniel B. Silver
1973 *Illness and Shamanistic Curing in Zinacantan: An Ethnomedical Analysis*. Stanford: Stanford University Press.

Feld, Steven
1982 *Sound and Sentiment*. Philadelphia: University of Pennsylvania Press.

Figueiredo, Christina
1996 "Identité et consitoyenneté: La réélaboration des rélations entre hommes et femmes aux marges de la société Kel Adagh (Mali)." In *Touaregs et autres Sahariens entre plusieurs mondes,* ed. Helene Claudot-Hawad. Aix-en-Provence: Edisud.

Figueiredo-Biton, Christina
2002 "Le Voyage en chaud et froid: conceptions thermiques des Touaregs." In *Voyager d'un point de vue nomade,* ed. Helene Claudot-Hawad, pp. 137–45. Paris: IR MAM, Éditions Paris-Méditerranée.

Finerman, Ruth Beth
1989 "The Forgotten Healers: Women as Family Healers in an Andean Indian Community." In *Women as Healers*, ed. Carol McClain, pp.24-42. New Brunswick: Rutgers University Press.

Fiore, Barbara, and Fadi Wallet Faqqi
1993 *Isefran (Illnesses): Maladies et soins en milieu Touareg*. Perugia, Italie, et Bandiagara, Mali: Éditions CRMT/PSMTM.

Fitz Poole, John
1981 "Female Mediators among the Bimin-Kouskousmin." In *Sexual Meanings*, ed. Sherry Ortner and Harriet Whitehead. Cambridge: Cambridge University Press.

Flax, Jane
1990 "Postmodernism and Gender Relations in Feminist Theory." In *Feminism/Postmodernism,* ed. Linda Nicholson, pp. 39–62. New York: Routledge.

Foster, George M.
　1976　"Disease Categories in Non-Western Medical Systems." *American Anthropologist* 78(4):773–81.

Fugelstad, Fin
　1983　*A History of Niger 1850–1960.* Cambridge: Cambridge University Press.

Gast, Marceau
　1992　"Rélations amoureuses chez les Kel Ahaggar." In Amour, *Phantasms et sociétés en Afrique du Nord et au Sahara,* ed. by Tassadit Yacine, pp. 151–73. Paris: l'Harmattan-Awal.

Goddale, Jane
　1980　*Tiwi Wives.* Seattle: University of Washington Press.

Good, Charles
　1987　*Ethnomedical Systems in Africa.* New York: Guilford Press.

Goodenough, Ruth, and Peggy Sanday
　1995　*Beyond the Second Sex.* Philadelphia: University of Pennsylvania Press.

Gottlieb, Alma
　1992　*Under the Kapok Tree.* Bloomington: Indiana University Press.

Green, Edward
　1999　*Indigenous Theories of Contagious Disease.* Walnut Creek, Calif.: AltaMira Press.

Greenwood, Bernard
　1981　"Cold or Spirits? Choice and Ambiguity in Morocco's Pluralistic Medical System." *Social Science and Medicine* 15B:219–35.

Harding, Sandra
　1987　*The Science Question in Feminism.* Ithaca: Cornell University Press.

Harner, Michael
　1990　*The Way of the Shaman.* San Francisco: Harper and Row.

Hawad, Makhmoudan
　1979　"La Tagdudt." *Tisuraf: Groupe d'études berbères.* Université de Paris 8(3):79–82.
　1989　*Testament nomade.* La Bouilladisse: Amara.

Herzfeld, Michael
　2001　*Anthropology.* Malden, Mass., and Oxford: Blackwell.

Hoch-Smith, Judith, and Anita Spring, eds.
　1978　*Women in Ritual and Symbolic Roles.* New York: Plenum Press.

Horton, Robin
　1967　"African Traditional Thought and Western Science." *Africa* 37(1):50–71 and (2):155–87.
　1982　*Patterns of Thought in Africa and the West.* Cambridge: Cambridge University Press.
　1993　"Traditional African Thought Re-visited." In *Rationality and Relativism,* ed. Martin Hollis and Steven Lukes.

Hureiki, Jacques
　1999　*Les médicines touaregues traditionelles.* Paris: l'Harmattan.

Hutson, Alaine
　1997　*We Are Many.* PhD diss., Indiana University.

Ikhiri, Khalid, Saadou Mahamane, and Garba Mounkaila
　1984　*Recherche sur la Pharmacopée au Niger.* Niamey: UNESCO, OAU, AND CELTHO.

Imperato, Pascale James
　1977　*African Folk Medicine: Practices and Beliefs of the Bambara and Other Peoples.* Baltimore: York Press.

Jackson, Michael
　1989　*Paths Toward a Clearing: Radical Empiricism and Ethnographic Inquiry.* Bloomington: Indiana University Press.

James, Wendy
  1988   *The Whispering Ebony.* Cambridge: Cambridge University Press.
Jordan, Brigitte
  1993 [1978]   *Birth in Four Cultures: A Cross-Cultural Investigation of Childbirth in Yu-catan, Holland, Sweden and the United States.* 4th ed., rev. and exp. R. Davis-Floyd. Prospect Heights, Ill.: Waveland Press.
  1997   "Authoritative Knowledge and Its Construction." In *Childbirth and Authoritative Knowledge,* ed. Robbie Davis-Floyd and Carolyn Sargent, pp. 55–80. Berkeley: University of California Press.
Karp, Ivan, and D. A. Masolo
  2002   *African Philosophy as Cultural Inquiry.* Bloomington: Indiana University Press.
Keenan, Jeremy
  1976   *The Tuareg: People of Ahaggar.* London: Allen Lane.
  2003   "The End of the Matriline? The Changing Roles of Women and Descent amongst the Algerian Tuareg." *The Journal of North African Studies* 8(3–4 / Autumn–Winter):121–62.
Kendall, Laurel
  1989   "Old Ghosts and Ungrateful Children: A Korean Shaman's Story." In *Women as Healers,* ed. Carol McClain, pp. 138–57. New Brunswick and London: Rutgers University Press.
Kennedy, John G.
  1977   "Nubian Zar Ceremonies as Psychotherapy." In *Culture, Disease, and Healing,* ed. David Landy, pp. 375–85. New York: Macmillan.
Kitzinger, Sheila
  1997   "Authoritative Touch in Childbirth: A Cross-Cultural Approach." In *Childbirth and Authoritative Knowledge,* ed. Robbie Davis-Floyd and Carolyn Sargent, pp. 209–29. Berkeley: University of California Press.
Lamb, Sarah
  2000   *White Saris and Sweet Mangoes.* Berkeley: University of California Press.
Lejean, Yannick
  1986   *Médicine traditionnelle en milieu nomade dans la région de Tombouctou.* Paris-Sud: Medical thesis.
Lepowsky, Maria
  1995   "Gender in an Egalitarian Society: A Case Study from the Coral Sea." In *Beyond the Second Sex,* ed. Ruth Goodenough and Peggy Sanday, pp. 169–225. Philadelphia: University of Pennsylvania Press.
Levi-Strauss, Claude
  1962   *The Savage Mind.* Chicago: University of Chicago Press.
Lewis, I. M.
  1971   *Ecstatic Religion.* Harmondsworth, UK: Penguin.
  1986   *Religion in Context: Cults and Charisma.* Cambridge: Cambridge University Press.
Lock, Margaret
  1993   *Encounters with Aging: Mythologies of Menopause in Japan and America.* Berkeley: University of California Press.
MacCormack, Carol, ed.
  1982 [1994]   *Ethnography of Fertility and Birth.* New York: Academic Press [Prospect Heights, Ill: Waveland Press].
MacCormack, Carol, and Marilyn Strathern
  1980   *Nature, Culture, and Gender.* Cambridge: Cambridge University Press.
MacLean, U.
  1982   *Magical Medicine: A Nigerian Case-study.* London: Allan Lane.

Malinowski, Bronislaw
    1948   *Magic, Science, and Religion.* Glencoe, Ill.: Free Press.
Malkki, Liisa
    1995   *Purity and Exile.* Chicago: University of Chicago Press.
Martin, Emily
    1994   *Flexible Bodies.* Boston: Beacon Press.
Martin, Phyllis, and Patrick O'Meara, eds.
    1995   *Africa.* Bloomington: Indiana University Press.
Masquelier, Adeline
    1993   "Narratives of Power, Images of Wealth: The Ritual Economy of Bori in the Market." In
            Modernity and Its Malcontents, ed. Jean and John Comaroff, pp. 3–24. Chicago:
            University of Chicago Press.
McCarthy-Brown, Karen
    1991   *Mama Lola: A Voodou Priestess in Brooklyn.* Berkeley: University of California Press.
McClain, Carol, ed.
    1989   *Women As Healers.* New Brunswick: Rutgers University Press.
McNaughton, Patrick
    1988   *Mande Blacksmiths.* Bloomington: Indiana University Press.
Mernissi, Fatima
    1987   *Behind the Veil: Male-Female Dynamics in Modern Muslim Society.* London: Al Saqi Books.
Michael, Henry N., ed.
    1963   *Studies in Siberian Shamanism.* Trans. Stephen and Ethel Dunn. Toronto: University
            of Toronto Press.
Mikell, Gwendolyn
    1997   *African Feminism.* Philadelphia: University of Pennsylvania Press.
Monnig-Atkinson, Jane
    1992   "Shamanisms Today." *Annual Review of Anthropology,* vol. 21.
Mudimbe, V. Y.
    1988   *The Invention of Africa.* Bloomington: Indiana University Press.
    1992   *Parables and Fables.* Madison: University of Wisconsin Press.
Murdock, George P.
    1980   *Theories of Illness: A World Survey.* Pittsburgh: University of Pittsburgh Press.
Murphy, Robert
    1964   "Social Distance and the Veil." *American Anthropologist* 66:1257–74.
    1967   "Tuareg Kinship." *American Anthropologist* 69:163–70.
Nasr, Seyyed Hossein
    1993   *An Introduction to Islamic Cosmological Doctrines.* Albany, N.Y.: SUNY Press.
Ngubane, H.
    1977   *Body and Mind in Zulu Medicine: An Ethnography of Health and Disease in Nyuswa
            and Zulu Thought and Practice.* New York: Academic Press.
Nicolaisen, Ida, and Johannes Nicolaisen
    1997   *The Pastoral Tuareg.* Copenhagen: Rhodos.
Nicolaisen, Johannes
    1961   "La Réligion et la magie touaregues." *Folk* 3:113–60.
Nicolas, Guy
    1975   *Dynamique Sociale et Apprehension du Monde au Sein d'une Société Hausa.* Paris: l'In-
            stitut d'Ethnologie.
Noel, Marie-France
    2002   "Cheminement thérapeutique: les Touaregs de l'Adagh entre savoir-être et savoir-
            faire." In *Voyager d'un point de vue nomade,* ed. Helene Claudot-Hawad, pp.
            145–59. Paris: IRMAM, Éditions Paris-Méditerranée.

Norris, H. T.
    1975   *The Tuareg: Their Islamic Legacy and its Diffusion in the Sahel.* London: Aris and Phillips.
    1990   *Sufi Mystics of the Niger Desert.* Oxford: Clarendon Press.
Olkes, Cheryl, and Paul Stoller
    1987   *In Sorcery's Shadow.* Chicago: University of Chicago Press.
Ong, Walter
    1982   *Orality and Literacy: The Technologizing of the World.* London: Methuen.   ·
Oosten, J. G.
    1985   *The War of the Gods: The Social Code.* London and Boston: Routledge and Kegan Paul.
Orion, Loretta
    1995   *Never Again the Burning Times.* Prospect Heights, Ill.: Waveland Press.
Ortner, Sherry
    1974   "Is Female to Male what Nature is to Culture?" In *Women, Culture, and Society,* ed. Michelle Zimbalist Rosaldo and Louise Lamphere, pp. 67–89. Stanford: Stanford University Press.
    1996   *Making Gender.* Boston: Beacon Press.
Oxby, Clare
    1990   "The 'Living Milk' Runs Dry: The Decline of a Form of Joint Ownership and Matrilineal Inheritance among the Twareg (Niger)." In *Property, Poverty and People: Changing Rights in Property and Problems of Pastoral Development,* ed. P. T. W. Baxter with Richard Hogg, pp. 222–28. Manchester: Manchester University Press.
Parkin, David
    1991   *The Sacred Void.* Cambridge: Cambridge University Press.
Perrone, Bobbette, H. Henrietta Stockel, and Victoria Krueger
    1989   *Medicine Women, Curanderas, and Women Doctors.* Norman and London: University of Oklahoma Press.
Peters, Larry
    1981   *Ecstasy and Healing in Nepal.* Malibu, Calif.: Undena Publications.
Randall, Sara C.
    1993   "Le sang est plus chaud que l'eau: utilization populaire du chaud et du froid dans la cure en médecine tamacheq." In *Se Soigner au Mali,* ed. Brunet-Jailly, pp. 126–49. Paris: Karthala.
Rasmussen, Susan
    1989   "Accounting for Belief: Causation, Misfortune, and Concepts of Evil in Tuareg Systems of Thought." *Journal of the Royal Anthropological Institute* 5(24):124–44.
    1991   "Lack of Prayer: Ritual Restrictions, Social Experience, and the Anthropology of Menstruation among the Tuareg." *American Ethnologist* 18(4):751–69.
    1992   "Ritual Specialists, Ambiguity, and Power in Tuareg Society." *Journal of the Royal Anthropological Institute* 27(1):105–28.
    1994   "Female Sexuality, Social Reproduction, and Medical Intervention: Kel Ewey Tuareg Perspectives." *Culture, Medicine, and Psychiatry* 18:433–62.
    1995   *Spirit Possession and Personhood among the Kel Ewey Tuareg.* Cambridge: Cambridge University Press.
    1997   *The Poetics and Politics of Tuareg Aging: Life Course and Personal Destiny in Niger.* DeKalb: Northern Illinois University Press.
    1998a   "Only Women Know Trees." *Journal of Anthropological Research* 54(2):147–71.
    1998b   "Ritual Powers and Social Tensions as Moral Discourse among the Tuareg." *American Anthropologist* 100(2):458–68.
    1999   "Making Better 'Scents' in Anthropology: Aroma in Tuareg Sociocultural Systems

and the Shaping of Ethnography." *Anthropological Quarterly* 72(2 / April):55–74.

2000   "From Child-Bearers to Culture-Bearers: Transition to Postchildbearing among Tuareg Women." *Medical Anthropology* 19:91–116.

2001a   *Healing in Community: Medicine, Contested Terrains, and Cultural Encounters among the Tuareg.* Westport, Conn.: Bergin & Garvey.

2001b   "Grief At Seeing a Daughter Leave Home: Weeping and Emotions in the Tuareg *Techawait* Ceremony." *Journal of American Folklore* 113(450):391–421.

2001c   "In the Shadow of Great Sheltering Trees (Songs)." *The Journal of American Semiotics* 17(4 / Winter):43–92.

2003   "Gendered Discourses and Mediated Modernities: Urban and Rural Performances of Tuareg Smith Women." *Journal of Anthropological Research* 59:487–509.

2004   "'These Are Dirty Times!' Transformations of Gendered Spaces and Islamic Ritual Protection." *Journal of Ritual Studies* 18(2):43–60.

Reiter, Rayna
1975   *Toward an Anthropology of Women.* New York: Monthly Review Press.

Rival, Laura, ed.
1998   *The Social Life of Trees: Anthropological Perspectives on Tree Symbolism.* Oxford and New York: Berg Press.

Rodd, Francis, Lord of Rennell
1926   *People of the Veil.* London: MacMillan Anthropological Publications.

Rosaldo, Michelle Zimbalist
1980   *Knowledge and Passion: Ilongot Notions of Self and Social Life.* Cambridge: Cambridge University Press.

Rosaldo, Michelle Zimbalist, and Louise Lamphere, eds.
1974   *Women, Culture, and Society.* Stanford: Stanford University Press.

Sáenz, Candelario
1991   They Have Eaten Our Grandfather! The Status of Tuareg Smiths. PhD diss., Columbia University

Said, Edward
1978   *Orientalism.* New York: Pantheon Press.

Saladin d'Anglure, Bernard
1994   "From Foetus to Shaman: The Construction of an Inuit Third Sex." In *Amerindian Rebirth,* ed. A. Mills and R. Slobodin, pp. 82–106. Toronto: University of Toronto Press.

1996   "Shamanism." In *Encyclopedia of Social and Cultural Anthropology,* ed. by Alan Barnard and Jonathan Spencer. New York: Routledge.

Sargent, Carolyn
1989   *Maternity, Medicine, and Power: Reproductive Decisions in Urban Benin.* Berkeley: University of California Press.

Sargent, Carolyn F., and Caroline B. Brettell
1996   *Gender and Health: An International Perspective.* Upper Saddle River, N.J.: Prentice Hall.

Schlegel, Alice, ed.
1972   *Sexual Stratification: A Cross-Cultural View.* New York: Columbia University Press.

Schmoll, Pamela
1993   "Black Stomachs, Beautiful Stones: Soul-Eating among Hausa in Niger." In *Modernity and Its Malcontents,* ed. Jean and John Comaroff, pp. 193–220. Chicago: University of Chicago Press.

Schulz, Erhard, and Aboubacar Adamou
1992   Nutzung von Pflanzen in der Sahara und ihren Randgebieten. Wurtzburg.

Scott, Joan
    1994   "Deconstructing Equality-Versus-Difference: Or the Uses of Poststructuralist The-
ory for Feminism." In *The Postmodern Turn: New Perspectives on Social Theory*, ed.
S. Seidman. Cambridge: Cambridge University Press.
Siikala, Anne-Leena, and Mihaly Hoppal, eds.
    1992   *Studies on Shamanism.* Helsinki: Finnish Anthropological Society.
Sokolovsky, Jay, ed.
    1989   *The Cultural Context of Aging.* Grandy, Mass.: Bergin & Garvey Press.
Sontag, Susan
    1978   *Illness as Metaphor.* New York: Farrar, Straus, and Giroux.
    1989   *AIDS and Its Metaphors.* New York: Farrar, Straus, and Giroux.
Spittler, Gerd
    1993   *Les Touaregs face aux sécheresses et aux famines.* Paris: Karthala.
Stoller, Paul
    1989   *The Taste of Ethnographic Things.* Philadelphia: University of Pennsylvania Press.
    1997   *Sensuous Scholarship.* Philadelphia: University of Pennsylvania Press.
    2004   *Stranger in the Village of the Sick: A Memoir of Cancer, Sorcery, and Healing.* Boston:
Beacon Press.
Strathern, Marilyn
    1981   "Self-Interest and the Social Good: Some Implications of Hagen Gender Ideology."
In *Sexual Meanings: The Cultural Construction of Gender and Sexuality*, ed. Sherry
Ortner and Harriet Whitehead, pp. 166–91. Cambridge: Cambridge University Press.
Szasz, Thomas
    1970   *The Manufacture of Madness.* New York: Delta Books.
Tambiah, Stanley
    1990   *Magic, Science, and Religion and the Scope of Rationality.* Cambridge: Cambridge
University Press.
Taussig, Michael
    1987   *Shamanism, Colonialism, and the Wild Man.* Chicago: University of Chicago Press.
    1993   *Mimesis and Alterity.* New York: Routledge.
Trudelle-Schwartz, Maureen
    2003   *Blood and Voice.* Tucson: University of Arizona Press.
Tsing, Anna
    1993   *In the Realm of the Diamond Queen.* Princeton: Princeton University Press.
Turner, Edith
    1996   *The Hands Feel It.* DeKalb: Northern Illinois University Press.
Turner, Victor
    1967   *The Drums of Affliction.* Ithaca: Cornell University Press.
    1968   *The Forest of Symbols.* Ithaca: Cornell University Press.
Tyler, Stephen
    1987   *The Unspeakable.* Madison: University of Wisconsin Press.
U.S. Department of State
    1994   *Background Notes: Niger.* July. Washington, D.C.
    2000   *Background Notes: Mali.* June. Washington, D.C.
Urban, Greg
    1998   *Metaphysical Community.* Philadelphia: University of Pennsylvania Press.
Walentowitz, Saskia
    2002   "Partir sans quitter: rites et gestes autour des déplacements féminins chez les Inesli-
men de l'Azawagh." In *Voyager d'un point de vue nomade*, ed. Helene Claudot-
Hawad, pp. 37–53. Paris: IRMAM, Éditions Paris-Méditerranée.

Weaver, Marcia, Holly Wong, Amadou Sekou Sako, Robert Simon, and Felix Lee
  1994   "Prospects for Reform of Hospital Fees in Sub-Saharan Africa: A Case Study of Niamey National Hospital in Niger." *Social Science and Medicine* 38(4):565–74.
Wedenoja, William
  1989   "Mothering and the Practice of Balm in Jamaica." In *Women as Healers,* ed. Carol McClain, pp. 76–98. New Brunswick: Rutgers University Press.
Winkelman, Michael
  1992   "Shamans, Priests, and Witches. A Cross-Cultural Study of Magico-Religious Practitioners." *Anthropoological Research Papers* #44. Tempe: Arizona State University.
  1999   "Altered States of Consciousness." In *Encyclopedia of Human Emotions,* ed. D. Levinson, J. Ponzetti, and P. Jorgensen, pp. 32–38. New York: Macmillan.
  2000   *Shamanism: The Neural Ecology of Consciousness and Healing.* Westport, Conn.: Bergin & Garvey.
  2001   "Alternative and Traditional Medicine Approaches for Substance Abuse Programs: A Shamanic Perspective." *International Journal of Drug Policy* 12:337–51.
  2002   Shamanism as Neurotheology and Evolutionary Psychology." *American Behavioral Scientist* 45(2):1875–87.
Winkelman, Michael, and D. White
  1987   "A Cross-Cultural Study of Magico-Religious Practitioners and Trance States: Database." In *HRAF,* ed. by Levinson and R. Wagner, vol. 3D. New Haven, Conn.: HRAF Press.
Wolf, Marjorie
  1992   "The Woman Who Didn't Become a Shaman." In *A Thrice-Told Tale: Feminism, Postmodernism, and Ethnographic Responsibility.* Palo Alto: Stanford University Press.
Wolff, Norma
  2000   "The Use of Human Images in Yoruba Medicines." *Ethnology* 39(3):205–25.
Wood, John
  1999   *When Men Are Women.* Madison: University of Wisconsin Press.
World Bank
  1989   *World Development Report.*
Worley, Barbara
  1991   Women's War Drum, Women's Wealth. PhD diss., Columbia University.
  1992   "Where All the Women Are Strong." *Natural History* 101(II):55–63.

Index

Aaneghale, 90

Abadayan, 124

Abaka, 125. *See also* trees

abaket (pl. *ibakaden*), 22, 82, 85, 101, 152. *See also* sin

Abardak, 139

Abdou Maghchare Al Falaki, 161

ablutions, 61, 68, 77, 130. See also *alwalla*

Aboubacar Adamou, 199

Abu-Lughod, Lila, 105, 177, 203

Acacia, 65, 138

Acacia epinee, 128. See also *atise;* trees

Acacia raddiana, 126. See also *afagag;* trees

Achterberg, Jean, 24, 203

adade. See finger

Adagh-n-Ifoghas, xi, 3, 77, 181

Adam, 155

Adana, 68. See also *arabaz;* massage

Adaras, 37. *See also* trees

Adaoula, 125

adeleb, 100. *See also* obedience

Adima, 179

adir adir, 57, 58, 117. *See also* medicines; tea

ado, 18, 155. *See also* illness; wind

adolescents, 102, 145

adoption, 94, 110

adoua, 137. *See also* trees

afa, 35, 43–45. *See also* moon(light); sun

afagag, 126. See also *Acacia raddiana;* trees

afalo, 37

afazo. See grasses; plants

Affassas, 37

affines, 105, 113–14, 201

Africa(n), viii, x, 9; gender in, 113, 115; healing in, 25, 87, 163; health care in, 184–85; Islam in, 194; philosophies, 16–19; tree symbols in, 121, 124

Afro-Asian, 26

afterlife, 90, 199

Ag Arias, Alitinine, xi

Ag Erless, Mohammed, xi, 46, 203

Ag Hamaday el Mehdi, 47, 203

Ag Solimane, Alhassane, xi, 119, 143–44, 203

Agadez, xi, 2, 46; artisanry in, 91, 145; divination in, 161–62; gender and sexuality in, 77; health care in, 38, 179–81, 187–92; herbalists in, 100; historical migrations in and around, 137, 139; Hospital, 38, 39, 108, 170, 181, 187; market, 30; religion in, 159; sultan of Aïr in, 201

Agala, 88, 201. *See also* South

Agalal, 125

agar, 124, 125. See also *Maerua crassifolia;* trees

age/aging, 74, 78; and local theories of menopause, 66, 96, 99, 103, 106; and marriage, 41, 43; of medicine women, 3, 8, 33–36, 80, 93–94, 100; and rites of passage, 121, 199; theories of female, 22–23; theories of healing, 71

aggag (fem. *taggagart*), 141

Aghaghagh, 80

Aghaly, 136–39, 155, 169

Aghatchere, 169

aghitiss, 32, 57. *See also* blood

aghuru, 32, 73. *See also* back

Ahaggar, 3. *See also* Algeria; Hoggar

Ahearn, Laura, 6, 195, 198, 203

Ahmed, 158–60

AIDS (SIDA), 96

Aïr, vii, viii, xi, 30, 33; climate and geography, 2–4; descent, kinship, and property in, 112; diets in, 31–32; gardening in, 28; healing clans in, 82; health-care collaboration programs in, 181; history of, 88, 91, 93, 136–37, 139; smiths' roles in, 50; song verse reference to, 125; Sultan of, 201

Ajirou, 5, 91, 167, 169

Akakou, 37

Akhmed, 158–60

Akhmed Mohammed, 84

akh ihuderan, vii, 27, 86, 113, 197. *See also* inheritance; milk; property

akkamum, 95. *See also* medicine; plants; trees

al baraka: in bones, 167; healers', 72, 101–2; in land, vii, 58, 120–21, 130, 132; leaders', 9,

29; marabouts', 156, 158; medicine women's conveying of, 135–47; threats to, 187, 189–90, 195. *See also* blessing

albarass, 160. *See also* flesh; skin

albourouj, 158. *See also* divination

al hima, 5, 85, 135–36, 141. *See also* sacred

al ladat, 120. *See also* widowhood

alafaz, 43, 103, 154, 180. *See also* blood; sourness

alanmawdragh, 37. *See also* medicine; trees

Alawa, 123

alekhustara, 108, 157, 161, 169. *See also* divination; Qur'anic

Aligouran (Adigouran), 35, 88, 90

Algeria, 25, 27, 36, 124, 183

alghod, 158. *See also* trees

Alghou, 124

Alghoumour, 161. *See also* divination; marabouts; Qur'anic

Alhassane, 90

Alhousseini, 90

aljen (pl. *eljenan*), 127–28, 164. *See also* spirits

allopathic, medicine, 4, 9, 171, 178, 192

Almoravid, 29

Almoustafa, 159

alms, offerings, and *al baraka*, 143; and divination, 168–69; and healing, marabouts', 160, 150–53, 155; medicine women's, 130; at memorial mortuary feasts, 69, 90, 92; in sacred places, 138

altered states, 5, 19, 131, 174–76

alternative scripts, 177

alwalla, 68. *See also* ablutions

amadal, 68–69. *See also* earth

amadas (fem. *tamadas*), 68–69. *See also* bones; bone-setting

amagal, vii, 30, 37, 57, 199. *See also* medicine

amagal n anna, 37. *See also* birth; medicine; *tishi*

amasur, 32. *See also* wrist

amezeghi, 62. *See also* bones

amaghres, 43. *See also* diet

aman iman, 120. *See also* water

Amazon(ian), 118

ambilineality, 62

amegazo, 161. *See also* diviners

amenukal, 26, 201. *See also* leaders; sultan

amerdio, 34. *See also* bloating; body; swelling

America(n), 25, 197, 64

amezeghi, 62. *See also* bones

Amina, 99, 148, 164

amizou, 34. *See also* medicine; *Mitragyna inermes*; trees

Amougai, 124

Amoumoun, 107–11, 113, 139, 145, 160

amulets: protective, 39, 67, 70; Qur'anic, 154–55, 160, 167; and trees, 120; and work, 146

Ana, vii, 84–85, 90

anagar, 68. *See also* contagion; infection; pollution

analogical thought in science, 75. *See also* metaphor

anatomy, 32. *See also* body

ancestors: matrilineal, 129–30; medicine women's, vii–viii, 3, 22–23, 81–86, 88–91; regional clans', 135, 140; stone ruins of, 153

androgynous, 23, 78, 100

anemia, 179, 184

anezun, 37

anger, 98; in pregnancy, 42, 96, 144, 166; and smiths, 18, 49–50, 170–71. *See also* *tezma*; *tourgoum*

anezum, 37. *See also* medicine; plants; trees

Anna, 139

anoughou, 5, 43, 50, 167. *See also* diet; illness

Anou-migrin, 125

Anourra, 123

Anta, 33, 43, 88–89, 150

anthropology: of aging, life course, and symbolism, xi; gender and healing studies, 21, 23; of gender, healing, and religion, vii–viii, 5–6, 9, 152; medical, 9, 18; nature/culture theories, 129;

anthropomorphism: 69–70, 121

antibiotics: local needs for, 48, 63, 167, 179–80, 190

anti-social conduct 32, 86, 149, 162

anulem, 34. *See also* amerdio; bloating; body

anzad, 100. *See also* music

aousa, 135. *See also* spleen

Apache, 70

apprenticeships: and authorization to practice, 32–33, 62; and changes, 146; informal cases of, 66, 81; and knowledge, 117, 135, 154; marabouts', 158, 160; medicine women's, 7, 89, 168, 187, 190–91

Arab: Chamba, 124; Chronicles, 26; Kunta, 201; medicine, 74; men's intermarriage with some Tuareg women, 145; relations with Tuareg, 27–29

Arabane, 136

arabaz, 57, 64, 68, 97, 117. *See also* massage

Arabic, ix, 45, 113, 148, 154, 156, 198, 201

arakab, 117. *See also* liver; massage

arankat, 37. *See also* medicine; trees

arassal, 32, 58, 89. *See also* origins

arboreal imagery, 117–32

Arctic, 19

Arens, William, 16, 111, 163, 203

Aristotle, 45, 76

ark echaghel, 35, 70, 149. *See also* sorcery

Arlit, 2, 108

art(ist), x, 7–8, 81, 122

arthritis, 62

asakalabo, 39. *See also* calabash; music

Asalo, 92, 191

asawad, 61, 72, 157, 167. *See also* divination; medicine: and medicine women; *tamaswad*

ashik najad, 153. *See also* trees

Asian, East, 19

asikulu, 43

Assadek, 123

assiwi, 57. *See also* cooking; *ilaten;* medicine

astrology, 161

astronomy, 161

asul, 39. *See also* dance; exorcism; possession; spirits

Ata, 123

atanin, 123. *See also* trees

atise, 126, 128. *See also* trees

atri (pl. *itran*), 161. *See also* divination; horoscope; stars

Atkaki, 136, 137–41

atri, 161. *See also* astrology; astronomy; divination; horoscope; stars

audene, 37. *See also* medicine; trees

Aujem, 123

aural (oral), 8; and relationship to other senses and science, 59, 72, 76, 79, 81; and relationship to written, 20; sources for Tuareg and Saharan history, 26

Australia(n): aborigines, 45, 119

authoritative, viii, ix, xi, 8–9, 11; and knowledge construction, gender, and science issues, 24; medicine women's, 27; mythicohistory as, 82; plural systems, 181; and

power struggles, 164–65, 187, 194; and touch, 71

authorization: and marabouts, 154, 158, 162; by older mentor, 33, 62, 66, 80, 99; and referrals, 117;

awal, 81. *See also* speaking

ax, 121, 130, 148

Aya, 117

aza, 34, 126, 128. *See also* medicine; trees

Azawak, 28, 144

Azday, 139

Azel, 91, 188

azni, 74, 125. *See also* blood

back: and dune's name, 138; illnesses and treatments, 32, 34, 53, 149; researcher's consultations for, 164, 67, 185; symbolism of, 73. See also *aghuru*

Baghdad, 138

Bagzan, Mount (Massif), vii, 2, 30, 33–34, 58, 69; maraboutique families around, 50; powers of plants on, 73; regional history of, 138–40; and role in origins of healing and sacredness, 62–63, 80, 82–84, 88–91, 99, 117–18

bajalica, 23. *See also* Serbian

Bakhtinian, post-, 90

balance: and Arab and Greek humoral/thermal and counteractive medical influences, 74, 76–77; bodily, 30, 45

Balanites aegyptiaca, 126. See also *tiboraq;* trees

Bali, 120

Bamako, xi

Bambara, 17, 183

Bamberger, Judith, viii, 82, 203

bandits, 131, 143

barber, 68

Bariba, 23

barks, vii–viii, 55; and origins of herbal uses in healing, 83–85, 131; restrictions in gathering, 58, 194; sources of, 129; and treatments, 94, 96, 167

barley, 31

bathing, 38, 46, 81, 179

bawre (wild fig), 37. *See also* fruits; medicine; trees

beans, 31, 110

beef, 46

Beisele, Megan, 196

belladonna, 24

belly button, 150. *See also* umbilical cord
Bemba, 17
Beng, 63, 106, 121
Beni Hilal, 198
Beni Sulaym, 198
Benin, 24, 185
Berber: history of peoples, 198, 201; language group, 26. *See also* Tamajaq; Tuareg
Bernus, Edmond, viii, 3, 26, 112, 187, 197, 199, 203
Biannu, 148, 152
bilateral, 26, 62
bile, 75
Bilma, 30, 90, 125
Bimin Kuskusmin, 163
binary, ix, 19–23, 100, 119, 129
biomedicine, viii; classification and translation issues of, 5, 8–9, 40, 48; doctors, 180; local access to, 129; medicine women's encounters and differences with, 25, 58, 178–92, 196; and touch controversies, 71; Tuareg attitudes toward, 37, 181–84. *See also* allopathic medicine; clinics; doctors; hospitals
birds, 18, 86, 122, 129, 137
birth, 22; beliefs concerning, 124, 189–90; defects, 35, 45, 164, 166, 173, 177, 179; difficult cases, 35–42, 44, 81; records, 199; ritual restrictions and precautions, 71, 102, 144–45; tearing during, 64
bitterness, 102, 138, 167
black, 58, 75, 125, 128, 148, 156
bladder, 32, 94, 109, 150
blame, 29, 38, 50, 111
Bledsoe, Caroline, 21, 23, 203
blessing (benediction), 29, 37, 64, 81, 87, 95, 118, 120, 136, 189. See also *al baraka*
bloating, 34, 69, 117, 128. See also *amerdio; anulem;* body
Bloch, Maurice, 122
blood: beliefs concerning, 34, 69, 74–76, 166, 168, 184; blood-letting in cutting treatment, 34; illnesses, 32, 41, 179; and kinship symbolism, 143
blue, 20, 156
Boddy, Janice, 23, 75, 174, 177, 198, 203
body: beliefs concerning, 30–32, 34–35, 46, 51, 111; and birth-related beliefs and practices, 39, 189–90; local categories of, 68–70; local theories of vulnerability of,

94, 106; and relationship to mind, ix–x, 22; thermal/humoral theories of, 73–79; touching of, 61–63, 154, 167, 180; and women's distinctiveness, 151
boka(ye), 3, 20, 73, 161–62, 168, 174. *See also* Hausa; sorcery
bones, 44, 62, 68
bone-setting, 63, 68–69
bori, 161. *See also* Hausa; possession; spirits
botanical, 5, 118
Boilley, Pierre, 203
Boulkhou, 91, 141
Bouman, Annemarie, 25, 27, 77–78, 103, 198–99, 203
boundaries, x–xi, 7, 22, 88, 130, 143
Bourgeot, Andre, 27, 203
Boyer, 120
branch, 39, 122. *See also* trees
bread, 88
breastfeeding, 143
breech-birth, 63
Brenner, Suzanne April, 21, 23, 203
Brettell, Caroline, 156, 211
bricolage, 128–29
bricoleur, 20, 30, 75, 172
bridewealth, 39, 80, 92, 103, 112, 199
broadcasting, 145
brothers, 112, 121; in folklore, 123–24, 126–29
Brown, Judith, 23, 101, 115, 204
Buckley, Thomas, 23, 101, 115, 200, 204
budgets (national), 186. *See also* Mali; nation; Niger
bunion, 64
burial, 85, 200
Burkina Faso, 2, 25
butter, 37, 41, 45–46

calabash: and medicine, 33–34; as musical instrument, 39, 70
caliphs, 138
Camel, Florence, 27
calling: spirit, 5
cameliers, 84
camels: lost, 169; in myths, 84–85, 88, 127–29; as property, 92, 97; in song verses, 124; in subsistence (caravanning and herding), 3, 30, 32
camphor, 81
cancer, 18, 51

caravanning: clothing from, 138; colonial and post-colonial government restrictions on, 129; origins of, to Bilma and Fatchi, 85; socioeconomic relationships with Hausa, 140; as subsistence, 25–26, 36, 200
Carrier, James, 15, 25, 204
carriers, 46
Casajus, Dominique, xi, 48, 163, 204
cases, 6, 33, 36, 200–201. *See also* methods
Castaneda, Carlos, 17
cauterization, 32, 34, 36
cereals, 87
Chamba, 124
chamin, 95. *See also* medicine; trees
change: social, 179–92
character, 74–76, 91, 167, 177
charcoal, 82, 83, 131
cheese: goat, 30, 41, 80, 100, 121
Chelala, Donna, 130, 204
Chesler, Phyllis, 156, 204
chewing, 58, 125
chicken, 46
chicken-pox, 179
chiefs, 65, 67, 80, 90–92, 138, 144
childbearing: and age-related beliefs, 75, 93; illnesses of, 41–42; in life course, 101–2; postpartum taboo against, 35. *See also* age-laging; birth and transitions, 22
childlessness, 35–36, 42, 93, 100, 107–11, 113, 163, 176
children: alms given to, 143; and birth-related practices, 71; and descent imagery, 112; disabled, 166; and foods, 125; and illnesses, 35–36; in life course, 104–5; medicine women's healing of, 88–89; and medico-ritual treatments, 54–56; and motherhood and healing, 93, 116; naming of, 62; and usefulness, 66
Childs, Larry, 130, 204
chills, 41
Chimo, 123, 190–92
Chite, 90
chloroform, 24
Chodorow, Nancy, 23, 116, 204
Christian, Church, 24, 156
chronotopes, 88, 129
circumcision, 68, 106. See also *wanzam*
clans, viii, 3, 31, 62, 82, 88–89, 91, 140, 201. *See also* descent; origins
Classen, Constance, 59, 72, 75–76, 78, 204

classification, cultural, ix, 15–18, 46–48, 57
Claudot-Hawad, Hélène, viii, xi, 3, 6, 26–27, 37, 45, 47–49, 76–77, 101, 112, 184, 187, 197–99, 204, 205, 209
clay, 4, 58, 87, 96, 148
client-patron, 25–26, 139–40. *See also* status; stratification
climate, 4, 45
clinics: access to and need for locally, 167; and collaboration in training programs, 65, 149, 179–81, 184–90; local attitudes toward, 47, 99; medicine women's relations with, 8, 24
cloth(es): changing attitudes and practices regarding, 138, 196; inheritance of, 112; and life course, 38, 103; measure, 58, 66, 157; medico-ritual use of, 95; as payment, 148;
CNRST, xi
cold: and bodily humoral balance, 73–79; illnesses, 44–48; in local humoral medical systems, ix, 8, 91–97, 108, 111, 125, 135
Coles, Catherine, 163, 204
colonialism, 25–27, 124, 129, 140, 188, 198
colors: in illness diagnosis, 20, 32, 37; and symbolism, 46, 58, 94, 96, 148; song references to, 127–29
Comaroff, Jean, 3, 17
Comaroff, John, 3, 17
commemoration, 22, 90, 114
commemorative memorial feasts, 61, 69
compensation, 21, 28, 61, 145
competition, 70, 152–53, 156, 162, 164
complementarity: in herbalist-marabout relationships, 138, 152–53, 162, 164
conception, 35, 66, 101
confederation, 26
conflict, 29. *See also* disputes
Connerton, Paul, 27
constipation, 34
consultations: Dabo, 188–89; Hadia, 97–99, 108, 185; Eliman, 107–11; Tana, 32–33; Tata, 35–43; Tema, 65–67; Tina, 167–68; Zara, 63
consummation, 35, 41
contagion, 15–19, 37, 43, 73, 108. *See also* pollution
contraception, 107
contradictions, viii, x; *al baraka*-related, 135, 145; in healers' roles, 19, 115, 129, 164; social-cultural, 100, 107, 123; writing-related, 155

cooking, 45, 116; of medicines, 12, 83, 121, 152; ritual restrictions concerning, 135

cooperatives 145

cosmologies: arboreal spirits in, 120, 124, 130; body in, 32, 68; disputed, 193; life course–related, 102, 104; menstrual, 200; myth-related in healing, 87, 90; official/popular Islamic, 29, 194; and ritual symbolism references, 140–42, 173

coude, 58, 157, 159. *See also* forearm

cough, 63

counteractive, 44–46, 74–76, 99. *See also* balance; cold; hot; medicine

courtship, 190

cousins, 28, 33, 39, 65, 97, 123, 182, 200. *See also* kinship; marriage

cow, 127; dung, 35

co-wives, 65–66, 97–99. *See also* polygyny

cowrie shells, 161–62, 167–68

Crapanzano, Vincent, 6, 16, 106, 200, 204

creativity, vii, x, 17, 132

Crick, Malcolm, 5, 16, 204

crow, 96, 128–29

cultural, x, 4, 8; and cosmological, 193; and natural, 21, 130–31; and religious, 152; re-localizing of global, 20; theories of, 15–16; values, 29, 86, 147, 176

culture, ix, 3, 17; and classification, 21; and ethnicity issues, 25; and gender, 115; and nature, 119, 122, 129; and religion, 152–53

Cuna, 70

cupping, 61

curandera, 82

cutting, 34, 63, 84

Dabo, 187–90

Damagaram, 201

Damargou, 201

dance, 39-40, 131; spirit, 73

danger, 25, 34, 74, 91, 141, 153–54

dates: alms offerings of, 90, 100, 120, 143; amulet uses of, 120; caravan trade of, 25, 30, 166, 200; consumption of, 41, hot humoral classification of, 46; palms as *akh huderan* property, 197

Davis, Donna, 16–17, 197, 204

Davis: Floyd, Robbie, viii, 24, 59, 181, 196, 205, 207

Dayak, Mano, 25, 130, 199, 200, 205

De Heusch, Luc, 176

death, viii, 85, 90, 125, 166

debt: national, 184

Decalo, Samuel, 26, 130, 205

deconstruction, 3, 5

Delaney, Carol, 105, 204

Department of State, 186

depression, 3, 8, 67, 97. *See also* emotions; *tamazai*

descent, 26–27; medicine from Prophet, 167; women's clans, 82, 85, 88; regional clans, 136–40; transformations and effects on property, 113–15. *See also* bilateral; clans; inheritance; matrilineal; patrilineal; origins

Devil, 101, 125, 127–28, 137. *See also* Iblis

Di Leonardo, Michaela, 21, 23, 115, 204

diagnosis, viii; of Amoumoun and Hadjiatou, 107–12; in collaborative programs, 186, 188; and divination, 167–68, 170, 173; of Mariama, 97–99; medicine women's techniques of, 32–35, 40, 50–51, 64, 151–53; and sensorium, 71, 73, 81, 95; of Tahirou, 149–50

dialects, xi, 4, 45, 57

dialogue, 81

diarrhea, 50, 99, 162

diet, 30–31; and illness causation, 43–44, 57, 94, 189–92

difference, x, 15, 196

dignity, 48, 60, 90

dirt, 85, 104, 188–92. *See also* contagion; danger; pollution

discourses: dissonant, 177

disputes, 26, 193; *boka*-related, 162; land and money, 66–67; marital, 65–66, 98–100; property, 112–14; well use, 183;

divination: *bokaye,* 162; dream and spirit-related, 147, 150, 166–78; medicine women's conventional techniques of, viii, 9, 49–51, 61, 67–68, 72; Qur'anic, 156–61;

diviners, 5, 59, 61, 68, 117, 150. *See also* marabouts; medicine: and medicine women; mediumship

divorce, 33, 50, 68, 200; attitudes toward, 92; diviners' rate of, 169, 171, 173; polygyny as women's motive for, 110, 113

doctors: biomedical, 30, 57, 167, 186

dogs, 4, 137

domestic, 3, 21, 23; dynamics, 113–15, 130, 153, 173

donkeys, 3, 129
Dosso, 2
Douglas, Mary, 15, 17, 19, 21, 23, 59, 114, 197, 205
doum palm, 31, 83, 96, 127, 138
Dow, James, 25
dowry, 197
dreaming: in divining, 72, 100, 166–67, 173, 201
drought, xi; and depletion of livestock, 36, 169; and effects on diet and pharmacopia, 31, 180, 182, 196; and effects on gendered property relations, 112, 129–31; and historical recurrence of in region, 136–38; and local interpretation of causes, 146
drum, 39, 122–24, 126, 128, 144; chiefs', 26. *See also* exorcism; possession; *tende*
dryness, 45, 75, 145
dunes, 45, 125, 138
Durkheim, Emile, 119, 205

ears, 36, 49; and infection, 44
earth: and association with *al baraka* and sacred places, 141, 144, 167; as focus of birth-related beliefs and rituals, 87; and illness from hot sand, 43; spirit of (Old Woman, Waddawa), 102, 124; touching of, in healing rituals, 64, 68–69, 97
East, 5, 136, 201
eating, 29–30, 57, 97; ritual to combat infertility, 108–9
Eaux et Forets, 121
Ebalaqan, 128
ebisgin, 125–26, 128. *See also* medicine; trees
École Nomade, 107. *See also* schools
ecology, 27, 118, 129
economic, 23, 25–28, 124, 129, 165, 186–87
edes, 65, 67. *See also* touch
eggs, 46, 101, 109, 129
eghajira (eghale), 41, 69, 97. *See also* food
eghef, 73. *See also* head
ehan n barar, 41. *See also* children; tent; uterus
El Kebir, 158
elderly/elders, vii, 90, 160; and aged status of medicine women as confidantes, 36, 80, 100, 114; and *al baraka* of some leaders, 135; and councils for dispute-adjudication, 26; and healing roles across cultures, 71, 163; and reserve toward parents-in-law and chiefs, 93; youths' rebellion against, 143. *See also* age

elephant dung, 96
Eliade, Mircea, 176, 205
Eliman, 108–9, 111
eljeangougou, 35. *See also* birth; children; consummation; spirits; taboo
eljenan (pl.), 29, 135, 148, 164. See also *aljen* Qur'anic; spirits
Emdigra, 123, 139
emic/etic, 47
emotions, 73, 77
Emoud, 68–70
endogamy, 26, 28, 35, 102. *See also* marriage
epistemologies, 22, 193
environmental policies, 31, 145, 197
essentialism, 21, 23
essuf, 38, 171–72. *See also* nostalgia; solitude; wild
ethnicity, 25, 161
ethnobotany, vii, 195
ethnographic, 6–8, 41, 93; background on Tuareg, 25–29
ethnoscience, 40
etiologies, 17–18, 108–9
euphemism, 36, 79, 164. *See also* speaking; *tangal*
euphoria, 77. See also *tadawit*
Euro-American, x, 4, 21, 75, 82, 122, 129, 171
Europe, 25, 75–76, 142, 156, 188
Evans-Pritchard, E. E., ix, 86, 205
evil, 173; eye/mouth, 48, 67, 151, 157, 159, 168. See also *togerchet*
evolutionary, 20
ewel, 73. *See also* heart
exile, 28, 46
exorcism, 39–40, 47, 98, 128, 163. *See also* possession; ritual
exoticism, x, 115
eyes, 43–44, 49, 58
ezin, 126, 128
ezziz, 45, 94. *See also* hot; illness; sand

Fabian, Johannes, xi
Fabrega, Horatio, 177, 178, 205
face-veil: men's, 29, 40, 102, 198
Fachi, 85, 90
facilitators, 109
falling, 32, 43, 180
famine, 91, 138–39
Fana, 58–59
fasting, 74

fat: rooster, 62; sheep, 62
Fatane, 85
fatherhood, 42
Fatima, 36–43, 47, 76, 81, 83, 96, 150, 160
Fatimata, 83, 167–68
fatness, 31, 43, 60, 78, 97, 103, 108, 117
Fatoni, 85
Feld, Steven, 122, 205
feminist, 29
Fernandez, James, 121
fertility: conflicts over, 29; fatness as sign of, 31, 60; ritual control of, 63, 104, 108, 193; symbolism, 71, 124, 162
festivals, 44, 100, 123
fetus, 89
fever, 38, 97, 99, 180; child's, 125; following birth, 41, 43–44, 76. See also *tenede*
Fez, 137
Fezzan, 25–26
fieldwork, 197. *See also* methods
Figueiredo-Biton, Christina, 27, 47, 76–77, 101, 103, 197, 205
Finerman, Ruth Beth, 21, 205
finger, 32, 89, 158. See also *adade*
Fiore, Barbara, viii, ix, 3, 36–37, 40–43, 45–46, 197, 205
fire, 49, 66, 75, 89, 125, 127, 164, 167–68
firstborn, 66, 71. See also *tinout*
Fitz Poole, John, 23, 100–101, 163, 205
flashlight, 44
Flax, Jane, 115, 205
flesh, 31. *See also* skin
fly-tox, 184
fonio, 45, 46
food, 30–32, 41, 43, 45–46, 51, 66, 69, 94, 97, 146, 170, 174, 189–90. *See also* diet; eating; ritual
forearm, 157, 108
Foster, George M., 69, 206
founder, 5, 135–38
France, 87, 188, 197
French: colonialism, 25–26; language, 77; manumission of slaves, 124; massacres and imprisonment of Tuareg by, 137–40; policies, 198; secular schools, 188; sedentarizing of Tuareg, 129
Friday, 89, 143, 148, 162, 166
fright, 149
fruits, 31, 37, 46, 123, 125, 128, 138
Fugelstad, Finn, 198, 206

Fulbright Hays, xi
functionaries, 131, 189

Gabra, 116
gado, 34. *See also* Hausa; inheritance
Galen, 45
Gao, 2, 184, 188
gardening, 4, 29–30, 107; and impact on gender and property, 112, 117, 130; and theories on relation to "shamanistic" cultural complexes, 174
Garrison, Vivian, 16, 204
gasoline, 184
Gast, Marceau, 131, 206
gathering, 33, 182; of barks, 55; changing role of, among Tuareg, 30, 174; during apprenticeships, 80, 94; rituals, 130–31, 141–44, 153; taboos regulating, 121, 136, 148, 150
gazelle, 128
gender, 114–16; and body and senses, 75–79; and life course, 96–103; and marriage, 42–43; nature and culture issues concerning, 18, 129–31; relation to aging and healing, 22, 28–29; and shamans, 173–75; among Tuareg, viii, 8–9
gender issues, 75, 82, 115; local, 173; medicine women's, 41, 73, 122, 148
genealogy, 91–92, 198
general practitioners, 57
genetic, 46
genitals: as "door," 78, 166, 169
German(y), 110
germs, 48, 51
gestures, 40, 60, 149. See also *sikbar*
ghuneb, 161. *See also* divination; horoscope
Giambelli, 120
global(ization), 15–16, 18, 152, 182
goat(s), 120, 145; head, 87, 89; hide, 13; livestock, 30–32, 87–89; meat, 46. *See also* herding
God: appeals to, by healers, 31–33, 62, 69, 124, 126, 146, 153, 194
Goddale, Jane, 21, 206
gonorrhea, 94
Good, Charles, 184, 206
Goodenough, Ruth, viii, 82, 115, 206
gossip, 50, 59
Gottlieb, Alma, 5, 17, 23, 63, 82, 101, 106, 115, 121, 200, 204, 206

goumaten, 74, 149, 151, 158. *See also* exorcism; possession; spirits; *tende n goumaten*
government, 23, 27–28, 65, 181, 186, 194
grandchildren, 93, 141
granddaughter, 150
grandmother, 37, 80, 113, 140. *See also* kinship
grandparents, 93
grasses, 31, 96, 136. *See also* herbalism; medicine; plants
graves, 73, 90
Greece, 45, 74
green, 32
Green, Edward, x, 15–17, 19, 184–85, 206
Greenwood, Bernard, 74, 206
greetings, 14, 60
groom-service, 39, 80, 103
guinea hen, 126–28. *See also* myth; *Tellilen*
guns, 110, 166
gynecological, 37, 41, 108, 114

Habsu, 123
Hadia, 92–94, 96–99, 102–3, 106, 108, 110–11, 136, 138–40, 144, 149–51, 160, 169–71, 174, 176, 185
Hadjiatou, 107–11, 145, 150, 160
Hageners, 114
hair, 38, 50, 126–29, 144, 199
Haiti, 22
Halalo, 179
Hamid, 32
hand: and diagnostic massage use by medicine women, 61, 63, 67, 149, 167; measuring use of 157; and relation to writing, 153–54. *See also* massage; touch
hardness, 67, 94
Harding, Sandra, 115, 206
Harner, Michael, 19, 206
Hausa, 3, 17, 117, 125, 137–40, 161, 163, 167, 199, 201; regions, 88, 91
Hawa Efanghela, 145
Hawad, Makhmoudan viii, 57, 172, 174–75, 198–99, 206
Haya, 159
head, 39, 63, 73, 80, 100; dance, 131, 143, 149, 163
headaches, 64, 97
head-covering (scarf): women's, 29, 34, 199
healers/healing, vii, ix, 3–8, 26, 30, 32–42; and gender theories, 21–25; diviners,

166–78; marabouts, 155–65; psychosocial, viii, 38, 42, 61, 72, 150, 176, 188; relations between medicine women and marabouts, 148–49; role of touch in, 69–73, 195; shamans, 19–20, 21–23; treating of childlessness, 108–10. *See also* diviners; doctors; marabouts; medicine: and medicine women
health care: biomedical, 180–90
heart, 38, 73, 154. *See also ewel*
heaviness, 117; from healing, 68, 97; in pregnancy and birth, 189–90
henna, 20, 177
herbalism, 3, 22, 41, 68, 71, 83–88, 94, 96, 117–18, 125–26, 148, 151, 154, 156, 166, 193–94
herbs, 136, 174. *See also* medicine; plants; trees
herding, 26; difficulties of, 28; gendered aspects of, 112, 130; historical trends in, 138; and "shamanistic" culture complexes, 174
heritage, 89, 91. *See also* inheritance; *gado*
hermaneutics, 195
hermaphrodite, 77, 121
Herr, Melody, xii
Herzfeld, Michael, 15–16, 193, 206
hiccoughs, 85
hierarchies, ix, 20, 160, 172
Hippocrates, 45
histories: life, 6–7, 91
history: of Aïr region Tuareg, 25–26, 129, 198; of Atkaki region in Aïr, 136–40; of herbal medicine, vii–viii, 81–94, 118; and myth, 7, 85, 88, 91;
Hoch-Smith, Judith, 114, 206
Hoggar, 124. *See also* Ahaggar
Hollis, Martin 15
homme-femme (man-woman), 77–78
honor, 42
Hoppal, Mihaly, 176, 211
horoscope, 108, 157–58, 160–61
Horton, Robin, ix–x, 15, 75, 196, 206
horse, 138
hospitals, 37, 43, 47, 147, 159, 179–92
hot, ix, 8; body, 73–79, 94, 96–97, 135, 149, 180; illnesses, 44–48
Houna, 30, 46, 57
household, 113–14, 173. *See also* domestic; public

hunger, 31, 65, 138–39
hunter-gatherers, 19
Hureiki, Jacques, 45, 206
husbands: bridewealth and groom-service ob-
    ligation of, 39; and marriage and sexuality,
    42, 96; in mythico-history of herbal medi-
    cine, viii, 82–87; and polygyny, 28, 162;
    and social relations with wives, 29; and
    spirit analogy in mediumship, 169; and
    taboos during wife's pregnancy, 144, 166
Hutson, Alaine, 3, 206
hygiene: and biomedical discourse, 189–90

ibedni, 74, 88, 153. See also ancestors; graves;
    tombs
Ibil, 84–85, 90
Iblis, 101. See also Devil
icherifan: al baraka of, 144; clans, 142; laying
    on, of hands, 63, 157; and medicine, 85;
    medicine women's relationships to, 167;
    origins of, 201. See also descent; prophet
ida, 120. See also al ladat; widowhood
Idougdougan, 124
Iferouan, 63, 125
Ifoghas, xi, 2, 4, 112
igazen, 161. See also divination
ighawalen, 26. See also client-patron; status;
    stratification
Ikazkazan, 138
Ikhiri, Khalid, 199
iklan, 26. See also slaves; stratification
ilaten, 3, 30, 68, 70, 99, 117, 191. See also
    herbalism; medicine; trees
iliuwaten (alilui sing.), 104. See also dryness;
    last-born
illegitimacy, 92, 114, 140, 141
illness, 4–5, 7–18, 36–42, 57–59, 96–99,
    146; cold/hot, 41–48, 96; theories of, x, 4,
    17–18, 42–44, 48, 70, 130, 195
imajeghen, 26. See also nobles; stratification
iman, 73. See also soul
imghad, 26, 137. See also stratification; tributaries
Imperato, Pascale, 17, 206
inaden, 26. See also smiths; stratification
incantations, 72, 81, 189
incense, 37, 73, 94, 96, 158
indigenous, 16, 19
indigestion, 32, 34, 43, 46, 58, 154. See also
    tezoufnene
indigo, 46, 85

ineslemen, 3, 151, 191. See also marabouts;
    Islam; Qur'anic
infection, 68. See also anagar
infertility, 29, 73–74, 100, 107, 109, 160
infrastructures, 25
infusion, 37, 41
inhalation, 17, 34, 125
inheritance (heritage): of medicine, 34, 61,
    80, 82, 89, 91, 92; and medicine
    women's profession, vii, 4, 34, 118, 130,
    135; in Tuareg communities, 26, 27, 29,
    112–13, 197
injections, 38, 41, 99, 180, 185
ink: vegetal, 83, 149, 157
insomniacs, 46
insult, 89
intermarriage, 25
International Monetary Fund, 186
interviews, 6. See also methods
intestines, 58, 74, 109
Inuit, 142
Iraq, 136
iron, 87, 130, 148, 194
irrigation, 4, 198
IRSH, xi
iskoki, 17. See also Hausa; spirits; wind
Islam(ic): amulets, 102; and life course in
    Muslim societies, 105; in local history
    and migrations, 135–39, 193–95;
    marabouts or Qur'anic scholars', ix, 62,
    70, 84, 92, 98; medicine women's rela-
    tionships with, 9, 148–65; and repro-
    ductive rights, 107; ritual restrictions on
    medicine women's practices, 89, 148; rit-
    ual restrictions, and precautions on
    childbearing women, 101; spirits of
    Qur'an, 33; among Tuareg, 29; women in
    Qur'anic scholarship, 3
Islamist (reformist), 152
Ismaghil, 150
Itesen, 136
itran, 157–58, 160. See also atri; divination;
    marabouts; Qur'anic; stars
izafnen, 81. See also germs; microbes

jackals, 4, 120
Jackson, Michael, 17, 19, 206
Jambai, 181
James, Wendy, 120, 207
jawed, 158. See also trees

jealousy, viii, 38–39, 48, 66, 71, 84, 86, 87, 100, 102

jergo(nen): wa jerga, ta jerga, 85, 104, 188–92. *See also* dirt; pollution

jewelry, 197

joints, 62, 69

joking, 60, 93, 99, 182, 189

Jordan, Brigitte, 24, 71, 207

kadenya, 167. *See also* trees

Kadi, 157

Kafe, 114

Kahena, 82

kalgo, 153. *See also* trees

Kaluli, 122

Kano, 2, 30, 125

Kaoussan, 93, 137–40, 200

karambaza, 49–50, 166, 176. *See also* anger; diarrhea; stomachaches

Karp, Ivan, vii, ix, 16, 20, 1111, 115, 163, 195, 203, 207

Katsina, 2

Kawar, 125, 138

Keenan, Jeremy, 6, 27, 41, 198, 200, 207

Kel Agatan: healing clans, 31, 32, 34; and mythico-history and origins in healing, 82, 88–90, 94

Kel Arou, 88, 90. *See also* ancestors; Kel Nad; People of Night; People of Past or Before

Kel Azanghaydan, 88

Kel Bagzan, 33–34, 88

Kel Ewey, viii, 112

Kel Fares, 139

Kel Ferwan, 187

Kel Geres, 112

Kel Igadmawen, 137

Kel Igurmadan, 61, 158, 167; chief, 65; healing clans, 34, 62; and mythico-history of healing, 82–86, 88–90, 99; and migrations, 139–40, 144; and relation to Kel Agatan, 31

Kel Nad, 35, 88, 90

Kel Nagarou, 137

Kel Tamajaq, 25–26. *See also* Berber; culture; language; Tuareg

Kel Tates, 125

Kel Zingifan, 138

Kendall, Laurel, 6, 23, 207

Kennedy, John G., 174, 207

Kerewsky-Halpern, Barbara, 23, 71

Kerns, Virginia, 23, 101, 115, 204

Kidal, xi, 2, 27, 181, 183–84, 201

kidney, 37

kinship, 26–27; Aïr region, 137; and flexibility, 112; and informal healing among kin, 38, 185–87; and mother-child ties, 131; and relations among herbal medicine women, 117; and significance in rites of passage, 121; and symbolism, 74

Kitzinger, Sheila, 59, 60, 71, 207

knees, 34, 127

knife, 85, 128

knowledge: age-related beliefs concerning, 100; approaches to, ix, x; authoritative, 24; medicinal, vii, viii, 8–9; multisensorial, 61; mythico-historical, 80–82, 85, 90, 92; and power, 160, 165, 192–95; specialized, 121

kohl, 74

Kojaja, 138. *See also* food; history; seasons

Korean, 23, 175

kourji, 179, 180. See also *lumat;* measles

Krueger, Victoria, 6, 7, 70, 82, 87, 209

kulan tessa, 98. See also *arabaz;* massage

kuwurna, 37. *See also* medicine; trees

Kwoth, 86

Kyadara, 127

labor, 37, 61, 71, 102

Lagos, 107

laho, 35. *See also* illness; shame

Lala, vii, 80, 83, 85, 117, 141, 143, 152, 170

lama, 117. *See also* heaviness; illness

lamb, 45, 46

Lamb, Sarah, 101, 207

lamentation, 118, 127–28, 141

Lamphere, Louise, viii, 21, 23, 82, 203, 210

land, 121, 123, 140; shortages, 28–29

language, 4, 19, 44, 60, 199

laser, 58

last-born, 71, 104

Latin, 118

Latin American, 44

law/legal, 27, 107, 129, 131, 198; Qur'anic, 165

leaders, 9, 20, 28, 80, 143, 145. See also *amenukal;* chiefs; sultan

leather, 29, 101, 102

leaves, vii–viii, 83–85, 129

Lee, Felix, 186, 212

legitimacy, 35, 100

Lejean, Yannick, 45, 207

Lemta, 198
Lepowsky, Maria, viii, 82, 207
leprosy, 18, 197
Lere, 27
Levine, Robert, xi
Levi-Strauss, Claude, 15, 20, 21, 75, 87, 115, 122, 129, 207
Lewis, Ian M., 174, 176, 198, 207
lexicon, 199
Libya, 2, 25, 36, 200
life course, 102–4
liminality, 35, 102
lion, 158
lisafe, 109, 161. *See also* divination; marabouts; Qur'anic
liver, 32, 41, 59, 73, 95, 97, 98, 145. See also *tessa*
Lock, Margaret, 69, 207
logic(al), 15–18, 196
Lourdes, 87
love: attitudes concerning, 42, 73, 98, 177; illicit, 199; in song verses, 124–25; unrequited, 38
luck, 34, 74, 137, 161; in marriages, 158
Lukes, Steven, 15
lumat, 179, 180. See also *kourji;* measles
lungs, 109
Lyotard, Francois, 15

macaroni, 30, 31
MacCormack, Carol, ix, 18, 21, 129, 181, 207
madness: and association with wild, 89; beliefs concerning causes of 74; cases of, 92, 167, 169, 191; marabouts' treatment of, 149
Maerua crassifolia, 124, 125. See also *agar; trees*
Maghrak, 124
Magi (broth) cubes: use in cures, 184
magic: as alternative source of power, 70–71; issues in anthropology of religion, 9, 17, 122; purchased, 168; and relation to authoritative knowledge and power, 20; "sympathetic," 87
Mahamane, Saadou, 199, 206
Majila, 127
Malam Moussa, 161, 176
malaria, 140, 180
Mali, vii, ix, xi, 2, 6; medicine women in, 4, 180–81, 183–84, 186–87, 197–98; tents in, 13; Tuareg in, 25, 27
Malinowski, Bronislaw, ix, 15, 87, 195

Malkki, Liisa, 17, 208
Mama, 183, 190
manioc, 31, 138
mansin, 23. *See also* Korean; shamans
manzakar, 158. *See also* trees
marabouts: *al baraka* of, 72, 135–39; and beliefs concerning medicine women's postchildbearing status, 74; divination by, 158–59, 161; healing of, 47, 57, 107–11, 157, 159; official authority of, 24–25; and origins of healing among Kel Igurmadan, 83; and Qur'anic scholarship, 3, 78; referral of patients to, 59, 154–55; and relationships with medicine women, 9, 147–65; and sacred places, 140–42, 191, 199, 201; women's attitudes toward, 113. See also *ineslemen;* Islam; healers; Qur'an
Maradi, 2
marginalization: issues in gender and healing studies, 19, 20, 22, 150; and medicine women's divination, 100; and medicine women's status, 92, 152; threats to medicine women, 165, 177, 194
Mariama, 97–98, 168
markets, 25, 26, 30, 129, 191
marriage: chiefly, 98; folklore motif, 129; and husband-wife relationships, 145; marabouts' roles in arranging, 158; medicine women's, 100; practices, 28, 35, 41–42, 62, 65–66, 200; to spirits in mediumship, 173, 175; and status, 102, 104–5
Martin, Emily, 15, 16, 17, 19, 197, 208
Martin, Phyllis, 186, 208
Maslow, 160
Masolo, D. A., vii, ix, 16, 20, 115, 195, 207
Masquelier, Adeline, 17
massacres, 27, 109, 140
massage: in medicine women's diagnosis and treatments, 32, 64, 66, 68, 179; of back and shoulders, 153; of liver, 117; of stomach, 97–98. See also *arabaz*
maternity services, 183–84
matriarchy: myths of, in anthropology, viii, 82
matrifocal household, 120; changes in, 131
matrilineal: in current bilateral system, 26–27; inheritance of medicine women's healing, vii–viii; inheritance of property *(akh ihuderan),* 111–13; origins of Tuareg groups, 200; relation to Islam, 163–64; stomach symbolism of, 32, 73; upheavals of, 131

Mauritania, 25, 183

Mauss, Marcel, 119, 205

Mayan, 177–78

Mayo Clinic, 87

McCarthy-Brown, Karen, 7, 22, 208

McClain, Carol, 3, 6, 8, 21–23, 70, 71, 87, 156, 207, 208, 212

McNaughton, Patrick, 119, 153, 163, 208

measles, 17, 180

measuring, 108, 109, 157–59

meat: animal sacrifice role of, 121; consumption, 30, 31; folktale reference to, 127; as "hot" food, 46; and medicinal use to fatten, 97, 117; for new mother, 41, 145; and wedding, 50

Mecca, 146, 200

mediating, 109, 116, 163

medicine: biomedical influence, 182–84, 192, 199; clan specialty, origin, and transmission, 62, 80, 83–87, 135; gender-distinct preparations, 96, 117–18; herbal, 11–12, 150; mother's following birth, 37; preparation, 57–59; and medicine women, 27, 30–31, 44–45, 80–89; trees, 125–26, 129, 130. See also healers; tinesefren; tinesmegelen

medicine, pot, 4, 65, 88, 117, 148, 149; rotating by medicine women in diagnosis/divination, 49–50, 57, 100, 166, 170. See also ten; takabar

medieval, 44, 71

mediums/mediumship, viii, 9; anthropological theories concerning, 5–6, 19–20; medicine women's specialized, 165, 173, 175–76; types of, among Tuareg, 150, 156

memory: cultural and social, 8, 27, 62; medicine women's roles in, 192–93; in mythico-history, 86–87, 135, 140

men: and experiences in social upheavals, 131; health compared to women's in beliefs of medicine woman, 57; and medicines, 96 and sensorium, 76–79

Mende 181

menopause, 22, 66

menstruation: and beliefs in local cosmology concerning purity/pollution, 66, 77, 78, 96, 101–6 141, 155, 169, 200; ritual restrictions concerning, 63, 135; symbolism of, 37

mental deficiency, 35

Mernissi, Fatima, 105, 208

metals, 130, 148, 150

metaphor: bodily, 103–5; logic in, 75; in medicinal and amulet protective significance, 37, 146; mythical, 86; in ritual therapy of possession songs, 39, 122–23; in speech, 163

methods, 6–8

metonym(y), 7, 59, 119

Mexico, 17, 177

microbes, 81. See also izafnen

microcosm, 70

midwives, 23, 24, 156, 179–84

migraines, 64

migrations: and labor, 25, 38, 66, 112, 182, 199; in regional history, 136–40

Mikell, Gwendolyn 21, 208

militia: ambiguous identity of, 142; difficulty of controlling, 183; in nationalist-separatist rebellion conflict, 109–10, 131

milk, 31, 41, 112

millet: as food staple, 25, 30–31, 136–37, 146; ritual uses of by medicine women, 56, 68, 130, 191; symbolism of, 143–44; treatments, 41, 46, 96

mimesis, 69–71, 87

Mina, 80, 130, 143, 152–54, 160, 170–71

mind, ix, 74, 149–52, 155

Ministry of Health, 186, 190

mirage, 171

miscarriage, 89, 144, 184

Mitragyna inermes, 34. See also amizou; medicine; plants; trees

mixing, 58

mnemonic, ix, 27

modernistic, 15

Mohammed (of Ibil), 84

Monday, 59, 166

money, 31, 32, 112, 146, 188

Monnig-Atkinson, Jane, 172, 174, 208

moon(light), 35, 36, 43, 135

Moorish, 44

Morgan, Henry L., 81

Morocco, 74, 106, 137

mortuary practices, 90, 199

mosque, 65, 77, 103–4, 130, 136, 140, 153

mother/motherhood: apprenticeships with, 66, 80, 98, 154; and descent, 113; maternal imagery and roles of, vii–viii, 6–7, 36–42, 48, 66, 131, 145; and residence, 131; significance of, 21, 100, 116; treatment of, following difficult birth, 36–42

motions, 20, 68, 71–72, 86
Mounkaila, Garba, 199, 206
mountains: attitudes of medicine women toward, vii, 3, 87–88, 118, 121, 137; gathering in, 153, 182
Moussa, 123
Moussasabka, 138
mouth: "evil mouth," 67; and power of words, 98; vulnerability of, 37, 48, 49, 57. See also *togerchet*
Mudimbe, V. Y., ix, x, 16, 20, 195, 208
murder, viii, 82, 86, 166
Murdock, George, 17, 208
Murphy, Robert, 6, 27, 42, 112, 198, 208
music, 62, 100, 199
Muslim, vii. *See also* Islam(ic); Qur'anic; religion
mutton, 45, 46
myth: and history, 7, 82; of matriarchy in anthropology, viii; and medicine women, 87–88, 90; and tree imagery, 120–21, 125–29, 131–32
mythico-history: medicine women's, 27, 29, 81–86, 92, 100; regional, 140–42, 147, 194; theories of, viii, 7

Nabarro, 139
name day, 38, 94, 105, 145, 198
names, 114
narratives, 7, 93, 79, 89, 182
Nasr, Seyyed Hossein, 74, 75, 208
nation (state): history of Mali and Niger, 20, 25, 27, 129; political-economy of, relevant to health issues, 182, 197–98
National Geographic Society, xi
Native American, 17
nature: anthropological theories of, in relation to culture, ix, 3, 21–22; medicine women's cultural work in, 115, 119, 122, 129
nausea, 32
Navajo, 70, 181
neck, 40, 152, 199
nephew, 112, 130
Nescafe, 184
New Guinea, 45, 114, 163
Newtonian, 24
NGO's (non-governmental agencies), health-care programs, 8, 9, 25, 31, 121, 145; medicine women's relationships with, 181, 184, 190, 192
Ngubane, H., 22, 23, 208

Niamey, xi, 2, 190
Nicolaisen, Ida and Johannes, viii, 3, 6, 26–29, 42, 60, 73, 112, 126, 141–42, 162, 164, 172, 198, 199, 208, 209
Nicolas, Guy, 17, 208
nieces, 130, 153
Niger, vii–viii, ix, xi, 2; health care in, 180–81, 183, 186–87, 191; history of, 197–98; medicine women in, 3; researcher's fieldwork in, 4, 7; tents in Aïr, 14; Tuareg in, 25, 27, 107
Nigeria, 2; trading with, 25; travel to, 107, 163, 168
noble(s), vii; contemporary relationships with other social strata, 161–62, 171, 187; cultural values of reserve, 60; gendered roles, 8, 102, 200; marriage of, women, 40–42; and precolonial social prestige, roles, relations, and status, 28. See also *imajeghen; status; stratification
Noel, Marie-France, viii, 3, 37, 45, 48, 49, 184, 187, 197, 208
nomadism: changes in, 31–32; spaces of, 171–72; subsistence patterns of, 26, 29, 138; symbolism of, 125
nonorganic, ix–x, 48, 87
Norris, H. T., 29, 200, 209
North, 82
nostalgia, 38, 171–72. See also *essuf;* solitude; spirits; wild
nose, 37; bleeds, 97; nostrils, 34
Nuer, 86
numbers: in measuring and timing, 64, 108–11, 158–59
nurturing, 21–23
Nusa Penida, 120
nutrition, 31

oases, 84; clinics in, 37, 179, 180; gardening on, 28–29, 112
obedience, 29, 99–100
Occidentalism, 15, 16
occupations: precolonial, 26
oil, 32, 43
ointment, 37, 64
okuf, 5, 34, 124. *See also* illness
olfactory, 59, 81. *See also* scent
Olkes, Cheryl, 6, 17, 59, 72, 93, 196, 209
O'Meara, Patrick, 186
Ong, Walter, 72, 209

onions, 31
oogun, 71. *See also* Wolff; Yoruba
Oosten, J. G., 142, 209
organic, ix–x, 42, 44, 48, 176
Orientalism, 15
origins, vii–viii, 7, 32, 58, 89, 200; of Hadia
    and Ahmed's village, 136–40; of herbal
    healing, 81–86; of Tuareg, 25–26
Orion, Loretta, 156, 209
orphanhood, 98
orthography, 26
Ortner, Sherry, 6, 18, 21, 100, 101, 114, 129,
    195, 209
Other, 16
Ouagdougou, 2
Ouma, 139
Oxby, Clare, 6, 27, 112, 209

panoptic (gaze), 165
Papua, 114
Parkin, David, 5, 15, 16, 141, 209
participant-observation, 6, 7
pastures, 30, 92, 138
patients, vii–viii, 132; Amoumoun and Hadi-
    jiatou, 107–11; diversity of, 88–89; Fa-
    tima, 32–36; Fatimata, 168; gendered dif-
    ferences in treatment of, 167; man in
    Agadez, 188; Mariama, 98–99; researcher,
    63–64, 67–68, 81; Takhia, 98–99
patrilineal, 27, 32, 83, 73, 164
payment (fees), 167; for hospital care, 186;
    and marabouts, 108; and medicine
    women, 58, 63, 64, 80, 89, 149
peace (accords), following Tuareg rebellion, 8,
    28, 65, 142, 181, 198
Peace Corps, 197
peanuts, 31
penicillin, 38
People of Night, 88, 90. *See also* Kel Nad
People of Past or Before, 35, 88, 90. *See also*
    Kel Arou
percale, 46
perfume, 73, 168, 199
Perrone, Bobbette, 6, 7, 70, 82, 87, 209
personalistic, x, 4, 43, 69–70
personhood, 38, 48, 51, 131–32
Peters, Larry, 93, 209
pharmacological, 87, 118
pharmacopia, 31, 115, 132
philosophy, 5, 9, 20

phlegm, 75
pilgrimages, 3, 98
pills: local attitudes toward, 50, 51, 180, 187
placenta, 37
places: and herbal healing, 8, 34, 36, 45, 74;
    sacred or "enchanted," 136–47, 152, 153;
    and symbolism in Saharan regions,
    118–19, 123–25, 130, 132; wild, 171–73
plants: knowledge of, 191; lexicons, 199; me-
    dicinal, viii–ix, 3, 11; sources of, 182–83;
    threats to, 30–31; uses in treatments,
    37–38, 40–42, 57–58, 64, 73, 87, 102.
    See also herbalism; medicine; trees
pluralism: medical, viii, 197
poet(ry), 146, 123, 131, 199
police, 46, 142
political/polity, 26–29, 46, 163
pollution: aging in relation to, 71, 85, 101;
    anthropology of, 15, 17–19, 22–23; gen-
    der in relation to, 114; ritual protection
    and, 37, 40, 140, 152, 188–92, 197. *See
    also* contagion; dirt; purity
polygraph, 61, 87
polygyny: practice of, 28, 42–43, 113, 177;
    women's opposition to, 65–66, 97–99, 110
possession, viii, 197; anthropological theories
    of, 22; body imagery surrounding, 32, 73;
    Fatima's, 39–47; Mariama's, 97–98; and
    matrilineal inheritance of possessing spir-
    its, 36; and medicine women's diagnosis
    and referrals to other healers, 163; mediu-
    mistic, 174–75; and relation to Islam,
    151; and significance among Tuareg, 29;
    spirits of, 201; symbolism of, 122–25,
    131; trance, 5. *See also* exorcism; ritual;
    spirits
post-childbearing: life course significance of,
    100–101, 103–6; healing significance of,
    141–43
postcolonial, 27, 129
post-menopausal, 23, 100, 103. *See also* post-
    childbearing
postpartum (restriction or taboo) 35, 37, 38, 44
potatoes, 31
poverty, 186–87
power, 8, 133; gendered, 122; medicine
    women's in relation to biomedicine, 181,
    196; medicine women's in relation to Is-
    lamic and marabouts', 147, 153, 160, 166,
    173, 174; precolonial types of, among

Tuareg, 26, 69; theories of, in healing cosmologies, 16, 63, 70–71
practice, x, 6–7, 116
praise, 29, 198
praxis, viii
prayers, 55, 89, 104. See also religion; ritual
pregnancy: medicine women's work with pregnant women, 105, 179, 189–90; in origins of herbal healing, 82–86; ritual precautions concerning, 102, 144–45, 166
prestige, 23, 26, 28, 65, 129
pricking, 59. See also back; liver
prison, 140
privatization, 184
Programme de Securite Alimentaire, 145
property, 28–29, 82, 98, 112–14, 163, 197
prophet, 28, 63, 159, 167, 201
protection, 37, 143, 147
protein, 31
pseudonyms, 8, 30
psychotherapists, 20
puberty, 76–77
public, 21, 23, 115
purgings, 149
purity: and relation to contagion and pollution, 101–2; relation to sacred, 136–37, 141; theories of, 15, 23, 77

Qur'an(ic), ix, 26–27, 33, 47, 131, 137; spirits, 29; verses, 98, 130. See also Islam; marabouts; versus

rabbit dung, 68, 96
Radio Kidal, xi
Rahma, 91–92, 191
Rahmou, 155
raiders, 94, 131
rains, 30
Ramadan, 74
Randall, Sara, 47, 74, 209
rape, viii, 131, 143
Rasmussen, Susan, viii, 3, 6, 8, 18, 23, 25–27, 32, 38, 39, 42, 43, 48, 57, 60, 61, 71, 73, 77–79, 83, 87, 101–5, 112–15, 119, 126, 130, 131, 141, 142, 144, 151, 153, 156, 162, 163, 172, 174, 175, 177, 181, 186, 187, 198, 199, 200, 201, 209–10
rationality, 15–18, 79, 193–96
razor, 34, 63
Rebellion (Tuareg), 8, 28, 88, 131, 181

rebels, 65, 142
recasting, 3, 5
red, 32, 37, 96, 128
referrals; medicine women's to other healers, 39, 73, 89, 114, 160, 162–63, 165, 169–70, 180. See also diagnosis; divination; marabouts; possession
refugees, 28, 146
regeneration, 153
Reiter, Rayna, 23, 114, 210
religion: anthropological theories of, 8, 9, 17; in relation to healing, 21, 105, 122, 136, 152. See also Islam; spirits
Renaissance, 76
repatriation, 28, 146. See also refugees
reproduction, 23, 29, 89, 95–96, 101, 107, 179
reserve: changes concerning, 146; between elders and youths, 36, 93; and men's face-veil, 198; between mother-in-law and son-in-law, 103, 105; noble cultural value, 22, 29, 60; and touch, 37, 71. See also takarakit
residence, 28–29; changes in postmarital, 68, 80, 112, 123, 131, 200–201
respect, 22, 29; healers' mutual, 152; male healers' toward Tagurmat, 68–69; social changes in, 146
respiratory, 97
restrictions: birth-related ritual precautions, 37, 63; Islamic-related, 152–53, 159–60, 162, 166, 169, 199; and menstrual cosmology, 77, 89, 101–5, 200; sacred and al baraka-related, 136, 141–45, 148, 150; social, 62
revitalization: cultural 28
rice, 31, 46
riddles, 81
Rinkidan, 118
rinsed, 77, 104, 106. See also children; dryness; last-born; post-menopausal
rites of passage: aging-related, 103–5, 199; name day, 37–39, 113, 121; puberty, 77, 102; wedding, 50
ritual, 195; blessing-conveying, 64, 152; commemorative, 114, 121; divination, 50; healing, 70; medicine gathering, 130–32; possession, 29, 39–40, 122, 150; sacred land-related, 140, 147
Rival, Laura, 119–22, 210

rock art, 26, 35
Rodd, Francis Lord of Rennell, 26, 85, 198, 200, 201, 210
roots vii, 96. *See also* herbalism; medicine; plants; trees
Rosaldo, Michelle Zimbalist, viii, 21, 23, 82, 203, 210

sa'a, 34. *See also* luck
sacred, 5; anthropological theories of, 8, 15; lands, 121, 135–47, 178, 191
sacrifice (animal): diviners', 169, 177; fertility promotion, 108–11; gendered, 119, 121; healing, 87; marabouts', 144; mortuary, 90, sacred land-related, 138
Sádik, 124
sadness, 77
Sáenz, Candelario, 163, 198, 210
Sahara, 3, 25–27, 35, 87, 118, 143, 200
Sahel, 3, 26–27
Said, Edward, x, 25, 210
Saint Bernadette, 87
Sako, Armadou Sekou, 186, 212
Saladin d'Anglure, 19, 210
salt, 25, 94, 128, 200
sand, 37, 125, 130, 161
Sanday, Peggy, viii, 82, 115, 206
Sande, 181
sandstorms, 4, 36, 159
Sargent, Carolyn, viii, 3, 23–24, 156, 181, 185, 196, 204, 207, 210
scent, 57, 72–73; and infertility, 160
Schlegel, Alice, 113, 210
Schmoll, Pamela, 3, 17, 210
schools: history of, among Tuareg, 65–66, 77, 107, 180, 188, 199, 200; nomadic boarding, 129–30
Schotz, Mohammed, 184, 199
Schulz, Erhard, 199, 210
science, 7, 9; anthropological theories of, in relation to religion and "magic," viii–x, 17, 129; conflicts between medicine women's and allopathic biomedical, 194–96
Scott, Joan, 15–16, 211
seasons, 4, 36, 38, 44–45
seclusion, 29, 37–38, 159
sedentarization, 24, 26, 28, 112–13, 129, 131, 146
semiotics, 118

Senoussi revolt, 93, 137, 140
Senses, 51, 57, 72–77, 81
Serbian, 23, 71
sexual(ity): and age, 66, 75–78, 93, 95; and family planning, 105, 173, 191; relations with spirits, 160, 173; "sex warfare" theories, 198; taboos, 35–36, 63
shamanism: anthropological theories of, 5–6, 9, 19–20; gender and healing issues concerning, 23, 24; Tuareg approximations to, 172–75. *See also* divination; mediumship
shamans, 3; theories of, 5, 6, 9, 19–20; Tuareg specialists approximating, 166, 175
shame(ful): and hospital attitudes, 180; illegitimacy-related, 114, 190–91; illnesses, 35–36, 38, 99; and reserve, 103, 105
sheep, 30, 145, 169
shivering, 135
shops, 31
shoulder: in healing, 32, 34, 39, 40, 64, 152, 185. *See also* body; *tarzak*
shrine: founder/ancestor's, 135–37, 152–53
Siberian, 19, 175
siblings: in folklore, 126–29
Sidi Mohammed, 136
Sierra Leone, 181
Siikala, Anne-Leena, 176, 211
sikbar, 60. *See also* gestures
Silver, Daniel, 177–78, 205
Simon, Robert, 186, 212
sin: and attitudes among medicine women, 22, 82, 85, 101, 143, 152
singlehood, 145
sinus, 64
sisters, 39, 66, 109, 112, 121, 123, 126–29, 167
skin, 49, 151, 160, 180. *See also* body; flesh
slaves: beliefs concerning, 78; and contemporary situation of descendants, 65–66, 169, 198; past roles of, 26, 34, 136–37; reference to, in noble naming, 62. *See also* history; *iklan;* stratification
smallpox, 17, 179
smiths: beliefs about, 32, 78, 87, 163–64, 170–71; and lack of reserve, 105; occupations, 120–21, 144–45; precolonial status and roles of, 18, 26; and relationships with nobles, 32, 37, 49–50. See also *inaden;* stratification

snakebite, 63
sneezing, 34
sociability, 31, 188
Social Science Research Council, xi
softness, 31, 94
Sokoto, 2
soldiers, 131
solitude, 38
Songhai, 201
songs: and imagery in verses, 123–25, 131, 132; possession ritual, 39, 98, 151, 199
Sontag, Susan, 18, 197, 211
sorcery, 32; association of some *bokaye* with, 161; case of, 149; causes of, 35; and diagnosis and referral by medicine women, 154–56; dissociation of medicine women from, 70–71
soul: beliefs regarding, 38, 48, 73, 90, 125, 132
sourness, 103
South, 129, 137; Hausaland, 32, 88, 89
Soviet Union, 20
Spanish, 45
speaking: knowledge forms, 81; in mediumship, 20; power of, 48; theories of aural/written relationship, 72. See also *awal;* gossip; *togerchet*
sperm, 75, 101
spices, 46
spirits: and diagnosis and referrals by medicine women, 148–51, 153–58; healing, 22, 49, 71, 94; and hot fire and smiths, 144; Islamic and popular/local, 29, 102; marabouts' treatment of, 160, 164; and matrilineal tree, vii–viii, 111, 120–28, 130, 153; mediumship pacts with, 61, 167–76; and possession, 19, 32, 39, 47, 73–74, 97–98, 197, 201; and wind, 17. See also *eljenan; goumaten; iskoki*spitting (to convey blessing), 108, 130, 158
Spittler, Gerd, 112, 146, 211
spleen, 135. See also *aousa*
spoilage, 50–51
sprains, 58
Spring, Anita, 114, 206
stars: and *al baraka,* 144; and body, 74; and maraboutique divination, 157, 160–61; and seasons, 4, 45
status: and age, 100, 116; changes concerning, 145, 199; of divorced women, 92; gender

and healing issues of, 22–23; in precolonial social relations, 26
steeping, 57
sterility, 29, 107
Stockel, H. Henrietta, 6, 7, 70, 82, 87, 209
Stoller, Paul, xi, 6, 17, 19, 59, 72, 93, 196, 198, 209, 211
stomach: and association with matriline, 73, 111–12; illnesses and treatments of, 32, 43–45, 94; male healers' refraining from touching, 68; medicine women's touching of, 193; and symbolism in medicine women's heritage, viii
stomachaches: causes, etiologies, and treatment of, 36, 49–51, 97, 99, 176
stones, 90, 87, 130, 148
stories, xii, 86, 124, 139
strata, 36, 31, 48, 78, 199
Strathern, Marilyn, ix, 18, 21, 114, 129, 207, 211
stratification, 26, 198–99
strength, 77, 96, 100, 104, 106
Streptococci, 81
stress, 43, 61
structuralism, 15, 21–22
subsistence, 25–26
Sudan (French), 26
suffering, 4, 38, 42, 49, 193
Sufism, 29, 75, 85, 137
sugar, 31, 43, 64, 94, 130, 153, 179
sultan, 26, 198, 201. See also *amenukal*
sun, 36, 43, 64, 94
Sunday, 59
superhuman, 48, 69, 71, 119
Surat, 157–58
surgery, 160, 183, 185
Swazi, 17
sweets, 30
swelling, 34, 69, 179. See also *amerdio; anulem*
sword, 39, 141, 150
symbol(ic)/symbolism: approaches and methods concerning, 7, 115; arboreal, 118–31; bodily, 111, 143; Islamic, medicine women's interpretation of Qur'anic, 152, 162; 116; mythical, 87; ritual, 98; shamanic, 20, 23
syphilis, 43, 188
Szasz, Thomas, 156, 211

Tabaidot, 118

Tabarakatine, 159. *See also* Qur'anic; Surat;
  verses
Tabelot, 180
taboo: and ritual precautions and restrictions, 48,
  92, 105, 143, 145, 148, 152; sexual, 35–36
taboutout, 150. *See also* belly button; umbilical
  cord
Tachida, 84
tachilchit, 34. *See also* medicine; plants; trees
tactile, 33, 79, 64. *See also* touch
tadawit, 77. *See also* euphoria
tadeine, 130. *See also* trees
Tadulafaye, 139
Tafadek, 155, 159
tafarchit, 96. *See also* incense
tagaye, 127. *See also* doum palm
taghrawe, 179. *See also* smallpox
Tagurmat: matrilineal clan ancestor and
  founder of herbal medicine, viii, 7, 62, 68,
  69; mytico-historical motifs of, 82–84,
  87–88, 90, 98
Tahirou, 149
Tahoua, 161
tailoring, 110
tajart, 41. *See also* medicine; plants; trees
tajiye n'assilimoumisse, 63. *See also* hands; healing; *icherifan*
takabar, 170. *See also* divination; pot
takachit, 27. *See also* inheritance; Qur'anic
takarakit, 36, 38. *See also* reserve
Takhia, 98–99, 144
Takibichere, 139
Taklilt, 62
takote, 80, 90. *See also* alms
Takriaz, 125
Talat, 139
talawankan, 123. *See also* songs
tamadas, 5. *See also* bone-setting
Tamajaq: culture, ethnicity, and language
  connections, 25–26, 161, 201; gendered
  tree names, 121, 124; kinship expressions,
  117; language barriers in clinics and hospitals, 181, 187; language terminology
  and translation problems, 40, 42, 91,
  169, 188, 189; plant lexicons, 199; Tifinagh script, 154
Tamalete, 170–71
tamanai, 5. *See also* diviners
Tamanrassat, 2
tamarind, 46

tamaswad, 5, 150, 162, 166. *See also* diviners;
  tamanai
tamat, 37. *See also* medicine; trees
tamazai, 38, 41, 67, 97. *See also* depression;
  emotions
Tambiah, Stanley, ix–x, 15, 17, 195, 211
Tamgak Mountains, 63, 85, 87, 90–91, 137
tamghart, 103. *See also* age/aging; elderly;
  women
Tana, 31, 33, 46, 57, 96, 138, 152, 166, 179,
  183
taneqait 113. *See also* rites of passage
tanesmegel , viii, 30, 34. *See also* herbalism;
  medicine: and medicine women
tangal, 36, 779, 163. *See also* metaphor; speaking
Tanike, 84
Tanou, 70, 83, 117, 150
Tanout, 137
tarama, 38
tarraf, 101. *See also* conception; sexuality
tarzak, 32, 57, 152. *See also* back; illness;
  shoulder
Tasakay, 124
tasemde ta n amnennad n ehan, 41. *See also*
  cold; illness
tasemde ta n aressud, 41. *See also* cold; illness
Tassili-n-Ajjer, 2
taste, 72
Tata, 33–40, 42, 44, 46, 48, 96, 150–52
Taussig, Michael, 19, 70, 87, 211
tawsit, 30, 85. *See also* clans; descent; wrist
tax revolt, 27
taxes, 138, 140, 198
taxonomies, viii, 40, 45, 47
tazagat, 85
tchidguite n tessa, 32, 59. *See also* back; illness
Tchighozerine, 136, 187–89
Tchiluzduk, 168
Tchin Tabaradan, 27
tchiquat, 32
tea, 31, 41, 43, 57, 64
tearing, 64. *See also* birth
tebaremt, 41. *See also* medicine; plants; trees
tebes, 35
tebillant, 60
techkout, 124. *See also* slaves; stratification
tedis, 32. *See also* stomach
Tedlock, Barbara, xii
tekaka, 166. *See also* trees

tekanawene, 84, 123. *See also* twins

teknonymy, 22

Tellilen, 126–28

Telwa, 123

Tema, 65–67, 70

temoust, 25. *See also* culture; Tuareg

ten, 4, 32, 117. *See also* medicine pot

tende, 39. *See also* drum; exorcism; possession

tende n goumaten: case of, 39–40; and ritual healing, 57, 73, 98, 149–51, 155, 174. *See also* exorcism; possession; ritual; spirits

tenderu, 88. *See also* food

tenede, 41, 43, 44, 99. *See also* fever

Tenere, 136, 137

tent: "child's," as euphemism for uterus or womb, 29, 41; in Mali, 13; in Niger, 14; as place of children's birth, 69; and relation to wild, 129, 171–72; as researcher's residence, 4; symbolism of, 115, 120; as women's property, 65, 197. *See also* household; reproduction

tessa, 73. *See also* liver

tessmut, 74, 135. *See also* cold; illness

Tessouat, 139

tetanus, 35

Tewar, 136

tezma, 50, 170–71, 176. *See also* anger; nobles; smiths

tezoufnene: medicine women's classification and etiology of, 32, 34, 46, 58, 89, 149, 154, 166. *See also* indigestion

tezzort, 49. *See also* suffering

theft, 80, 143, 162, 166, 200; of *al baraka*, 189–90

thinness, 57, 69, 184

t-hum-a-hum, 39, 124. *See also* exorcism; possession; spirits

Thursday, 89, 148, 152, 162, 166

tiboraq, 126. *See also* Balanites aegyptiaca; trees

tichgar, 126, 128. *See also* medicine; trees

Tifinagh, 88, 154, 156. *See also* Tamajaq; writing

tifo temoya, 17

Tilia, 169

tilwayen 44. *See also* bones; illness

timazzujen, 44. *See also* ears; infection

Timia, 34, 84, 90

Tin Hinan, 82

Tina, 84, 166–68, 173–75

tinesefren, 4, 57. *See also* Mali: medicine women in

tinesmegelen (sing., *tanesmegel*), viii, 3, 57, 143, 161. *See also* Niger: medicine women in

tinout, 66. *See also* children; firstborn

tishi, 37. See also *amagal;* medicine; mother

toberas, 196. *See also* medicine; trees

togerchet, 48, 67, 151, 157, 168. *See also* evil: eye/mouth; gossip; mouth; speaking

tomatoes, 31, 138, 43

Tombouctou, 2

tombs: ancestral, 135; founder/marabout's, 137–38, 140; marabouts', 36, 90

totems, 119

Toua, 139, 169–71, 173, 175

touch: diagnostic, 32–34, 53, 148, 167–68; by herbal medicine women and bone-setters, viii, 4, 157, 199; massage specialties of, 117; origins of, 83; ritual motions of, 95; significance of, 57–66, 71–76

tourgoum, 42, 96, 98, 166, 177. *See also* anger; disputes; husbands; pregnancy

tourists, 110, 143

trading, 25, 200

trance, 174–75. *See also* mediumship; possession

transition, 35, 38

translation: of botanical terminology, 199; of illness terminology, 40–41, 44, 58, 66; issues in anthropology of healing, religion, and science, 4, 5, 16, 19, 20, 44, 195–96; of Qur'an, 158

trapezoids, 32

travel: gendered aspects, 76–78, 201; for medical attention, 36, symbolism of, 132, 141

treatments, 32–35; for birth difficulties, 39–47; of children, 53–54; and collaborative programs at hospital, 189–90; for depression, 97–99, 188; herbal, 117–18; for hot/cold humoral imbalances, 94–95; for *karambaza* from *tezma*, 50; and possession ritual, 125–26; Qur'anic/maraboutique, 157–61

trees: gathering from, 30–31, 55; lexicons for, 199; rituals surrounding, 152–54; as symbols, 117–32; uses of by medicine women, vii–ix, 57–58

tributaries, 26

Tripolitania, 198

tropes (healing), 22, 71, 111, 118; arboreal, 117–32

trucks, 4, 180, 182

Trudelle-Schwartz, Maureen, 6, 7, 70, 181, 211

trust, 86–87

Tsing, Anna, 23, 211

Tuareg: and age and gender in healing, 93, 94, 105, 115, 116; cultural healing classifications, 18–23, 193–96; diviners among, 171, 173; environment, 118–22; folklore, 124–26, 129; history, economics, and ethnography, 25–29, 197–201; humoral/thermal system, 43, 46, 49; Islam among, 152, 156, 159, 162–65; matrilineal myths, 82, 87–88; medicine women among, iii, vii, viii, ix, x, xi, 3, 5, 8, 15–16; mortuary practices, 90–91; political oppression, 131; property, 112; position in nation-states, 181–89; regional history, 137–40; religion, 141–42, 145–46; sensorium, 70–79; and tuberculosis, 17, 18, 197

Tubu: relations with Tuareg, 84, 88, 107, 125, 137, 138, 140, 200, 201

tuksi, 44, 94, 135, 149, 180. See also hot; illness

turhena, 77

Turkey, 136, 201

Turner, Edith, 6, 7, 19, 59, 71, 212

tuwila, 153. See also trees

twins: beliefs concerning, 123, 124; in mythico-history of medicine women, viii, 81–86, 90

Tyler, Stephen, 59, 212

Uduk, 120

umbilical cord, 37, 85

unemployment, 27

United Nations, 145

United States, 51, 181, 197, 212

universe, 72, 74

urban, 24, 201

Urban, Greg, 25, 26, 211

urination, 34, 179

usufruct, 26

uterus, 29, 41

uxorilocality, 29, 39, 80, 131

vanity, 78

veil: in possession ritual dress, 40. See also face-veil; men's; covering, women's

veins, 69

verses (Qur'anic), 98, 130, 149, 151; in song, 98, 123–25; uses of, 156–58, 162, 164, 168, 201;

veterinary, viii, 41

Victorians, 73

violence, viii, 87

virilocal, 123

visual, 70, 72, 76, 81

vitamins, 125

voice(s), 6

vomiting, 32, 94, 89, 149, 154, 166

Waddawa, 68, 102, 124. See also birth; earth; spirits

Wagner, Roy, xi

Walentowitz, Saskia, 71, 112, 212

Wallet Faqqi, Fadi, viii–ix, 3, 36, 37, 40, 41, 42, 43, 45, 46, 187, 205

wanzam, 68. See also barber; circumcision

wars: Chamba Arabs, 124; French, 137–40; rebellion, 131; Tubu, 94, 137–40

Wasu, 80–81, 83, 170–71

water: conditions of, 46, 75, 120, 137, 143; conflicts over, 183–84

weakness, 66–67, 97

Weaver, Marcia, 186, 212

Weberian, 16

weddings, 35, 50, 102, 129

Wedenoja, William, 21, 212

Wednesday, 35, 124

wellness: humoral balance, 47–49, 77; in life course, 104, 106; medicine women's ideas concerning, 4–5, 8, 30, 34

wells: conflicts surrounding, 142, 145, 183–84; ritual restrictions concerning, 136, 137; sacred, 138; symbolism of, 121, 127

Wenner Gren Foundation, xi

wet(ness), 75, 78, 119

wheat, 110

white, 40, 46, 129, 137

Whitehead, Harriet, 23, 100, 101, 114, 163, 211

widowhood, 92, 68, 120

wife-beating, viii, 42

wild: and nature/culture contextual transformations, 129, 130; as place of ambiguity and transition, 120, 122; as place of gathering medicines, 34, 100, 153; as psychosocial condition of possession, 38; spirits of, 71, 81, 171–72. See also *essuf*

wind: and climate, 4; humoral imbalance, 45; illnesses, 17, 18, 64; spirits, 36, 172, 179; and symbol in possession, 123, 131; women's vulnerability to, 94, 155

Winkelman, Michael, 3, 5, 6, 19, 20, 172, 212

wives, 25, 29, 62, 74, 152

Wolff, Norma, 69, 70, 71, 212

womb, 29

women: and descent and property, 112–16; as different from men, 96; as diviners, 173–75; and medicine, vii–viii; and referrals to marabouts, 57, 151; and sensorium beliefs concerning body, 76–79

Wong, Holly, 186–212

Wood, John, 23, 116, 212

World Bank, 186, 212

Worley, Barbara, 6, 27, 60, 71, 77, 101, 102, 198, 200, 212

wrestling, 60

wrist, 30, 32. See also *amasur;* body; clans; descent

writing: in divination, 39, 157–60, 162, 164, 169; marabouts' and Qur'anic Arabic, 87, 149, 151–54; and relation to aural, 20, 72

x-ray, 58

Yacine, Tossadit, 131

Yaguiji, 139

Yaqui, 17

yellow, 75, 32, 124

Yemen, 25

Yoruba, 69–71, 87, 201

youths, 74, 138, 146, 160, 163, 182

Zambia, 17

Zara, 61–64, 166, 179

Zarawa, 198

Zarma, 191, 199

Zinacantan, 177

Zinder, 2, 139

Zulu, 22, 23

Lightning Source UK Ltd.
Milton Keynes UK
UKHW010706250421
382482UK00014B/401